ASSESSING AND TREATING
Youth Exposed to
Traumatic Stress

ASSESSING AND TREATING
Youth Exposed to Traumatic Stress

Edited by

Victor G. Carrión, M.D.

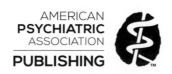

AMERICAN
PSYCHIATRIC
ASSOCIATION
PUBLISHING

Copyright © 2019 American Psychiatric Association Publishing
ALL RIGHTS RESERVED
First Edition
Manufactured in the United States of America on acid-free paper
22   21   20   19   18   5   4   3   2   1
American Psychiatric Association Publishing
800 Maine Avenue SW
Suite 900
Washington, DC 20024-2812
www.appi.org
Library of Congress Cataloging-in-Publication Data
Names: Carrión, Victor G., editor. | American Psychiatric Association Publishing, issuing body.
Title: Assessing and treating youth exposed to traumatic stress / edited by Victor G. Carrión.
Description: First edition. | Washington, D.C. : American Psychiatric Association Publishing, [2019] | Includes bibliographical references and index.
Identifiers: LCCN 2018032009| ISBN 9781615371426 (pbk : alk. paper) | ISBN 9781615372164 (E-ISBN)
Subjects: | MESH: Stress Disorders, Post-Traumatic—diagnosis | Stress Disorders, Post-Traumatic—therapy | Psychotherapy—methods | Child | Adolescent | Young Adult
Classification: LCC RJ506.P66 | NLM WM 172.5 | DDC 618.92/8521—dc23
LC record available at https://lccn.loc.gov/2018032009
British Library Cataloguing in Publication Data
A CIP record is available from the British Library.

Contents

PART 1

Assessment

PART II
Treatment

PART III

Associated Clinical Issues

PART IV

Systems of Care

Contributors

Brian Allen, Psy.D.
Associate Professor, Department of Pediatrics/Department of Psychiatry, Penn State College of Medicine, Hershey, Pennsylvania

Antra Bami, M.D.
Chief Fellow, Section of Child and Adolescent Psychiatry, Geisel School of Medicine at Dartmouth, Dartmouth-Hitchcock Medical Center, Lebanon, New Hampshire

Brian Bauer, M.S.
Department of Clinical Psychology, University of Southern Mississippi, Hattiesburg, Mississippi

Heather Bensman, Psy.D.
Assistant Professor, Department of Pediatrics, University of Cincinnati College of Medicine, Cincinnati, Ohio

Daniel W. Capron, Ph.D.
Nina Bell Suggs Professor of Psychology, Department of Clinical Psychology, University of Southern Mississippi, Hattiesburg, Mississippi

Victor G. Carrión, M.D.
John A. Turner, M.D. Endowed Chair of Child and Adolescent Psychiatry; Professor and Vice-Chair, Department of Psychiatry and Behavioral Sciences; and Director, Early Life Stress and Pediatric Anxiety Program, Stanford University, Stanford, California

Stephanie Clarke, Ph.D.
Clinical Instructor, Department of Child and Adolescent Psychiatry, Stanford University School of Medicine, Stanford, California

Simone Conde
Research Assistant, Stanford University, Stanford, California

Michael D. De Bellis, M.D., M.P.H.
Professor of Psychiatry and Behavioral Sciences and Director, Duke Healthy Childhood Brain Development Developmental Traumatology Research Program, Department of Psychiatry and Behavioral Sciences, Duke University School of Medicine, Durham, North Carolina

Miriam Hernandez Dimmler, Ph.D.
Associate Clinical Professor, Department of Psychiatry, University of California, San Francisco; Associate Director and Director of Community Partnerships, Child Trauma Research Program, Zuckerberg San Francisco General Hospital, San Francisco, California

Craig L. Donnelly, M.D.
Professor of Psychiatry and Pediatrics, Geisel School of Medicine at Dartmouth, Dartmouth-Hitchcock Medical Center, Lebanon, New Hampshire

Joyce Dorado, Ph.D.
Clinical Professor, University of California, San Francisco, Zuckerberg General Hospital, Division of Infant, Child, and Adolescent Psychiatry, San Francisco, California

Flint M. Espil, Ph.D.
Instructor, Department of Psychiatry and Behavioral Sciences, Stanford University, Stanford, California

Chandra Ghosh Ippen, Ph.D.
Department of Psychiatry, University of California, San Francisco; Associate Director and Director of Dissemination, Child Trauma Research Program, Zuckerberg San Francisco General Hospital, San Francisco, California

Chelsea N. Grefe, Psy.D.
Psychologist, UPMC Children's Hospital of Pittsburgh, Pittsburgh, Pennsylvania

Jessica L. Griffin, Psy.D.
Associate Professor, Department of Psychiatry, University of Massachusetts Medical School, Worcester, Massachusetts

David S. Grunwald, M.D., M.S.
Child and Adolescent Psychiatry Fellow (Community Track), Stanford University School of Medicine, Stanford, California

Laura D. Heintz, Psy.D.
Chief Executive Officer, Stanford Youth Solutions, Sacramento, California

Sara Blythe Heron, M.D.
Child, Adolescent, and Adult Psychiatrist, Bay Area Clinical Associates, Oakland, California

Sheryl H. Kataoka, M.D., M.S.H.S.
Professor, UCLA Semel Institute for Neuroscience and Human Behavior, Los Angeles, California

Michael Kelly, M.D.
Staff Psychiatrist, San Quentin State Prison, San Quentin, California

Moira Kessler, M.D.
Clinical Assistant Professor, Department of Psychiatry and Behavioral Sciences, Stanford University School of Medicine, Stanford, California

Christina Tara Khan, M.D., Ph.D.
Clinical Assistant Professor, Department of Psychiatry and Behavioral Sciences, Stanford University School of Medicine, Stanford, California, and Research Associate, National Center for Posttraumatic Stress Disorder, Veterans Affairs Palo Alto Health Care System, Palo Alto, California

Hilit Kletter, Ph.D.
Clinical Assistant Professor and Director of Trauma Program, Division of Child and Adolescent Psychiatry, Stanford University School of Medicine, Stanford, California

Julia LaMotte, M.S.
Doctoral candidate, Department of Psychology, University of Georgia, Athens, Georgia

Alicia F. Lieberman, Ph.D.
Irving B. Harris Endowed Chair in Infant Mental Health and Professor and Vice Chair for Faculty Development, Department of Psychiatry, University of California, San Francisco; Director, Child Trauma Research Program, Zuckerberg San Francisco General Hospital, San Francisco, California

Roy Lubit M.D., Ph.D.
Private practice, New York, New York

Rachel L. Martin, B.A.
Department of Clinical Psychology, University of Southern Mississippi, Hattiesburg, Mississippi

Ryan B. Matlow, Ph.D.
Director of Community Programs, Department of Psychiatry and Behavioral Sciences, Stanford University School of Medicine, Stanford, California

Anne B. McBride, M.D.
Assistant Professor of Clinical Psychiatry and Program Director, Child and Adolescent Psychiatry Residency, Department of Psychiatry and Behavioral Sciences, University of California, Davis, Sacramento, California

Martha Merchant, Psy.D.
Psychologist, University of California, San Francisco, Zuckerberg General Hospital, Division of Infant, Child, and Adolescent Psychiatry, San Francisco, California

Kate B. Nooner, Ph.D.
Associate Professor of Psychology, Director of the Trauma and Resilience Laboratory, Department of Psychology, University of North Carolina Wilmington, Wilmington, North Carolina

Michelle Primeau, M.D.
Staff Physician, Palo Alto Medical Foundation, Department of Sleep Medicine, Stanford University School of Medicine, Stanford, California

Nicole Quiterio, M.D.
Clinical Director, Bay Area Clinical Associates, Oakland, California

Shayne N. Ragbeer, Ph.D.
Instructor in Clinical Psychology (in Psychiatry), Columbia University College of Physicians and Surgeons, Department of Psychiatry, Division of Child and Adolescent Psychiatry, Columbia University Medical Center, New York, New York

John P. Rettger, Ph.D.
Director of Mindfulness Program, Early Life Stress and Pediatric Anxiety Program, Department of Psychiatry and Behavioral Sciences, School of Medicine, Stanford University, Stanford, California

Jared T. Ritter, M.D., FAPA
Clinical Assistant Professor, Department of Psychiatry, Florida State University College of Medicine, Tallahassee, Florida

Chad Shenk, Ph.D.
Associate Professor, Department of Human Development and Family Studies/Department of Pediatrics, Pennsylvania State University, State College, Pennsylvania

Pamela J. Shime, J.D., M.A.
Neuro-Tech and Game Designer, University Lecturer, and 2016–2108 Research Associate, Early Life Stress and Pediatric Anxiety Program, Department of Psychiatry and Behavioral Sciences, Stanford University, Stanford, California

Karen Smith, Ph.D.
Adjunct Assistant Professor, Department of Psychology, University of Georgia; School Counselor, Alps Road Elementary School, Athens, Georgia

Bradley D. Stein, M.D., Ph.D.
Senior Natural Scientist, RAND Corporation, Pittsburgh, Pennsylvania

Steven Sust, M.D.
Clinical Instructor, Psychiatry and Behavioral Sciences, Stanford University School of Medicine, Stanford, California

Pamela Vona, M.P.H., M.A.
Research Associate, USC Suzanne Dworak-Peck School of Social Work, Los Angeles, California

Elizabeth Weiss, Psy.D.
Palo Alto, California

Jessica Wozniak, Psy.D.
Assistant Professor, Department of Psychiatry, University of Massachusetts Medical School—Baystate, Springfield, Massachusetts

Sanno E. Zack, Ph.D.
Clinical Associate Professor, Department of Child and Adolescent Psychiatry, Stanford University School of Medicine, Stanford, California

DISCLOSURE OF INTERESTS

The following contributors to this book have indicated a financial interest in or other affiliation with a commercial supporter, a manufacturer of a commercial product, a provider of a commercial service, a nongovernmental organization, and/or a government agency, as listed below:

Michelle Primeau, M.D.   *Speaker:* Merck

John P. Rettger, Ph.D.   *Paid contributor:* Sonima.com; *Consultant:* Pure Edge, Inc.

Jessica Wozniak, Psy.D.   *Funding:* SAMHSA

The following contributors have indicated that they have no financial interests or other affiliations that represent or could appear to represent a competing interest with the contributions to this book:

Victor G. Carrión, M.D.; Michael D. De Bellis, M.D., M.P.H.; Joyce Dorado, Ph.D.; Flint M. Espil, Ph.D.; Chelsea N. Grefe, Psy.D.; David S. Grunwald, M.D., M.S.; Laura D. Heintz, Psy.D.; Sheryl H. Kataoka, M.D., M.S.H.S.; Michael Kelly, M.D.; Moira Kessler, M.D.; Christina Tara Khan, M.D. Ph.D.; Hilit Kletter, Ph.D.; Julia LaMotte, M.S.; Martha Merchant, Psy.D.; Kate B. Nooner, Ph.D.; Nicole Quiterio, M.D.; Chad Shenk, Ph.D.; Pamela J. Shime, J.D., M.A.; Karen Smith, Ph.D.; Steven Sust, M.D.; Sanno E. Zack, Ph.D.

International Editorial Board

Ruth Pat-Horenczyk, Ph.D.
Associate Professor, Paul Baerwald School of Social Work and Social Welfare, Hebrew University of Jerusalem

Nuria A. Sabaté, M.D., FAPA
Director, Child and Adolescent Psychiatry Program, and Chair, Wellness Center Research Committee, Ponce Health Sciences University

Brandon G. Scott, Ph.D.
Assistant Professor and Graduate Coordinator, Director of the Child and Adolescent Anxiety Lab of Montana (CAALM), Department of Psychology, Montana State University

Thomas Paul Tarshis, M.D., M.P.H.
Founder and Executive Director, Bay Area Children's Association; Adjunct Clinical Assistant Professor, Stanford University

Carl Weems, Ph.D.
Professor and Chair, Human Development and Family Studies, Iowa State University

Preface

Victor G. Carrión, M.D.

WE ARE ALL the sum of our experiences. For most of us, enriching, safe, nurturing, and learning experiences outweigh those underscored by adversity, disenfranchisement, disrespect, and threat. Many children, however, live lives in which they feel—and are—in constant threat, fear, and confusion. Many of these children also experience neglect, either physical or emotional, and they are not given opportunities for positive social interactions, stimulation, and empowerment. When negative experiences outweigh positive ones, this takes a toll on an individual's adaptive mechanisms, both biological and psychological. This allostatic load, to use a term coined by Bruce McEwen from Rockefeller University, has a physiological impact that results in the behaviors and emotional and cognitive challenges we find in children who have been traumatized.

Posttraumatic stress disorder (PTSD) has been a useful anchor for studying, evaluating, and treating children who experience trauma. But trauma itself is a significant stressor to the body and may lead to any disorder a particular individual may be vulnerable to developing. Most of us would develop PTSD symptoms under the right circumstances (e.g., torture), suggesting to many that, perhaps, the correct nomenclature should be posttraumatic stress injury, reflecting the vulnerability of the autonomic and fear systems and their propensity to recover. The diagnosis is further challenged by research and clinical findings that subthreshold symptoms of PTSD may lead to the same functional disability as the full diagnosis.

Being sensitive and inquisitive about the individual life narratives of young children may be the most important requirements for obtaining detailed histories of the impact that trauma has had in their development. Yet children may be particularly limited in offering these histories because of their concrete thinking and limited vocabulary. Becoming sensitive to these issues, Michael Scheeringa and Charles Zeanah conducted research that eventually influenced the addition of a separate posttraumatic diagnosis for preschool children in the most recent version of the Diagnostic and Statistical Manual of Mental Disorders (DSM-5). These developmentally sensitive criteria anchor on behavioral symptoms. For older children, the criteria are similar to those of adults (see Chapter 1, "The Clinical Interview").

This book is divided into four parts. The first two parts address assessment and treatment. When assessing youth with PTSD, two points are critical: First, rarely does PTSD exist alone; comorbidity (the presence of other diagnoses) is the norm. Second, the population that fulfills criteria for the diagnosis is highly heterogeneous in terms of presentation and target symptoms.

Comorbidity may reflect a number of clinical scenarios. It may be the overlap of symptoms with other conditions or the true presence of separate conditions, such as depression, anxiety, or attention-deficit/hyperactivity disorder. It may also reflect our lack of specificity in fully understanding this syndrome in children. All these possibilities have some clinical and research support, and since the diagnosis of PTSD first appeared in DSM in 1980, new editions have been increasingly adaptive in reflecting the true posttraumatic experience of children.

Suggestions on how to manage challenging issues surrounding comorbidity are offered in Chapter 15, "Addressing Comorbidity." The heterogeneity of PTSD can be attributed to differences in the type of trauma, duration of trauma, accumulation of trauma, age of insult, stress vulnerability, family history, and other individual factors. The interplay among these factors may result in emotional numbness and dissociative states in some youth (see Chapter 16, "Dissociation") but increased arousability in others. A third group of children may combine aspects of both dissociation and hypervigilance. The traumatic insult in the development of different branches of the autonomic nervous system may play a role on this differentiation. Individual differences are critical in the assessment because they will influence the course of treatment. Chapter 10, "Cue-Centered Therapy," presents our approach at Stanford in treating children with a history of trauma and underscores the importance of identifying individual cues or triggers that may precipitate the symptoms. Self-empowerment in addressing how the youth's own experience is understood, manifested, and addressed is the cornerstone of the cue-centered therapy approach.

Because of the heterogeneity of this population, more treatments are needed. Currently, we are limited to a handful of approaches. In Part II, we present the principles behind trauma-focused cognitive-behavioral therapy (Chapter 9) and a treatment for younger children and their caretakers (Chapter 11, "Child-Parent Psychotherapy"). General principles of psychotherapy (Chapter 5) and play therapy (Chapter 6) are also discussed. Whenever appropriate, the authors of these chapters take a developmental approach to illustrate how these techniques are applied to preschoolers, school-age children, adolescents, and transitional-age youth.

Even when psychosocial interventions are the first line of intervention when treating youth with PTSD symptoms, there is a role for pharmacological treatment. The use of medications is discussed in Chapter 14, "Psychopharmacology." Medication use is limited to a number of clinical scenarios, such as treating symptoms (PTSD or comorbid) that interfere with the proper use of psychotherapy (e.g., persistent agitation that limits therapeutic progress, difficulties with attention that limit the acquisition of cognitive tools).

Perhaps the best approach to ameliorating the academic, cognitive, and emotional sequelae of trauma is to address trauma *before* these impairments manifest. Preventative approaches include the use of school-based interventions; for an example, see Chapter 8, "UCSF Healthy Environments and Response to Trauma in Schools (HEARTS)." Assessing vulnerable populations—those who are known to have experienced human-made disasters (e.g., school shooting, terrorist attack) or natural disasters (e.g., fire, earthquake, hurricane) and those involved with the justice system (e.g., probation)—is a sound approach to reaching kids early. Suggestions on how to conduct such assessments are offered in Chapter 2, "Assessment in Schools or Other Large Groups," Chapter 3, "Assessment of Individuals," and Chapter 4, "The Forensic Evaluation." There are also approaches that can be taken even before a traumatic event occurs. More recently, the application of yoga and mindfulness in school settings has been gaining momentum. Our group, for example, is concluding a 3-year, multimethod assessment of the Pure Edge curriculum for application of yoga and mindfulness in physical education. In Chapter 13, "Mindfulness and Yoga," the author discusses the application of yoga and mindfulness in youth, specifically in those who have experienced traumatic events.

In Part III, we address associated clinical issues that may influence the manifestation of pediatric PTSD: dissociation, problems with sleep, self-injurious behaviors, suicidality, and substance use. The fight-or-flight response in children is inhibited by children's physical limitations and their limited ability to avoid certain situations; hence, a natural response is to pretend that what is happening is not really happening, or to dissociate.

This coping mechanism in young people may take a life of its own very early in their development or in those who need to use it with more frequency, and it may pose therapeutic challenges (Chapter 16). For those who tend to be more aroused than dissociated, nighttime can be particularly difficult. Difficulties with or during sleep (e.g., insomnia, enuresis, nightmares) have always been part of the pediatric PTSD picture. Lately, however, we have been acquiring a better understanding of how these sleep problems may not necessarily be sequelae of trauma and that abnormalities with sleep architecture may, in fact, precede PTSD as a risk factor. In these instances, treating sleep abnormalities may prevent the development of PTSD symptoms (see Chapter 17, "Sleep").

Self-injury may develop as a means to deter an uncomfortable state of dissociation. In others, it may develop as a means to reach that state. Once again, these differences highlight the importance of assessing individual experience in symptom presentation (see Chapter 18, "Self-Injurious Behaviors and Suicidality"). Although suicidality is clinically distinct from self-injury, we include it in Chapter 18 because PTSD increases the risk of suicidality, probably through a number of different mechanisms. Preventing PTSD can prevent suicide. In order to prevent PTSD, the trauma must be confronted and approached rather than avoided. PTSD feeds on avoidance. Therapy relies on approach. Substance use (Chapter 19), either primary or secondary (as a consequence of PTSD), can foster avoidance.

There is nothing in the scientific literature that supports the idea that children are resilient by virtue of being children. In fact, the opposite idea has more scientific validity. It stands to reason that while the brain and physiology are developing in a young child, there is an inherent risk in normative development secondary to traumatic injury. Behaviorally, we see this in children's limitations in using play to assist their development. Trauma can rob children of their play, making this activity one that is nonjoyful and repetitive. The child then needs individual help, in addition to support from the system that extends his or her existence and experience: family, school, and society. This ecological approach is the foundation of trauma treatment, and policy is a means to engage this broader system. Although psychosocial intervention for children addresses the impact of trauma, trauma itself is a social ill, not the children's ill; hence, the treatment needs to be geared toward the system that maintains it. Accordingly, in Part IV, we conclude the book with a discussion of systems of care, acknowledging that an ecological approach is needed when treating posttraumatic conditions in children and adolescents.

A "whatever it takes" treatment method is presented in Chapter 20, "Full Spectrum of Care," by introducing a model of care that is comprehensive in its approach. Delivery of such a method, or some of its aspects, may eventually become more easily distributed by the inclusion of new technologies that aim at facilitating dissemination and adherence to treatment (see Chapter 23, "Technology-Facilitated Interventions"). Development of technology-facilitated interventions is crucial in our attempt to tackle the limited workforce predicament of the field. Not having enough pediatric therapists for the number of children who need them also has been addressed through partnerships with primary care. In Chapter 21, "Integrated Models," we discuss the role of integrated care models in treating trauma in youth. In Chapter 22, "Global Mental Health and Trauma," assessment and treatment principles are applied to work with world populations afflicted by trauma.

As advocates for children, adolescents, and survivors of trauma, therapists must break out of silos and engage collaboratively with other stakeholders. Children do not vote and do not hire lobbyists to represent their needs. Society, as a whole, has a tremendous stake in the well-being of younger generations. We must procure health for children who face adversity and promote opportunities for them to develop to their full potential.

Dedication and Acknowledgments

THIS BOOK is dedicated to the new wave of youth who have taken leadership in recognizing the impact of trauma in society. Active youth from the Black Lives Matter movement to Parkland, Florida have recognized the importance of working together, using approach rather than avoidance, and informing rather than confusing society. Youth who do not make the news fight battles alone every day and struggle for opportunities, having a voice, and developing resilience, and they inspire our work. This book is dedicated to all youth struggling to maintain a world where empathy, justice, and humanity prevail.

I thank American Psychiatric Association Publishing and its Editor-in-Chief, Dr. Laura Roberts, for having the vision to value a contribution in the area of trauma and recovery in youth. I also thank Ms. Elizabeth Santana, whose support and guidance to all contributors made this volume possible.

Victor G. Carrión, M.D.
June 2018

PART I
Assessment

1

The Clinical Interview

Sara Blythe Heron, M.D.

THERE ARE VARYING TYPES of trauma and various ways in which patients experience and cope with trauma. Trauma can be a single occurrence, such as a natural or man-made disaster, or it can be experienced in a repeated fashion over many months or years before coming to the attention of a mental health professional. Patients who experience trauma may present for the initial interview in a variety of settings, including the emergency department, a pediatrician's office, or an outpatient mental health clinic, or they may even present to a school counselor or other school authority. When a child or teenager is the patient, he or she may have been referred or brought in for a treatment by an adult rather than of his or her own accord. In fact, sometimes the patient will not understand why he or she has been brought in for an evaluation, the purpose of the session, or the role of the clinician. In this chapter, I explore the clinical interview in detail, reviewing the key components of the interview, providing clinical examples, and addressing ways to prepare for and deal with common obstacles.

Building Rapport

The most important initial step of the first encounter is to establish rapport with the patient. The strength of the therapeutic alliance is vital in gathering critical and sensitive information and also sets the tone for progress in the therapy that follows the initial interview. The clinician will establish rapport in different ways, depending on the age of the patient and the type of therapy, and these will be elaborated in further detail later in this chapter and in the book. The clinician should give an introduction of his or her role and prepare the patient for what will happen during the course of the initial session (King et al. 1997; Stubbe 2007). Many mental health professionals will forgo their traditional title followed by last name and use only their first name to help put younger patients at ease. Other providers feel that using their title, such as "doctor," actually allows the patient to feel more secure, knowing they are talking to a person whom they can trust and who is designated to help.

Choosing a setting for the session that helps the patient to feel calm and safe is ideal although not always possible. The intention is to reassure the patient that he or she will be accepted so that the patient can share any of his or her thoughts and feelings without fear of judgment, criticism, shame, or stigmatization. Projecting a feeling of warmth, empathy, and sensitivity is essential and is done with both verbal and nonverbal communication (Manley 2000). The patient should be informed of the benefits and bounds of confidentiality so that he or she may speak freely. The clinician should allow the patient to initiate the exchange, following his or her lead, and encouraging further elaboration with open-ended questions (Carlat 2012). Younger patients may need the clinician to initiate the discussion or begin with a game, activity, or free play. Sometimes, a clinician will conduct the interview independently, but in other settings a multidisciplinary team, including a psychologist, social worker, marriage and family therapist, and/or psychiatrist will conduct the interview together. Obviously, the number of clinicians in the room at a given time can have an impact on rapport, and this should be taken into consideration.

Gathering a Thorough History

Obtaining a Patient's History

During the initial clinical interview, it is important to obtain a detailed history of the patient's background, both biological and psychosocial. When working with children and teenagers, information from parents, guardians, or other adults involved in their lives (e.g., teachers, pediatrician) will be vital. The purpose of meeting with the parent or guardian is not only to obtain details about the patient's current functioning and history but also to better assess the functioning of the parents and family as a whole (King et al. 1997). For younger children, gathering history from the parent(s) or guardian should be completed first. For teenagers, the decision of whom to meet with first will vary on the basis of the patient's comfort and maturity level. Patients should always be given time to meet with the clinician individually because there may be information that the patient does not feel comfortable disclosing in front of the parent or guardian. Discrepancies between the parent and child perspectives should be noted and explored further.

Items of history that should be covered in the initial intake are detailed in the following subsection, and clinical examples will be provided later in the chapter. It is worth noting that this information need not be covered in exactly this order nor in a single session, but obtaining basic information early in the course of treatment will help in clarifying the diagnosis and determining the best initial plan for ongoing care. Additionally, the clinician need not cover every symptom in the fifth edition of the *Diagnostic and Statistical Manual of Mental Disorders* (DSM-5; American Psychiatric Association 2013) but rather should begin with basic screening questions and use his or her judgment to further pursue areas that seem most relevant (King et al. 1997). In addition to the clinical interview, the clinician may also choose to administer other screening or assessment tools as part of the initial assessment.

Key Elements of the Patient's History

- *History of the present illness:* The clinician should obtain further details about the patient's primary complaint or reason for seeking treatment.
- *Previous psychiatric history:* The clinician should gather information about previous courses of psychotherapy, any previous psychiatric hospitalizations or suicide attempts, and any previous trials of psychotropic medication (including details about efficacy of medication and any adverse reactions).
- *Past medical history:* Often elicited by a psychiatrist or other medical doctor, the past medical history includes information about any acute, chronic, or severe physical illnesses; surgical procedures; or head injuries. In addition, information about over-the-counter medicines or

supplements, non-psychotropic medications, and allergies is also reviewed.

- *Family history:* The presence of mental health disorders or symptoms, including a history of trauma, in any family members is also important to obtain because both environmental and genetic factors can influence the patient's symptoms and response to treatment.

- *Birth and development:* Information about the health and care of the mother of the patient during pregnancy, as well as any complications or concerns that occurred during delivery, should be recorded. Notable pieces of the patient's early development such as temperament as a baby, feeding (including whether or not the patient was breastfed and the duration), motor and speech development, and challenges with separation from primary caregiver(s) are important as well. This information may not be available depending on the age of the patient and whether or not the biological parents are still involved in the patient's care.

- *Social history:* The social history includes information about where and with whom the patient resides, including any changes in residence or caregivers. Identification of key social supports (both family and community) and quality of friendships and peer relationships is useful. For children and adolescents, the clinician should obtain an educational history, including where the patient attends school, his or her current grade, and current academic standing. For adult patients or parents of younger patients, information about occupation and financial stability are relevant. Information about any extracurricular activities, hobbies, and cultural or religious affiliations also provides a picture of who the patient is and how he or she relates to the surrounding social environment. If the patient or family has any legal history or current involvement with the legal system, this would also be important to document.

- *Trauma history:* Although some patients come to the clinic specifically seeking support related to a traumatic experience and reveal this at the outset, it is not uncommon for patients to refrain from revealing any history of traumatic events until later in the course of treatment. Given the sensitivity of the topic, it is often necessary to establish trust between the patient and therapist before the patient feels comfortable disclosing a trauma history. Regardless, the clinician should inquire about a history of trauma during the initial clinical session. The clinician must find a balance between directness and softness when asking about trauma so as not to stigmatize patients while also helping them feel reassured that therapy will be a safe place to talk about anything.

- *Substance use:* Use of illicit substances (alcohol, street drugs) or misuse of prescription drugs can co-occur with other mental health symptoms. It is necessary to know which substances the patient uses currently or has tried in the past and the frequency and duration with which each substance is or was used.

Assessing the Patient's Mental State

The Mental Status Examination

In addition to a thorough history, observations about the patient's mental state should be recorded. As a complement to the history, the mental status examination gives the practitioner a picture of who the patient is and how he or she interacts with the surrounding world. The key elements of the examination, as detailed by Manley (2000), are listed in the following subsection. The clinician can use the examination to determine whether or not the patient is behaving in a developmentally appropriate way. Abnormalities in the mental status examination may be suggestive of a trauma history, even if the history is not obviously concerning, and warrants further clinical assessment. The mental status examination is of particular importance in patients who, because of age (or other reasons), are unable to thoroughly articulate a trauma history in words. Clinical examples of mental status examinations will be provided later in the chapter.

Key Elements of the Mental Status Examination

- *Appearance:* Important information about the patient can be obtained by simply taking note of his or her attire, grooming, and hygiene. The patient's general weight and stature, as well as whether or not his or her appearance matches the stated biological age, should also be noted.
- *Speech:* The clinician should observe the tone, rate, volume, and amount of the patient's speech as well as whether the patient's speech is spontaneous or whether he or she only gives brief responses to questions without elaboration or detail. The patient's speech may be pressured, making it difficult for the clinician to speak or interrupt, or there may be a delay in responses for a variety of reasons. The prosody,

or patterns of intonation, is also important. The patient's vocabulary is worth noting because, again, it can provide clues about the patient's developmental age and whether or not it appropriately matches the biological age.

- *Behavior:* The patient's movements, facial expression, and eye contact are key components of behavior that need to be documented. If the patient is fidgeting or unable to sit still or if he or she moves slowly or minimally, with a downcast gaze and no eye contact throughout the session, these items would be important to note as well as whether these behaviors occur throughout the session or only when discussing particular topics.
- *Affect:* Noting affect requires the clinician to infer the internal emotion of the patient on the basis of the patient's demeanor, facial expression, and other objective observations.
- *Mood:* The clinician should note the patient's subjectively stated emotions.
- *Thought:* The clinician needs to note both the patient's thought process, whether linear and logical or aberrant (e.g., following tangents with or without returning to the topic of discussion, moving quickly from one idea to another, jumping from one topic to another without any clear association), and the content of the thought, including suicidal or homicidal thoughts, bizarre or paranoid delusions, or any obsessions.
- *Perception:* The clinician should note how the patient perceives the world around him or her. This includes instances in which the patient perceives things that are not real as if they were real, as with auditory and visual hallucinations, illusions, and perceptions that others are not who they say they are or are reading or controlling the patient's mind.
- *Cognition:* Components of the patient's cognition include orientation (to his or her own person, current location, and current time), memory (immediate, recent, and remote), concentration (ability to attend to the session and engage in the interview without distraction), abstract reasoning (ability to apply general concepts to specific situations), and fund of knowledge (which will vary with age).
- *Insight:* The clinician should be able to assess the patient's ability to "recognize and understand his or her own symptoms" via direct questioning and/or observation over the course of the clinical interview (Manley 2000).
- *Judgment:* Through both questions and observation, the clinician should try to determine the patient's level of judgment. This is the pa-

tient's ability to make and follow through on appropriate and safe choices about a particular course of action, using whatever information is available to him or her. Like affect, assessment of a patient's judgment is generally inferred rather than directly measured.

Family Evaluation

In addition to meeting with the patient and caregivers individually, the clinician should meet with the entire family together, which also provides useful information. It is important to observe the interaction between each caregiver and the child and between caregivers in the child's presence. Things to pay close attention to include how attuned the caregivers are to the child, whether or not they are able to show empathy for and curiosity about their child, and whether they allow space for the child to express himself or herself without intrusion or censorship. The interviewer can observe the child's attachment to the caregiver, which is expected to be different at various developmental stages. For example, a preschoolage child would be expected to explore the surrounding environment while intermittently looking to the caregiver for his or her involvement and feedback, whereas an adolescent may be more withdrawn and less talkative when a caregiver is present. It is important to note how the caregiver responds to high expressed emotion in the child and if the caregiver is able to manage his or her own emotions in that context. If there are concerns during the evaluation of the family, this can inform decisions about future treatment, including the need for individual or couples therapy for caregivers, dyadic therapy with the caregiver and child, or family therapy.

Assessing the family as a whole also aids in screening other members of the family for symptoms of posttraumatic stress disorder (PTSD), particularly if they were exposed to the same trauma as the patient (Box 1–1). If PTSD in the caregivers is missed, it can impact the progress of treatment for the patient because healthy caregivers and a stable home environment are essential to the child's mental health. If there are siblings or other extended family members living in the home who are involved in the patient's life, their participation in the assessment process may also be valuable, although this can happen at a later stage in the treatment. With young adults, the patient's autonomy and independence must be recognized and prioritized, but it may be appropriate to involve family members in the evaluation of these patients as well, particularly if the young adult is still living at home with his or her nuclear family.

Diagnostic Criteria

Although the initial interview should be comprehensive, for the purpose of this book it is worth reviewing the DSM-5 criteria for posttraumatic stress disorder (Box 1–1).

Box 1–1.   DSM-5 Diagnostic Criteria for Posttraumatic Stress Disorder

---

Posttraumatic Stress Disorder

Note: The following criteria apply to adults, adolescents, and children older than 6 years. For children 6 years and younger, see corresponding criteria below.

A. Exposure to actual or threatened death, serious injury, or sexual violence in one (or more) of the following ways:

1. Directly experiencing the traumatic event(s).
2. Witnessing, in person, the event(s) as it occurred to others.
3. Learning that the traumatic event(s) occurred to a close family member or close friend. In cases of actual or threatened death of a family member or friend, the event(s) must have been violent or accidental.
4. Experiencing repeated or extreme exposure to aversive details of the traumatic event(s) (e.g., first responders collecting human remains; police officers repeatedly exposed to details of child abuse).

   Note: Criterion A4 does not apply to exposure through electronic media, television, movies, or pictures, unless this exposure is work related.

B. Presence of one (or more) of the following intrusion symptoms associated with the traumatic event(s), beginning after the traumatic event(s) occurred:

1. Recurrent, involuntary, and intrusive distressing memories of the traumatic event(s).

   Note: In children older than 6 years, repetitive play may occur in which themes or aspects of the traumatic event(s) are expressed.
2. Recurrent distressing dreams in which the content and/or affect of the dream are related to the traumatic event(s).

   Note: In children, there may be frightening dreams without recognizable content.
3. Dissociative reactions (e.g., flashbacks) in which the individual feels or acts as if the traumatic event(s) were recurring. (Such reactions may occur on a continuum, with the most extreme expression being a complete loss of awareness of present surroundings.)

   Note: In children, trauma-specific reenactment may occur in play.

 4. Intense or prolonged psychological distress at exposure to internal or external cues that symbolize or resemble an aspect of the traumatic event(s).
 5. Marked physiological reactions to internal or external cues that symbolize or resemble an aspect of the traumatic event(s).

C. Persistent avoidance of stimuli associated with the traumatic event(s), beginning after the traumatic event(s) occurred, as evidenced by one or both of the following:

 1. Avoidance of or efforts to avoid distressing memories, thoughts, or feelings about or closely associated with the traumatic event(s).
 2. Avoidance of or efforts to avoid external reminders (people, places, conversations, activities, objects, situations) that arouse distressing memories, thoughts, or feelings about or closely associated with the traumatic event(s).

D. Negative alterations in cognitions and mood associated with the traumatic event(s), beginning or worsening after the traumatic event(s) occurred, as evidenced by two (or more) of the following:

 1. Inability to remember an important aspect of the traumatic event(s) (typically due to dissociative amnesia and not to other factors such as head injury, alcohol, or drugs).
 2. Persistent and exaggerated negative beliefs or expectations about oneself, others, or the world (e.g., "I am bad," "No one can be trusted," "The world is completely dangerous," "My whole nervous system is permanently ruined").
 3. Persistent, distorted cognitions about the cause or consequences of the traumatic event(s) that lead the individual to blame himself/herself or others.
 4. Persistent negative emotional state (e.g., fear, horror, anger, guilt, or shame).
 5. Markedly diminished interest or participation in significant activities.
 6. Feelings of detachment or estrangement from others.
 7. Persistent inability to experience positive emotions (e.g., inability to experience happiness, satisfaction, or loving feelings).

E. Marked alterations in arousal and reactivity associated with the traumatic event(s), beginning or worsening after the traumatic event(s) occurred, as evidenced by two (or more) of the following:

 1. Irritable behavior and angry outbursts (with little or no provocation) typically expressed as verbal or physical aggression toward people or objects.
 2. Reckless or self-destructive behavior.
 3. Hypervigilance.
 4. Exaggerated startle response.
 5. Problems with concentration.

6. Sleep disturbance (e.g., difficulty falling or staying asleep or restless sleep).

F. Duration of the disturbance (Criteria B, C, D, and E) is more than 1 month.

G. The disturbance causes clinically significant distress or impairment in social, occupational, or other important areas of functioning.

H. The disturbance is not attributable to the physiological effects of a substance (e.g., medication, alcohol) or another medical condition.

Specify whether:

With dissociative symptoms: The individual's symptoms meet the criteria for posttraumatic stress disorder, and in addition, in response to the stressor, the individual experiences persistent or recurrent symptoms of either of the following:

1. **Depersonalization:** Persistent or recurrent experiences of feeling detached from, and as if one were an outside observer of, one's mental processes or body (e.g., feeling as though one were in a dream; feeling a sense of unreality of self or body or of time moving slowly).

2. **Derealization:** Persistent or recurrent experiences of unreality of surroundings (e.g., the world around the individual is experienced as unreal, dreamlike, distant, or distorted).

Note: To use this subtype, the dissociative symptoms must not be attributable to the physiological effects of a substance (e.g., blackouts, behavior during alcohol intoxication) or another medical condition (e.g., complex partial seizures).

Specify if:

With delayed expression: If the full diagnostic criteria are not met until at least 6 months after the event (although the onset and expression of some symptoms may be immediate).

Posttraumatic Stress Disorder for Children 6 Years and Younger

A. In children 6 years and younger, exposure to actual or threatened death, serious injury, or sexual violence in one (or more) of the following ways:

1. Directly experiencing the traumatic event(s).

2. Witnessing, in person, the event(s) as it occurred to others, especially primary caregivers.

   Note: Witnessing does not include events that are witnessed only in electronic media, television, movies, or pictures.

3. Learning that the traumatic event(s) occurred to a parent or caregiving figure.

B. Presence of one (or more) of the following intrusion symptoms associated with the traumatic event(s), beginning after the traumatic event(s) occurred:

1. Recurrent, involuntary, and intrusive distressing memories of the traumatic event(s).

Note: Spontaneous and intrusive memories may not necessarily appear distressing and may be expressed as play reenactment.

2. Recurrent distressing dreams in which the content and/or affect of the dream are related to the traumatic event(s).

   Note: It may not be possible to ascertain that the frightening content is related to the traumatic event.

3. Dissociative reactions (e.g., flashbacks) in which the child feels or acts as if the traumatic event(s) were recurring. (Such reactions may occur on a continuum, with the most extreme expression being a complete loss of awareness of present surroundings.) Such trauma-specific reenactment may occur in play.

4. Intense or prolonged psychological distress at exposure to internal or external cues that symbolize or resemble an aspect of the traumatic event(s).

5. Marked physiological reactions to reminders of the traumatic event(s).

C. One (or more) of the following symptoms, representing either persistent avoidance of stimuli associated with the traumatic event(s) or negative alterations in cognitions and mood associated with the traumatic event(s), must be present, beginning after the event(s) or worsening after the event(s):

Persistent Avoidance of Stimuli

1. Avoidance of or efforts to avoid activities, places, or physical reminders that arouse recollections of the traumatic event(s).

2. Avoidance of or efforts to avoid people, conversations, or interpersonal situations that arouse recollections of the traumatic event(s).

Negative Alterations in Cognitions

3. Substantially increased frequency of negative emotional states (e.g., fear, guilt, sadness, shame, confusion).

4. Markedly diminished interest or participation in significant activities, including constriction of play.

5. Socially withdrawn behavior.

6. Persistent reduction in expression of positive emotions.

D. Alterations in arousal and reactivity associated with the traumatic event(s), beginning or worsening after the traumatic event(s) occurred, as evidenced by two (or more) of the following:

1. Irritable behavior and angry outbursts (with little or no provocation) typically expressed as verbal or physical aggression toward people or objects (including extreme temper tantrums).

2. Hypervigilance.

3. Exaggerated startle response.

4. Problems with concentration.

5. Sleep disturbance (e.g., difficulty falling or staying asleep or restless sleep).

E. The duration of the disturbance is more than 1 month.

F. The disturbance causes clinically significant distress or impairment in relationships with parents, siblings, peers, or other caregivers or with school behavior.

G. The disturbance is not attributable to the physiological effects of a substance (e.g., medication or alcohol) or another medical condition.

Specify whether:

With dissociative symptoms: The individual's symptoms meet the criteria for posttraumatic stress disorder, and the individual experiences persistent or recurrent symptoms of either of the following:

1. **Depersonalization:** Persistent or recurrent experiences of feeling detached from, and as if one were an outside observer of, one's mental processes or body (e.g., feeling as though one were in a dream; feeling a sense of unreality of self or body or of time moving slowly).

2. **Derealization:** Persistent or recurrent experiences of unreality of surroundings (e.g., the world around the individual is experienced as unreal, dreamlike, distant, or distorted).

Note: To use this subtype, the dissociative symptoms must not be attributable to the physiological effects of a substance (e.g., blackouts) or another medical condition (e.g., complex partial seizures).

Specify if:

With delayed expression: If the full diagnostic criteria are not met until at least 6 months after the event (although the onset and expression of some symptoms may be immediate).

In the following section, we will explore the finer points of the different ways in which children, adolescents, and young adults present with symptoms of PTSD.

The Clinical Interview at Different Developmental Stages

Review of Development

Prior to moving on, it is worth reviewing the typical developmental stages in order to understand what differences the clinician might observe in children who have been exposed to trauma. Table 1–1 provides a summary of the key characteristics of development that are expected in each age group along with relevant trauma correlates.

Preschool and School-Age Children

For young children, dyadic sessions and collateral information from the caregiver(s) are essential because young children often cannot give a detailed account of their history or the specifics of a traumatic event. Additionally, dyadic sessions can be useful in observing how the patient interacts with the caregiver because this interaction is likely to be quite different from the interaction with the clinician, who is unknown to the patient.

When meeting with the patient individually, the clinician should incorporate play therapy, which is an important technique for obtaining history about the traumatic event and the patient's symptoms. Having a room equipped with a reasonable selection of toys—simple board games, a deck of cards, a ball, dolls or action figures, paper and other art materials—is useful for the initial interview with the child. Children use play as a way of expressing emotion, thoughts, desire, and conflicts. Using symbolism, patients may reveal important details about a traumatic incident and their thoughts and feelings about it. In addition to attending to the content of the play, the clinician should pay attention to the process of the play, including repetition or play disruptions. This allows the clinician to surmise the patient's inner state—how the patient experiences and relates to the surrounding world. The clinician should note the patient's desire for order or control, his or her ability to respect limits set by the clinician, aggression, imaginative play, disorganization or messiness, inhibition versus impulsivity and disregard for safety, and trust and involvement of the therapist in the play versus isolation and withdrawal. In observing and interacting with a child through play, the clinician can also assess whether the child is developing as expected; significant differences from developmentally expected behaviors could be indicative of trauma.

TABLE 1–1.   Trauma exposure at different developmental stages

Age	Key developmental characteristics (Stubbe 2007)	Trauma correlate
Infancy	• Dependence on the caregiver • Developing a sense of security based on the caregiver's ability to meet the physical and emotional needs of the infant • Recognizing the permanence of an object even when it is out of view (by 6 months) • Preference for known caregivers and stranger anxiety (by 9 months) • Inference of cause and effect and organization of memories (by 1–2 years)	Trauma during infancy and early childhood would negatively impact the patient's sense of safety in the world. Inattentiveness, unavailability, or loss of a caregiver would be particularly traumatic. The patient would remember a trauma and draw conclusions, although not necessarily accurate, about the causes of the trauma. Particularly problematic is the limited language available to the patient at this stage, making it difficult, if not impossible, to verbally encode and express these thoughts and memories.
Preschool	• Desire for control and order • Development of self-esteem • Feelings of shame, guilt, and self-doubt • Identification with the same sex parent • Transductive reasoning (belief that incidents occurring in close temporal or spatial proximity are causally related) • Magical thinking • Egocentricity • Language development • Ability to use symbolism	The perfect storm of egocentricity, guilt, shame, magical thinking, and transductive reasoning results in patients at this developmental stage more frequently believing that any traumatic events are somehow their fault. Having language and the ability to use symbolism does provide different opportunities for assessment and therapy that are not available at earlier stages of development.

TABLE 1–1. **Trauma exposure at different developmental stages** *(continued)*

Age	Key developmental characteristics (Stubbe 2007)	Trauma correlate
School age	• A sense of accomplishment with creation and participation in socially appropriate activities (school, extracurricular activities) • Feelings of inferiority or inadequacy • Development of basic logic • Understanding of cause and effect • Recognition of the unique perspective and separate mind of the other	As children enter school, symptoms of trauma that went unrecognized at earlier stages may become more apparent. Significant challenges with structure, learning, and socialization with peers would warrant further evaluation. Occasionally, these symptoms are erroneously presumed to be related to other diagnoses, such as learning disorders, attention-deficit/hyperactivity disorder, social anxiety disorder (social phobia), or oppositional defiant disorder, when they are actually a consequence of trauma. Any abrupt change in behavior or functioning at school is a red flag. Somatic symptoms or physical illness without a clear etiology and resulting in missed days of school should also raise concern.

TABLE 1–1.   Trauma exposure at different developmental stages *(continued)*

Age	Key developmental characteristics (Stubbe 2007)	Trauma correlate
Adolescence	• Self-reliance • Sexual maturation • Identity formation and development of values and goals • Separation from family and increased identification with peers • Emotional reactivity • Hypothetical and deductive abstract reasoning • Increased risk-taking behavior	As adolescents distance themselves from their family of origin and venture into the world, they are likely to engage in more risk-taking behaviors, including drug and alcohol use. This places them at greater risk of exposure to traumatic experiences, including accidents, physical violence, and sexual assault. Unlike school-age children, emotionality and stress in this age group sometimes are overlooked as "hormonal" or "just being a teenager," and a diagnosis of acute stress disorder or posttraumatic stress disorder is missed. Trauma can have a significant negative impact on the development of an adolescent patient's identity and values and view of himself or herself. The risk of suicide is also increased in this age group (Skehan and Davis 2017).

TABLE 1–1. Trauma exposure at different developmental stages *(continued)*

Age	Key developmental characteristics (Stubbe 2007)	Trauma correlate
Young adulthood	• Development of increased insight • Ability to predict the outcome of decisions and less reliance on peers with regard to decision making • Increased autonomy and independence (from family) • Refining social relationships with a focus on intimacy and loyalty • Navigating sexual relationships and solidifying personal sexual orientation and gender identity • Increased empathy and focus on community as greater than self	Considering that a primary developmental goal of this stage is to establish more trust and intimacy between oneself and the surrounding community, turning away from the egocentrism and self-reliance of earlier stages, we can easily understand how trauma that is experienced interpersonally or as a result of man-made disasters would be disruptive to healthy development of the young adult. Trauma may leave the patient feeling more isolated and can interfere with intimacy in relationships. Where a history of sexual abuse or assault is involved, the ability to negotiate sexual relationships and find a sense of comfort with one's own sexual preferences may also be disrupted.

At other times, when the patient is able to be more expressive, play is used simply to create a fun and relaxed environment and to provide opportunities for the patient to talk with the clinician (Kernberg et al. 2012).

Projective techniques can also be useful in assessing the patient's inner state. The clinician might ask the patient to draw something of his or her choice or give more specific instructions (e.g., a house, tree, and a person or the patient's family). Winnicott's "squiggle" drawing game, in which the patient and clinician take turns in adding onto a line that can go in various directions, allows the patient and clinician to participate together in creating or imagining something (Winnicott 1990). The clinician might also ask the child to tell a story, share a dream, or talk about a movie or television show he or she has seen recently (King et al. 1997). What the patient chooses to share and how he or she conveys this information helps the clinician assess the child's developmental skills; get a sense of the patient's thoughts, ideas, and conflicts; and build rapport.

Like unstructured play, projective questions provide more information about the child's inner state. Some examples include the following questions: "If you could be any animal, what would you be?" "What do you want to be when you grow up?" "If you had three wishes, what would you wish for?" (King et al. 1997). A child who has been traumatized might identify with a more vulnerable animal, reflective of his or her own feeling of insecurity, or may choose to be a strong and powerful animal, reflective of a desire to protect himself or herself. A child who has been traumatized may not have any hopes for the future or may not be able to envision himself or herself as "a grown-up." Direct questions about the traumatic incident may be less effective. The clinician should ensure that the language used with the child is developmentally appropriate given his or her age. Younger children may be more suggestible and may provide answers they believe the clinician is seeking, whether true or false, whereas older children may feel too anxious or vulnerable and thus may avoid discussing negative feelings or topics. It is necessary to state that observations made using play therapy and projective techniques are not, in and of themselves, diagnostic of trauma. As with other screening tools, they must be used in conjunction with other, objective information obtained during the assessment.

Clinical Vignette 1

The following are process notes from a session with Lily, a 5-year-old girl who presented after the death of her sibling. She talked about the incident as we sat and played together with "magic sand." Of note, prior to the death of her sibling, Lily already had an extensive trauma history, including separation and reunification with her biological parents following incidents of physical abuse.

> Lily reported that she had been feeling sad and tired recently. She said that she had been feeling sad because her brother, Dylan, died. She said that the other day her mother said that she and her sister, Julia, should go to the park, but they did not want to because that was "Dylan's favorite place." Lily said she didn't want to leave him behind. She said that Dylan had been stung by a bee and "got a big bump on his back." Then, for several days she said he kept getting "fatter and fatter." Lily said she saw her brother in the hospital, and, when he was dead, he was getting skinnier. She said that when they were riding home in the car, Julia was crying and

screaming, "This can't be! This can't be! Why did this happen?" Lily said that when her brother Dylan "got fat," he also had trouble talking and walking.

Lily told me that when people die they might not be bloody, they might just look like they are asleep but you can't wake them up. She said that a person's spirit is what makes them speak and move their body. She said that Dylan's spirit went up to the sky with God. I asked her how she knew all of these things about what happens when a person dies, and she said that she just knew them.

Lily then went on to talk about her uncle seeing "the devil" in Mexico. She said that the devil is a man with big horns who is red and under the ground. She said that sometimes the devil will come up from the ground and take humans underground and feed them to his friends. She said Julia told her this. Julia also told her that she should listen to only what she hears in her right ear and "do what this hand (pointing to her right hand) does." Julia said that Lily should not do what her left ear hears or what her left hand does. Lily told me that the devil is very powerful and has a lot of friends, but God is more powerful. She said that in order to go and be with God you have to be good. I asked Lily what happens if someone makes a mistake. She responded that it would be OK, and the person would get to try again.

Clinical Vignette 2

The following is an example of a complete initial clinical interview with Anthony, 7-year-old boy who was receiving mental health services in a counseling-enriched classroom at his school. The complete clinical interview took place over two separate sessions, the first with the patient alone and the second with his caregivers.

Patient Session

History of the Present Illness

Anthony's initial assessment included both a classroom observation and an individual interview. During the classroom observation, Anthony was at times calm and cooperative, busy doing his work. When he attempted to interact with staff and didn't receive the response he wanted, Anthony became irritable and would begin cursing. He also demonstrated some physically aggressive behaviors, for example, throwing a glue stick at the basket it was to be placed in. Anthony was then given a 3-minute time-out, which seemed to cause more frustration. He initially refused to comply with the time-out but was eventually able to do so with calm guidance from staff.

During the individual session, Anthony was calm, cooperative, and engaged. He told me that he lives with his brother, who is a surgeon. Anthony reported that he was doing well. He reported that activities such as coming to school, playing video games, doing his work, and coloring help make him feel happy. He reported that he is sad a lot since his mom died and said that his older brother died as well. He reported feeling sad when he thinks about missing his mom. He reported that he used to think that he would be better off dead when she died and wanted his teacher to get something to kill him with. He also reported that he gets scared sometimes at night when he has nightmares (e.g., of being kidnapped) but had a difficult time quantifying how often he has nightmares. He also reported that he sees "stuff" at night such as zombies and that this makes sleeping difficult. He reported that he gets tired a lot and sometimes has headaches and stomachaches due to his medicine, but he did not recall the name of the medication. Anthony reported that things that make him angry include when he gets punished and when he does not get to use the computer.

When Anthony was asked what he would wish for if he had three wishes, he responded that he would wish for his mom to come back to life, to be rich, and to be in the NBA. Anthony also talked about wanting to be a rapper or an actor when he grows up. He reported not having many friends.

Mental Status Examination

Anthony appeared casually dressed and was clean and well groomed. He was slender and appeared slightly younger than his stated age. He had some problems with articulation of speech, but his speech was intelligible. At times he was physically agitated and notably tense, but otherwise his activity level was as expected for his age without hyperactivity or psychomotor retardation. No abnormalities were observed in his gait. His eye contact varied; at times he was able to make good eye contact, and other times he looked away or was attending to other things around the room. His attention and concentration were generally good and appropriate for his age. He described his mood as "good," and his affect ranged from irritable to euthymic to anxious. His thought process was linear and concrete. He did not report any thoughts of harming himself or others, nor were there any delusions or other abnormal thoughts present. He denied any hallucinations or other perceptual disturbances. His insight was age appropriate, and his judgment was fair.

Caregiver Session

History of the Present Illness

Anthony's current caregivers were also involved in his initial assessment, including his adoptive brother, Russell, and Russell's wife, Monica. They reported that Anthony has had a history of verbal and physical aggression at home and at school since he was in pre-kindergarten. They reported that Anthony has been in his current counseling-enriched classroom since last year. They reported that Anthony has already been expelled from three different schools because of aggression toward peers and teachers. Russell reported that Anthony's behavioral issues are not present at his home because he and Monica are very stern and consistent with Anthony and the other children in their home, ensuring that there are clear rules, consequences, and rewards. They reported that Anthony did have behavioral issues when living with his adoptive mother and that this was exacerbated by her declining health.

Russell and Monica reported that it is difficult to assess Anthony's mood because he does not express much to them. They reported that he does not describe feeling sad or worried, but he has told them he has nightmares. They said that Anthony will either respond with few words after a long pause or will not respond at all. They reported that he appears to have a good time when interacting with other children, but there are times when Anthony appears to prefer being left alone. When they pick him up from his after-school program, they sometimes find him waiting in the same spot, by himself, looking out the window.

Russell reported other symptoms he has observed, including that Anthony seems easily distractible, is avoidant of tasks that require sustained effort, and has difficulty completing tasks efficiently. Russell reported that Anthony is very active but does not feel that he is hyperactive.

Past Psychiatric History

Russell and Monica reported that Anthony was previously diagnosed with attention-deficit/hyperactivity disorder (ADHD) and is currently prescribed methylphenidate 10 mg/day and guanfacine 1 mg/day. Russell reported that Anthony takes his stimulant medication only during the school week and not on the weekend. Russell reported that he has not noticed a significant difference in Anthony's behavior with or without the medication. Anthony has complained of some stomachaches and headaches with the medication.

Past Medical History

Anthony has a diagnosis of asthma, but symptoms are currently well controlled.

Family History

Because Anthony was adopted and his adoptive mother is now deceased, Russell and Monica were unable to provide any information about Anthony's biological family's mental health history.

Birth and Development

Anthony's biological mother abused unknown substances during her pregnancy. Anthony was removed from her care at the time of birth and placed with his adoptive mother within a few days. His current caregivers do not have additional information about Anthony's motor, speech, or social early development. Anthony does not have any contact with his biological mother.

Social History

Anthony's adoptive mother was a single parent, with the exception of a brief marriage lasting from the time Anthony was 1 year old until he was 4 years old. Anthony's adoptive mother also adopted five other boys, now between ages 7 and 15 years, with the exception of her eldest adopted son, who was murdered when Anthony was 5 years old. The death of her eldest adopted son reportedly took a significant toll on her emotional and physical health.

Anthony's adoptive mother had one biological son, Russell, who is 41 years old. Russell and Monica are now the primary caregivers for Anthony. They also took in Anthony's adoptive brothers. They have struggled to provide care for them given that the services and resources that Russell's mother was receiving ended when she passed away. They were ultimately able to place two of the boys back with their biological families. Russell and Monica also have three of their own children between the ages of 2 and 9 years. Anthony gets along well with his adoptive nieces and nephews. Russell works as a physician's assistant, and Monica is employed as an engineer.

Trauma History

Anthony has experienced multiple losses and transitions in attachment figures as detailed in the social history. Russell denies abuse of any kind that he knows of but does report two prior unfounded child protective services reports against his mother for spanking.

Adolescents

Respecting adolescent patients' autonomy and privacy is particularly important as they are beginning to develop their own identity and to differentiate themselves from their parents. A clear explanation of what will and will not remain confidential is essential at the time of the initial interview. It requires nuance to involve the parents in the clinical interview without disrupting rapport with the patient, but parents often have relevant information that the teenager may avoid or omit. Additionally, parents are less likely to be engaged in treatment (and continue to bring the adolescent for care) if they feel alienated by the clinician. The clinician must maintain a delicate balance. If the intake is scheduled for a single session, it is preferable to meet first with the adolescent, then with the parents, and then with the entire family together. On some occasions, the intake may be scheduled as several separate sessions over a period of days or weeks. In this scenario, meeting with the parents first may be more appropriate.

Developing an alliance with an adolescent patient can be challenging because there may be a negative transference to the provider, who appears to be more aligned with the patient's parents or caregiver. Connecting with the patient first around his or her interests rather than jumping directly into a symptom checklist may help the patient to feel more relaxed and willing to open up. The clinician can aim to find commonalities between himself or herself and the patient, using appropriate judgment about personal disclosure, or can take an alternative route of using some mildly self-deprecating humor about the clinician's level of "uncoolness" and ask the patient to educate him or her about what it is like to be a teenager. Questions about sexual activity and substance use may feel uncomfortable, for the patient and clinician alike, but they are vital. Depending on the patient, a direct approach may be effective—asking the questions in a very matter-of-fact or medically focused way so as to normalize them—whereas for other patients, beginning by asking about drug use or dating at their school or among peers may be a prelude to asking more personal questions (Carlat 2012).

Clinical Vignette 3

The following are clinical notes from an initial visit with Blake, a 15-year-old male who was in foster care for several years because of chronic and repeated physical abuse by his father. Important pieces of history include that Blake's father had a substance abuse problem and was also a victim of physical abuse when he was a child. The abuse was reported by a teacher when Blake was in elementary school, and child protective services became involved. However, Blake remained in the home, and the abuse persisted for several more years despite therapeutic interventions with the family. Blake ran away from home several times, began using drugs and alcohol, was placed in several group homes, and was also in juvenile hall for several months prior to finally returning to live with his biological family.

> Blake entered the room and immediately slouched in the chair, playing music loudly from his headphones. I asked him if he could turn the volume down a bit, explaining that I have a hard time concentrating with too many distractions. Blake respectfully turned off the music without protest. His parents were unable to attend the session, and therefore his case manager had provided transportation. I asked Blake if he wanted to meet with his case manager present or wanted to meet individually, and he responded, "Whatever. I don't care." I recommended that he and I meet alone and that we could have his case manager join the session at the end.
>
> Despite his apparent indifference to being at the clinic, Blake was readily open in sharing his history, likely because he has been through this process several times in the past. He revealed details of horrific abuse by his father in an unexpectedly casual manner, explaining that "pain doesn't bother me" because he has learned that it "only lasts for a little bit." Blake spoke of his experiences in group homes and juvenile hall with some bravado, saying, "Fuck group homes" because "they make you do chores,

and I don't do chores." He bragged about running away and using drugs and alcohol with older peers and adults. However, he did add that he wished he could have stayed in juvenile hall until he completed high school because he liked the food, and the academic program there helped him accrue credits quickly.

Blake described his mood as "generally pissed" and "fuck everything" but is not seeking treatment for this and does not have much hope that these feelings will change. His chief complaint was insomnia, and he was anxious to obtain a medication to address this problem. He did not, on his own, relate his insomnia to his past trauma experiences. As he described significant symptoms of hypervigilance, always feeling vulnerable, threatened, and having to be aware of his surroundings and ready to defend himself, I reflected that perhaps this contributed to his difficulty sleeping, and he agreed.

Blake was frank in saying that he is unable to and never will trust anyone because he has always been let down. He said this, too, in a very matter-of-fact way, with an air of nonchalance. He did not seem, as one might have expected, discouraged or saddened by being unable to rely on anyone. He said that he has had too many experiences of telling people things and then being "put back in the system" because they are "mandated reporters." He reported feeling that some clinicians want to help but that others are "just in it for the money."

Blake talked about Max, a staff member at his last group home with whom he did connect with and still talks. Blake said that Max is the only person he trusts and is fully open with. He said that Max also had a hard life growing up and therefore was relatable. Blake explained that Max was able to listen without "tattling" and would provide "consequences" for negative behaviors but not "punishments." Blake felt that he actually learned and grew from these consequences. Blake aspires to having a life and change in course like Max, who he said now has a good job, money, a beautiful wife, and a nice car and home and is happy. Blake said Max is also a priest. Blake said he tried God himself and really wanted it to work, but it didn't. He said God never listened to him or helped him with anything.

Blake demonstrated some positive prognostic signs, including a sense of humor, the ability to articulate his thoughts and emotions, and a willingness to open up while maintaining some control and boundaries. His past experiences have definitely colored how he interacts with others, particularly mental health professionals, but he has had at least one positive experience with a trustworthy adult and expresses some future orientation and aspirations.

Transitional-Age Youth

As expected, developmentally, a young adult patient is able to better articulate his or her feelings and thoughts about various experiences that have occurred over the course of life than is a younger patient. This allows for more direct questioning in order to obtain key pieces of historical information. Nevertheless, the topic of trauma remains sensitive regardless of the patient's age, and rapport is no less important in this patient group. The clinician must consider that for some patients, the trauma may be proximal to the initial clinical interview and the primary reason that the patient is seeking care. For other patients, the trauma may be more remote, and these patients can be further categorized into 1) patients who have received therapy previously and have already had practice at revealing and working through trauma and 2) patients who experienced trauma several years ago but either never sought care or have been in care but never disclosed their trauma history. Another important distinction between young adults and younger children is the lack of collateral information obtained from parents and other family members because these people are rarely interviewed when working with patients older than 18 years.

Clinical Vignette 4

The following vignette consists of pertinent excerpts from a clinical interview with a young adult, 25 years old, named Grace. The history was obtained across three sessions, each lasting 45–60 minutes, and this will be indicated in the vignette in order to highlight how it is often challenging to obtain all relevant information in the first interview because of constraints of time and the patient's level of comfort. Sometimes, pertinent history of trauma is not obtained until several weeks to months into treatment because these topics are quite sensitive and require a significant level of trust. You will see that there are notable differences in the information obtained, particularly the social and developmental history, from this patient versus the younger patient in Clinical Vignette 3.

First Session

Grace presented to the clinic with uncertainty about her diagnosis and the medications (an atypical antipsychotic and an antiepileptic mood stabilizer) she had been prescribed. She reported being diagnosed with bipolar disorder by a previous provider and was seeking a second opinion about her diagnosis and treatment. Grace reported that she began feeling depressed 2 years ago. She reported being unable to get out of bed or leave the house and said she was "addicted" to TV. At the time of presentation, she reported current depressive symptoms, including spending a lot of time at home, social withdrawal, anhedonia, hypersomnia and insomnia, poor appetite, and occasional suicidal thoughts without any specific plan. She also described difficulty following through on things once she starts them.

Grace was born and raised in the South. She reported that her father was in the military and was gone for several months at a time. Her mother would become emotionally and behaviorally dysregulated (for example, throwing Grace's father's belongings into the front yard) during these absences. Grace's parents divorced when she was 6 years old, at which point she said she closed herself off emotionally. She recalled her parents fighting prior to the divorce and said that her brother, who is 6 years older, tried to shield her from the fighting.

Grace described her father as "a wonderful human being," whereas she described her mother as "crazy," with her mood fluctuating "on a whim." She reported that her mother struggled with mental illness, with a possible diagnosis of bipolar disorder. She also reported a history of alcohol abuse on both the maternal and paternal sides of her family. Grace reported a good relationship with her brother, whom she described as "successful but unemotional." Both of Grace's parents remarried. Grace lived primarily with her mother, stepfather, and half-sister, who is 13 years her junior, after her parents' divorce. As an older teenager, Grace moved in with her father and stepmother.

Grace described her stepmother as "cool" and "having good moral character" but described her stepfather as "a sociopath." She described initially having a good relationship with her stepfather, but when they moved to yet another new state when Grace was in middle school and her younger sister was born, her stepfather's behavior changed. Grace reported one incident of physical abuse by her stepfather when she was 11 years old in which her stepfather put his hands around her neck. She could not recall what prompted this behavior, but she remembers it being for something like "talking back" to him. Grace said she never reported the incident to anyone outside the home. She also witnessed her mother and stepfather physically fighting while her mother was holding her younger sister in her arms.

Grace reported performing very well academically throughout school. She said that school provided useful structure for her, and she immersed herself in academics as an escape from stress at home. She was engaged in sports and music but said she has since given up these activities. She described her social life as a contrast to her academic life. She reported that she began hanging out with the "misfits," sneaking around and using substances, all while maintaining the facade of "the perfect student."

Grace attended a 4-year college in the Northwest. She reported having a lot of freedom there, but the school was so accepting of differences among students that it "almost glorified mental illness." Since college, Grace has worked at three different jobs and lived in three different cities over the course of 4 years. Her jobs were not related to her major in college, and she admitted she was not sure what she wanted to do. The first two jobs were in teaching; she was fired from one and elected to leave the other because of low salary and lack of structure. She reported that she currently is employed at a tech company and works from home.

Grace reported having questions about her sexuality. She said that in relationships she tends to become quickly attached and "obsessive," even if the feeling is not reciprocated. She reported several sexual partners during college. She reported that her most recent relationship lasted 2 years, ending 1 month ago. She had been living with her boyfriend but currently lives in the home of her friend's mother. Grace is able to live there rent free and lives alone because her friend's mother lives in a skilled nursing facility.

Grace reported using marijuana, alcohol, and cigarettes from the time she was 13 years old. She reported that she currently uses marijuana and alcohol (1–2 glasses of wine) daily and smokes cigarettes occasionally. She reported that alcohol had been a problem in the past, with episodes of binge drinking and getting into fights, and having many sexual experiences while intoxicated. She reported a brief period of sobriety from marijuana and said during that time she noticed that her friendships improved and she had more time and motivation to engage in other activities. She reported that sometimes marijuana makes her feel more anxious. She also reported experimentation with mushrooms, cocaine, and "Molly."

Second Session

Grace opened up more about her current symptoms, talking about feelings of loneliness and isolation. She reported that she rarely leaves her house. She was tearful during the session in recounting how things in her life are piling up and beginning to feel unmanageable. She reported that her house is messy and many things are broken, but she feels hopeless and too unmotivated to address these problems. She said that she has not been grocery shopping and has not been eating regularly. She endorsed low mood and energy and variable sleep, at times sleeping too much and at other times being unable to sleep. She reported feeling insecure and having low self-esteem. She described a feeling of "being in the muck."

Grace talked about chaotic relationships in her life. She described both seeking connection with others and rejecting it because relationships inevitably unravel. She described feeling rejected or emotionally overwhelmed by the other person in the relationship. She talked about dating and about someone she recently met on a dating website. She reported that things were going well after a couple of dates. She felt that she was "following the rules" and "had the upper hand" but then noticed herself intentionally distancing herself from him, and the tables quickly turned. She talked about feeling "needy" and having difficulty being single. She talked more about her most recent relationship and said it was the only long-term relationship she had ever had. Although Grace described the relationship as chaotic, she also reported feeling bored and wanting more excitement. She tried to push the relationship to be polyamorous, and although her boyfriend was reluctant, she engaged with several other sexual partners in addition to her boyfriend.

Third Session

(*Note the significant traumatic incident that is not reported until this session.*) Grace talked more about her childhood and her lack of good social supports. She stated that her mother did lose legal custody of the children at one point, although she is not entirely sure of the reason. After her parents divorced, Grace transferred to a different school for third grade. She attended a Pentecostal school, which she described as oppressive. She reported that the school permitted corporal punishment, but her parents did not approve it, so instead she was placed in detention daily for refusing to wear a skirt and electing to wear pants instead. She said her parents chose the school only because it was equidistant from their homes. Grace lived with her paternal grandmother in fourth grade, but when her father was called away again for work, her mother and her mother's boyfriend "kidnapped" the children and took them to another state. Grace said that she continued to have occasional visits with her father, but custody, as per the divorce agreement, was never restored.

Grace reported having sex with a young adult male when she was 13 years old. She reported that she met him at the pool in her apartment complex and he invited her to his apartment, where she also used marijuana and alcohol for the first time. Grace said that she returned to the man's apartment the next day and they again had sex. She described repeating the act as a way of convincing herself that the sex was consensual and something that she wanted rather than rape. Grace told her mom that she was raped but fabricated a story about being kidnapped on the way home and being raped behind a building. The police were called, and Grace reported the same fabrication to them. Grace said that nothing happened after the report. Her mother and stepfather separated, and Grace, her mother, and her half-sister relocated to another state.

Shortly thereafter, an incident occurred that prompted Grace to go and live with her father. Grace had a fight with her mother, who hit Grace on the face and then called Grace's father to come and pick her up. Grace said that her father drove for 13 hours to get her, and she lived with him for the remainder of high school. She reported engaging in sexual activity with different partners and using drugs throughout that time. Grace reported that she came to view herself as a manipulative person who could get whatever she wanted.

Summary

As demonstrated by the clinical vignettes, patients of varying ages and developmental stages present differently during the initial visit(s). This includes if, how, and when they begin revealing details about any traumatic experiences. Table 1–2 provides a summary of the major differences in initial clinical presentation and interview techniques needed at varying ages, and Table 1–3 provides a list of sample interview questions to use based on the age and developmental stage of the patient.

TABLE 1–2.   Summary of developmental differences in initial assessment of trauma

	Young children	Adolescents	Transitional-age youth
Key differences in presentation at initial interview	During the initial clinical assessment, symptoms of trauma may appear as extreme shyness or inhibition, with limited engagement in play (independently and/or with the therapist) and minimal verbal communication or complete refusal to talk. Alternatively, the patient may interact with the therapist in an overly familiar manner, exhibiting little to no caution despite the clinician being a stranger. The patient may exhibit aggressive behavior (throwing or breaking toys), a high level of activity (inability to sit and focus on a single activity for more than a few minutes), emotional dysregulation, or affective lability (yelling or crying).	Commonly, adolescent patients are reticent to share any personal information and may minimize symptoms. They deny having any idea why they have been brought to the clinic, responding with "I don't know" to many questions asked by the interviewer, particularly when the questions have high emotional content. They may appear tense, hypervigilant, and restless. They may avoid direct eye contact. Alternatively, they may be overly agreeable or accommodating, trying to answer questions on the basis of what they perceive or imagine the interviewer wants to hear. Still other patients may present as sullen, irritable, defiant, or aggressive.	Young adult patients generally present to the initial session of their own accord. Some may begin talking about traumatic events during the first session, but more often, the chief complaint will not be directly related to trauma. Instead, patients may begin by reporting problems at work or with their social or romantic relationships. As with other age groups, the affective and behavioral presentation of the patient can vary greatly, and patients may present as guarded, anxious, depressed, dissociated, disinhibited, or agitated. If the patient is more resilient and mentally healthy, he or she may be open and insightful, even at the outset of treatment.

TABLE 1–2.   Summary of developmental differences in initial assessment of trauma *(continued)*

	Young children	Adolescents	Transitional-age youth
Key differences in interview technique	Because of limited language abilities at this developmental stage, direct questions tend to be less effective in obtaining necessary history. Instead, the clinician often uses play as a way to infer the child's view of himself or herself and his or her experience of the world. Young children use play to express emotion, thought, desire, and conflict. Play can also help provide a relaxed environment to help the child feel comfortable and develop trust with the clinician. More information is needed from caregivers, and dyadic sessions in which the clinician observes interactions between patients and caregivers are helpful. Birth, early development, and family history can be limited in cases where the patient is in foster or adoptive care.	Giving the adolescent patient control over what topics are discussed is useful considering the importance of autonomy and independence for patients at this developmental stage. Helpful techniques include expressing curiosity and interest about the adolescent's hobbies and social life, rather than running through a checklist of symptoms, and thoughtful self-disclosure on the part of the clinician in an effort to connect and find common ground. The clinician must not avoid questions about sexual activity and substance use, even if such questioning makes the patient and/or clinician uncomfortable. Another major challenge for the clinician is being able to maintain the adolescent's confidentiality while still involving caregivers in the assessment process.	The assessment of young adults is unique in that the clinician generally does not have the input of caregivers and the history is primarily, if not solely, dependent on the memory and openness of the individual patient. Trauma history may be more remote, and thus subsequent experiences and the course of the patient's life may have been altered or impacted by a traumatic incident occurring several years prior to the patient's presentation to the clinic. Questions about birth, early development, and family history can be more challenging than when answers are not provided by a parent. The social history also becomes more complex, often including occupational history, economic and housing stressors, romantic relationships, and the patient's own children.

TABLE 1–3. Sample interview questions by developmental stage

	Young children	Adolescents	Transitional-age youth and caregivers
History of the present illness	*How old you are? What is the best thing about being ___ years old? What's the worst thing about being ___ years old?*	The clinician may begin by gathering the social history (see below) and come back to the history of the present illness later in the session.	*Can you tell me about why have you come (brought your child) into the clinic today? What current problems are you (is your child) struggling with? In what settings are these problems occurring? When did these problems or symptoms first begin? Have they gotten better or worse over time?*
	What would you like to do today? We have lots of different toys to play with. Does anything look fun or interesting to you?	*Can you tell me something about yourself? I noticed you have your headphones in; what were you listening to? Have you ever been to any live concerts?*	
		What does your shirt say? I don't know that reference; what does it mean?	
		You look sort of tired today. What time did you have to wake up to get to the clinic today? Are you missing any school to be here? How do you feel about missing school?	

TABLE 1–3.   Sample interview questions by developmental stage *(continued)*

	Young children	Adolescents	Transitional-age youth and caregivers
History of the present illness *(continued)*	Following these initial questions, much of the session might involve the therapist commenting on the child's activities; making observations; and offering ideas about emotional content, fantasies, or conflicts coming up in the play. For example, if the patient picks up two action figures, one large and one small, and pretends that they are fighting with one another, the therapist might comment, *One of those guys is much bigger than the other. This fight might not be very fair. Wow, that big guy hits very hard! Ouch! That looked like it hurt! I wonder if the smaller guy feels afraid of the bigger guy. Do you think he needs a doctor? I wonder if there is anyone who can help. I wonder if we need a referee.*	*You seem a bit annoyed. Did your parents explain that you would be coming to meet with me today? What did they tell you about it? Whose idea was it to come to the clinic to meet with me? Why did your parents think that you needed to see a mental health provider? Is there anything in your life that you think could be better?*	

TABLE 1–3. Sample interview questions by developmental stage (*continued*)

	Young children	Adolescents	Transitional-age youth and caregivers
History of the present illness (*continued*)	The therapist might also ask questions to clarify and understand what the patient might be thinking as he or she makes certain choices in the play. For example, if a patient draws a picture, the therapist could ask, *What is happening in your picture? What is going to happen next? How are the people in the picture feeling? What are the people in the picture thinking?*		

TABLE 1–3.   Sample interview questions by developmental stage (continued)

	Young children	Adolescents	Transitional-age youth and caregivers
Previous psychiatric history	Have you ever met with someone like me before? Have you ever talked and played with someone like this before? Do you take any medicines to help you with anything? What do they help you with? Do you take any medicines when you feel sad or worried or to help your body and mind be more calm and relaxed? Is there anything about the medicine that you don't like or that makes you feel sick?	Have you ever met with a therapist or counselor before? What was that like? Were there things about it that you didn't like? Some people take medicines to help with their mood or their anxiety. Have you ever taken any medicines? What are your thoughts on medications in general? Do you know anyone else who has ever taken medication? What have they said about their experience?	Have you (has your child) ever met with a mental health professional before? What was that experience like? What was helpful? Was there anything about the experience that you did not like or that you would have wanted to be different? Have you (has your child) ever been to a psychiatric hospital? How many times? What were the reasons you were (your child was) admitted? Have you (has your child) ever been on any medications to address mental health symptoms? Were any of the medications effective? Did you (does your child) experience any side effects?

TABLE 1–3. Sample interview questions by developmental stage *(continued)*

	Young children	Adolescents	Transitional-age youth and caregivers
Past medical history	Unless there is a known history, it is generally not necessary to screen for medical problems in the initial interview. The clinician can ask some general medical questions: *Do you ever have problems sleeping? Do you ever have problems with tummy aches or your head hurting? What are your favorite foods? Do you ever have problems with eating? Do you ever eat more and more even after you are full? Are there times when your mom or dad makes you something to eat, but you don't feel like eating it?*	The clinician does not need to routinely screen for medical history unless the caregiver has already reported a significant medical or surgical history. For patients with chronic medical illness, adolescence can be a time when teenagers begin to take on more of a role in their own treatment and can also be a time of increased noncompliance with treatment. *How were you first diagnosed? How does your medical diagnosis interfere with your daily life or with being a teenager? Do you feel that your doctors and other people around you understand your experience? Who is most supportive when you are feeling physically ill? Do you ever intentionally miss medical appointments or skip your medications? Why?*	Important things to screen for include medical hospitalizations or surgeries; current medications; allergies; head injuries or concussions; injuries related to physical abuse or assault; traumatic medical experiences and life-threatening medical diagnoses; menarche and regularity of menstrual cycles; and pregnancies, miscarriages, or abortions.

TABLE 1–3.   Sample interview questions by developmental stage *(continued)*

	Young children	Adolescents	Transitional-age youth and caregivers
Past medical history *(continued)*	If there is a known, significant medical or surgical history, the clinician should be aware of any references to this in the child's play or, if appropriate, may ask direct questions. The clinician may have toys available that would allow the patient to engage in pretend play as a doctor, nurse, or patient, such as a toy first aid kit or toy medical equipment.	*Who helps take care of you when you are sick? Is there anything scary about going to the doctor? Have you ever been so sick that you had to sleep in a hospital? Have you ever hit your head so hard that you felt funny, couldn't talk clearly, or couldn't remember things? Have you ever gotten hurt so badly that you had to wear a cast or use crutches to help you walk?*	

TABLE 1–3. Sample interview questions by developmental stage *(continued)*

	Young children	Adolescents	Transitional-age youth and caregivers
Past medical history *(continued)*	Some patients may present with chronic medical illnesses, and inquiry about multiple medical visits or daily treatments may be appropriate. Again, looking for or bringing up the topic via play may be more appropriate than asking direct questions.		
Social history	*Who do you live with? What is your house like? Where do you sleep? Do you have your own room? What things do you like to do at home? Do you have a favorite game? Who do you like to play with at home?*	The clinician should attempt to engage casually with the adolescent, expressing a genuine curiosity about what is important and interesting to the teenager.	*Who lives in your home? Do you (does your child) share a room or bed with anyone else? How are you (is the family) financially supported?*

TABLE 1–3.   Sample interview questions by developmental stage *(continued)*

	Young children	Adolescents	Transitional-age youth and caregivers
Social history *(continued)*	*Do you go to school? What is your favorite thing to do at school? Is there anything you don't like about school? Do you have friends or a best friend? Does anyone at school say mean things to you or hurt you? What do you do when that happens? What is your teacher like?*	*What school do you go to? What is your least favorite thing about school? What is the most difficult thing about school? Is school important to you? Is school important to your parents? How do you react when you get a bad grade? How do your parents react when you get a bad grade? Do you have ideas about what you want to do after high school?* *Do you do any activities at or outside of school? What is your favorite thing to do in your free time?*	*For the caregiver: What school does your child attend and what grade is he or she in? How does your child do in school, academically and socially? Has your child ever been suspended or expelled? Has your child ever been bullied? Does your child ever miss school? How often?*

TABLE 1–3. **Sample interview questions by developmental stage** *(continued)*

Young children	Adolescents	Transitional-age youth and caregivers
Social history *(continued)*	*Do you have friends? Do you have a best friend? Do you ever get into arguments with friends? What are they about? How do they get resolved? Have you ever been bullied? Have you ever bullied anyone else? Are you dating or thinking about dating? Are you interested in boys, girls, or both?*	*For the youth: Did you complete high school? Did you attend any college or graduate schools? Are you currently employed? Do you enjoy your job? Do you ever miss work? How often? What do you do for fun? What is your social support system like? Do you have any romantic partners currently? Are you sexually active? How many partners have you had? Do you use protection? Do you enjoy sex? Have you ever been pregnant? Have you ever had a miscarriage or abortion? Do you currently have any children? What is your relationship like with your children?*

TABLE 1–3. Sample interview questions by developmental stage *(continued)*

Young children	Adolescents	Transitional-age youth and caregivers
Social history *(continued)*	The clinician should try to assess the developmental appropriateness of taking a sexual history on the basis of the age and maturity level of the adolescent. That is, the clinician should be aware of the developmental differences between a typical 13-year-old and a typical 17-year-old while also considering variability in experiences even between two adolescents of the same age. The sexual history can be asked as part of social or medical history: *Have you ever been sexually active? How old were you when you lost your virginity? What was that experience like for you? What have subsequent sexual experiences been like? How many partners have you had? Do you use protection? Do you enjoy sex?*	

TABLE 1–3. Sample interview questions by developmental stage (*continued*)

	Young children	Adolescents	Transitional-age youth and caregivers
Trauma history	*Has anything very scary ever happened in your life, to you, or to someone you know? What do you remember? Are there things you are afraid of now? Do you ever feel worried about someone hurting you? Has anyone ever hurt you in the past? Do you ever have scary dreams? Can you tell me about a scary dream you had?*	*Has anything really scary ever happened to you or someone you know? Has anyone ever physically hurt you? Has anyone ever touched you in a way that felt uncomfortable or that you did not consent to?*	*Have you (has your child) ever experienced any traumatic events? This could be anything very scary that happened to you (your child) or that you (your child) witnessed. Did your (your child's) mood or behavior change after this traumatic event? Have you (has your child) had any nightmares or frequent memories of the incident? Are you (is your child) more fearful or on edge? Do you (does your child) feel numb or without a normal range of emotions? Do you (does your child) make comments or have feelings that you (he or she) won't live a full life? Do you (does your child) avoid things that remind you (him or her) of the incident?*

TABLE 1–3. Sample interview questions by developmental stage *(continued)*

	Young children	Adolescents	Transitional-age youth and caregivers
Substance use	Generally not applicable.	The clinician can begin by talking about the patient's exposure to substance use before asking him or her directly about his or her own use. *Do you know anyone at your school who uses drugs or alcohol? Have you ever tried alcohol or marijuana? What was it like when you tried it? Were there things that you liked about it? Was there anything you didn't like about it? Have you experimented with any other drugs, including prescription drugs? What have you tried?*	For the caregiver: *Do you have any concerns about your child using drugs or alcohol? Do you know what (s)he has tried? Has (s)he ever become so intoxicated that (s)he was in medical danger? Has (s)he had any traumatic experiences, for example, being sexually assaulted, while intoxicated? Has (s)he ever been in legal trouble as a result of drug use?*

TABLE 1–3. Sample interview questions by developmental stage *(continued)*

Young children	Adolescents	Transitional-age youth and caregivers
Substance use *(continued)*	If possible, the clinician should try to get as much detail as possible, including when the substance was first and last used; how often it was used; and any consequences, legal or medical, of use. *Did you ever black out or not remember something you did while you were drunk or high? Did anything scary or dangerous ever happen while you were intoxicated?*	For the youth: *Have you ever experimented with drugs or alcohol, including prescription drugs? What have you tried?* If possible, the clinician should try to get as much detail as possible, including when the substance was first and last used; how often it was used; and any consequences, legal or medical, of use.

Potential Obstacles

Misdiagnoses and Comorbidities

One of the challenges of trauma is that the presenting symptoms can mimic symptoms of other mental health disorders, including affective and anxiety disorders, ADHD, oppositional defiant disorder, and psychotic disorders. This is even more complex in children and adolescents. For example, problems with concentration and hyperactivity are symptoms of ADHD, but these symptoms can also be observed in children with a trauma history. Irritability, sadness, hopelessness, and impaired sleep are symptoms of both depression and PTSD. Hypersexuality and aggression may be misperceived as symptoms of mania if the clinician misses a history of physical or sexual abuse. Intense fearfulness of certain people or places may be precipitated by a trauma experience but be incorrectly diagnosed as social anxiety or panic disorder (Cohen et al. 2010). When misdiagnosis occurs, it is not uncommon for patients to be prescribed medications that are inappropriate for the treatment of trauma. Tragically, as symptoms persist, medications may be deemed ineffective and doses increased, putting patients at greater risk of experiencing adverse reactions.

Further complicating the situation, some patients do have true comorbid diagnoses. Often, but not always, a thorough history, with a clear chronology of when symptoms began (particularly before or after a traumatic incident) can help determine whether the patient has PTSD alone or PTSD in addition to another psychiatric disorder. Substance abuse is one of the most common comorbidities, with a peak in the young adult population, where comorbid substance use and mental health disorders exist in 36% of patients (Skehan and Davis 2017). In the context of PTSD, patients may use drugs or alcohol as a way to avoid intrusive, traumatic memories or to numb feelings of anxiety, sadness, or irritability.

Symptoms of PTSD also may resemble those of some physical illnesses. Children with exposure to trauma may present not to mental health providers but to their pediatrician with somatic complaints (e.g., headaches or stomachaches), as the only symptoms. A full physical examination may uncover clear signs of abuse. However, not having physical evidence of abuse does not mean that abuse is not occurring. Medical providers, such as pediatricians, emergency department physicians, and nurses, need to be able to perform a basic mental health assessment so as not to miss a diagnosis of PTSD. The somatic symptoms may be solely an expression of psychological distress, but trauma can also result in true physical ailments. Comorbid physical illness can occur with and as a result of trauma and needs to be addressed (Cohen et al. 2010).

Temporality of Trauma

The clinician needs to keep in mind that the interview will need to be adapted on the basis of when the trauma occurred. For example, mental health clinicians acting as first responders in the context of a natural disaster or terrorist attack will likely not perform the thorough, in-depth assessment described earlier in the section "Gathering a Thorough History." They may focus on ensuring that there are no medical emergencies and on reconnecting the patient with family members, with a primary goal of providing a sense of comfort and safety.

In other situations, the patient may present with trauma that is ongoing, such as domestic violence, sexual or physical abuse, or neglect. Although it can be disruptive to rapport, the clinician, as a mandated reporter, needs to be prepared to file a child protective services report if an incident of past or ongoing child abuse is reported for the first time during the initial visit. Depending on the situation, the report may be completed with the patient and caregivers in the room. Sometimes this can help to maintain alliance with the patient and caregiver(s) because the involvement of child protective services is presented as a way for the family to get much needed help and support. At other times (e.g., if the caregiver is the perpetrator of the trauma), completing the report with the family present may be damaging, or even dangerous, for the clinician and patient. It will be important to inform child protective services about any imminent danger so that alternative placement can be found if the child is unsafe in the home. Many patients, especially younger children, may be reluctant to divulge information because they may feel protective of their caregivers, may fear retaliation or punishment by the perpetrator, or may fear that they will be separated from their family.

Suicidality and Homicidality

Patients with exposure to trauma may engage in self-injurious or suicidal behaviors. Even without taking trauma history into account, suicide rates are highest among adolescents and young adults, ages 15–24 (Fliege et al. 2009). For patients with PTSD, the rates of deliberate self-harm have been found to be as high as 50%, with increased likelihood of suicidal ideation and attempts (Dixon-Gordon et al. 2014). It has been suggested that self-harm is used as a way to cope with intrusive thoughts and painful negative emotions or to manage feelings of numbness that can occur in PTSD

(Smith et al. 2014). Self-injury, both nonsuicidal and suicidal, needs to be assessed when gathering the past psychiatric history and as a part of the mental status examination. Active suicidal thoughts with clear plan, intent, and means require psychiatric hospitalization. Some behaviors, such as cutting or other forms of self-mutilation, may not require psychiatric hospitalization but certainly require close monitoring by both the clinician and other adults in the patient's life. Removal of access to means of self-harm, particularly guns but also knives, prescription and over-the-counter medications, and toxic household items, is also important to help maintain the patient's safety.

If the patient voices an intention to seriously harm another person (e.g., the perpetrator of the trauma), this may also warrant psychiatric hospitalization. In most areas of the United States, when homicidal thoughts involve a clearly identified victim, as well as a plan and the capacity to carry it out, the clinician has a duty to warn the potential victim, even though this means breaking confidentiality.

Multiple Providers and Continuity of Care

Ideally, there are multiple people supporting a child or adolescent receiving care for trauma. This team generally includes an individual therapist for the patient, a therapist for the caregiver(s), a therapist to work with the family, and possibly a psychiatrist. (On some occasions, the psychiatrist also does individual therapy with the patient.) Adults at the patient's school (e.g., teachers, a school counselor), a pediatrician, and case workers or support staff at a group home or residential facility might be part of this team as well.

A large, multidisciplinary team has benefits but also disadvantages. It can be difficult to ensure that all parties are communicating and collaborating effectively, particularly when multiple systems or agencies are involved, each with its own policies and procedures, including different systems of documentation and maintaining records. It can also be overwhelming for the patient, particularly if the role of each member of the team is not clear. Additionally, patients, particularly those who have experienced abuse in their primary families, may already be experiencing frequent transitions in caregivers, residences, and geographic locations. Changes in insurance can also be disruptive to care and may require a change in providers. It is not uncommon to be engaged in an interview with the patient or family and hear the complaint, "I just told my entire life story to Dr. So-and-So, and now I have to start all over with you!"

Whenever possible, it is desirable to find a clinic or agency where there are multiple resources in one location. This enhances continuity of care for the patient because there is some assurance that the providers are communicating with one another if they are at the same clinic and sharing the same electronic medical record system. If it is not overwhelming for the patient or family, having core members of the multidisciplinary team meet the patient and family during the initial interview can be helpful. This provides an opportunity to explain the role of each team member. As treatment proceeds, reminders will likely be necessary to help the family know who they should turn to for what. To further simplify things for the family, having a clear team lead who organizes and communicates with all members of the team and who acts as a liaison between the patient and family and the team is helpful. Once the patient and family establish care with a particular team, it is preferable that they remain with these providers until treatment is complete because starting over and rebuilding the alliance can slow the process of recovery.

Sociocultural Factors

Every patient wants to feel understood, and it is the clinician's responsibility to foster an environment of acceptance. The clinician should make an effort to have a baseline knowledge of the social and cultural identities most prevalent in his or her community. However, every individual patient is unique, and the clinician is not expected to have a detailed understanding of the customs and histories of all cultures and social groups. If the clinician expresses a willingness to learn from and understand the patient, this can have a significant impact on the treatment, and this tone can be set during the first encounter.

Differences in culture can impact trauma in several ways, including how the patient perceives and interprets the traumatic event, what symptoms are exhibited, if and how the trauma is addressed by the family and community, and the ways in which the patient engages in and responds to different forms of treatment (Nader 2007). With regard to the initial intake, it is important for the clinician to obtain, by observation and direct questions, information about the patient's racial, ethnic, socioeconomic, and religious background, as well as his or her gender identity and sexual orientation. It is not enough to simply record how the patient identifies himself or herself; it is also necessary to understand the impacts on and what role these influences play in the patient's life. Two patients may both identify as "Christian," but one patient may attend church every Sunday, participate in a weekly youth group and Bible study, and pray nightly, whereas the other may follow particular moral codes set forth by the religion but may not regularly visit a place of worship or be actively affiliated with a religious community. For some cultures or racial groups, there is an association to a historical trauma that is remembered by the community as a whole, even if the patient never directly experienced the initial traumatic event (Nader 2007).

During the initial assessment, the clinician should be conscious of different customs that may influence interactions between the patient, caregivers, and clinician. Some parents or families may not feel comfortable with the clinician meeting with their child without them present. Some cultures have different norms or perspectives with regard to gender roles and familial hierarchy. Cultural background may impact behavior and disclosure, particularly around more sensitive issues (Vasquez 2007). The clinician should be aware that individuals from certain cultures and racial groups may be more prone to feelings of mistrust of medical or mental health providers. This can also impact access to care because some of these patients may never present to the clinic. Community outreach measures and mental health services available in schools can help with this problem.

In certain cultures, the patient and family may be deferential and accommodating to the clinician as a figure of authority. If the patient and family perceive that the clinician is of a similar cultural background, they may not provide detailed and important information because of a false assumption that the clinician already knows or understands certain elements of the patient's background, when in fact the clinician may have no knowledge of these elements. The clinician should be careful, too, of falling into this trap, being sure to follow up on things that might, on the surface, seem obvious or apparent. The clinician needs to be attentive to his or her own biases, prejudgments, and countertransferences when working with patients of both the same and different backgrounds.

Assessment of socioeconomic status is particularly important because low-income, inner-city populations are at higher risk of PTSD (Gillespie et al. 2009). In addition, lack of transportation, lack of insurance, or an inability to pay for treatment may impede access to care. Socioeconomic status can be difficult to assess directly because it may feel invasive to ask a family or patient for their annual household income. Indirectly, socioeconomic status can be assessed by observing the patient closely or by asking questions about whether or not the family has what is needed in terms of basic necessities: Are the patient's clothes tattered or unwashed? Does the patient ever go without eating? Is the patient or caregiver employed and in what field? How many members of the family are in the home? Is there adequate living space for each individual? Is or has the patient ever been homeless?

Unique populations include foster youth, who have been removed from the care of their biological parents, generally because of child endangerment. There are different legal and governmental supports in place with the aim to ensure that foster youth are provided with sufficient and ethical care. Lesbian, gay, bisexual, and transgender patients are also at increased risk of victimization and trauma, and thorough assessment of safety and acceptance in the home as well as any history of bullying by peers should be obtained.

Conclusion

When meeting a patient and family for the first time, the primary goal is to put them at ease. Particularly when trauma is one of the presenting symptoms, the clinician should aim to provide an atmosphere where the patient can feel safe and reassured that he or she is surrounded by people who want to listen, understand, and help. In this chapter, I reviewed some of the ways in which a clinician can achieve this type of atmosphere and how techniques vary on the basis of the patient's stage of development. Regardless of whether this is the patient's first contact with the mental health care system or he or she has received treatment previously, the initial visit is a crucial opportunity for the clinician to set the stage for ongoing treatment.

KEY CONCEPTS

- After reading this chapter, you should have knowledge of the following:
  - A complete mental health assessment interview, including obtaining a thorough history and assessing the patient's mental state
  - Unique aspects of interviewing a patient with a trauma history, including creating a welcoming and safe environment for the patient and family, as well as making necessary adaptations to history taking based on the patient's age and developmental stage
  - Potential obstacles to be aware of and address during the initial interview such as comorbid diagnoses, temporality of the trauma, suicidality and homicidality, and complex systems of care
  - Sociocultural factors that may impact the patient's experience of trauma and how they relate to or interact with the interviewing clinician

Discussion Questions

1. What techniques might a clinician use to develop rapport with patients of the following age groups: preschool age, school age, adolescents, and young adults?

2. What safety concerns requiring immediate attention and action could arise in the initial clinical encounter?

3. What are the potential pitfalls of having multiple providers involved in a patient's care and how can a clinician guard against them to ensure continuity of care?

4. What are three important things for a clinician to remember when working with a patient whose social or cultural customs are different from his or her own?

Suggested Readings

Carlat DJ: The Psychiatric Interview: A Practical Guide, 3rd Edition. Philadelphia, PA, Lippincott Williams & Wilkins, 2012

Nader K: Culture and the assessment of trauma, in Youths in Cross-Cultural Assessment of Psychological Trauma and PTSD. Edited by Wilson JP, So-Kum Tang CC. New York, Springer, 2007, pp 169–196

Stubbe D: Child and Adolescent Psychiatry: A Practical Guide. Philadelphia, PA, Lippincott Williams & Wilkins, 2007, pp 2–32

Vasquez MJ: Cultural difference and the therapeutic alliance: an evidence-based analysis. Am Psychol 62(8):878–885, 2007

References

American Psychiatric Association: Diagnostic and Statistical Manual of Mental Disorders, 5th Edition. Arlington, VA, American Psychiatric Association, 2013

Carlat DJ: Psychiatric Interview: A Practical Guide, 3rd Edition. Philadelphia, PA, Lippincott Williams & Wilkins, 2012

Cohen JA, Bukstein O, Walter H, et al: Practice parameter for the assessment and treatment of children and adolescents with posttraumatic stress disorder. J Am Acad Child Adolesc Psychiatry 49(4):414–430, 2010, 20410735

Dixon-Gordon KL, Tull MT, Gratz KL: Self-injurious behaviors in posttraumatic stress disorder: an examination of potential moderators. J Affect Disord 166:359–367, 2014 24981133

Fliege H, Lee JR, Grimm A, et al: Risk factors and correlates of deliberate self-harm behavior: a systematic review. J Psychosom Res 66(6):477–493, 2009 19446707

Gillespie CF, Bradley B, Mercer K, et al: Trauma exposure and stress-related disorders in inner city primary care patients. Gen Hospital Psychiatry 31(6):505–514, 2009 19892208

Kernberg PF, Ritvo R, Keable H, et al: Practice parameter for psychodynamic psychotherapy with children. J Am Acad Child Adolesc Psychiatry 51(5):541–557, 2012 22525961

King CA, Hovey JD, Brand E, et al: Prediction of positive outcomes for adolescent psychiatric inpatients. J Am Acad Child Adolesc Psychiatry 36(10)(supplement):1434–1442, 1997 9334557

Manley MRS: Psychiatric interview, history, and mental status exam, in Kaplan and Sadock's Comprehensive Textbook of Psychiatry, 7th Edition. Edited by Sadock BJ, Sadock VA. Philadelphia, PA, Lippincott Williams & Wilkins, 2000, pp 1426–1455

Nader K: Culture and the assessment of trauma, in Youths in Cross-Cultural Assessment of Psychological Trauma and PTSD. Edited by Wilson JP, So-Kum Tang CC. New York, Springer, 2007, pp 169–196

National Conference of State Legislatures: Mental Health Professionals' Duty to Warn. Washington, DC, National Conference of State Legislatures, September 28, 2015. Available at: www.ncsl.org/research/health/mental-health-professionals-duty-to-warn.aspx. Accessed March 13, 2018.

Skehan B, Davis M: Aligning mental health treatments with the developmental stage and needs of late adolescents and young adults. Child Adolesc Psychiatr Clin North Am 26(2):177–190, 2017 28314449

Smith NB, Kouros CD, Meuret AE: The role of trauma symptoms in nonsuicidal self-injury. Trauma Violence Abuse 15(1):41–56, 2014 23878154

Stubbe D: Child and Adolescent Psychiatry: A Practical Guide. Philadelphia, PA, Lippincott Williams & Wilkins, 2007, pp 2–32

Vasquez MJ: Cultural difference and the therapeutic alliance: an evidence-based analysis. Am Psychol 62(8):878–885, 2007, 18020774

Winnicott DW: Therapeutic Consultations in Child Psychiatry. New York, Basic Books, 1990

2

Assessment in Schools or Other Large Groups

Nicole Quiterio, M.D.
Jared T. Ritter, M.D., FAPA

> I was really frightened, thinking that everything and everyone around me was going to die. The ground was shaking all around...it made such a loud noise. I couldn't sleep the whole night.

Traumatic events can affect age-appropriate developmental tasks and trajectory. Resilience has been defined as an "active process resulting in positive adaptation in the face of major adversity" (Fayyad et al. 2017, p. 191) and as "the capacity to rebound and to restore pre-disaster psychological equilibrium" (Pfefferbaum et al. 2013, p. 1231). Man-made and natural disasters have the potential to expose large groups to traumatic stress. Assessing large groups of youth involves an understanding of the protective and risk factors that impact the group's resilience and likelihood of developing posttraumatic sequelae.

In this chapter, we first describe developmental differences to consider when assessing groups of children and adolescents of varying ages postdisaster. In the second part of the chapter, we focus on potential challenges when assessing large groups. We explore the obstacles that emergency department physicians and first responders face with the pediatric population and offer guidance regarding screening and triaging. Policy and sociocultural factors influencing pediatric disaster preparedness are also discussed.

Developmental Approaches: Preschoolers, School-Age Children, and Adolescents

Trauma literature suggests that children and adolescents' stress reactions and symptom manifestation vary according to developmental age (Dogan-Ates 2010; Scheeringa et al. 2012). Maturity can influence a youth's ability to understand the nature of a traumatic event and his or her sense of involvement within it. Table 2–1 lists age-specific reactions that are common for preschoolers, school-age children, and adolescents from somatic, cognitive, emotional, and behavioral viewpoints.

Postdisaster Reactions of Preschoolers

Following a disaster, preschoolers may show generalized or specific fears, loss of language skills, behavior problems (e.g., temper tantrums, aggression), dependency, separation anxiety, irritability, nightmares, posttraumatic play, behavioral reenactments, and specific regressive behaviors (e.g., thumb sucking, enuresis, tics).

Saylor et al. (1992) conducted a study involving 238 families and 278 children after a major hurricane in South Carolina in 1989. Parents reported that children had many new and unusual fears such as fears of storms and water after the hurricane. Some children even refused to take baths because of their fear of water. Other children personified Hurricane Hugo in their play. One set of parents reported their two-and-a-half-year-old daughter believing "Hugo was a real person—a very bad [person] who destroyed everything and then died." There was a significant increase in the number and severity of children's behaviors before and after the hurricane per parents' reports. Sleeping problems, dependent behavior, frustration, temper tantrums, and whining were the most frequently reported problems. There were reports of nervous behaviors such as twisting hair or biting fingernails. Fourteen months after the hurricane, the parents of 161 preschool children were resurveyed (Swenson et al. 1996). The findings showed that 9% of the children continued to play hurricane games, and 14% showed fear of storms or reminders of the hurricane. When compared with 170 children of similar age from Massachusetts and Utah who were not exposed to natural disasters, the postdisaster children showed significantly greater problematic behaviors than their peers in the control group.

Preschoolers exposed to disasters display more dependency behaviors following a disaster, including clinging to parents, wanting to remain

TABLE 2–1. **Common age-specific reactions of youth postdisaster**

	Preschoolers (ages 2–5)	School-age children (ages 6–11)	Adolescents (ages 12–18)
Somatic reactions	Sleep disturbances, eating issues, dizziness	Energy loss, somatic complaints, sleep disturbances	Eating issues, energy loss, pain, nausea, dizziness, fainting, sleep disturbances
Cognitive reactions	Magical explanations of the event, repeated retelling of the disaster, unpleasant memories of the disaster, persistent fears	Beliefs in supernatural or powerful forces, distractibility, distortions, intrusions of unwanted images, impaired concentration, poor school performance, reoccurrence of symptoms around disaster anniversary	Impaired concentration, poor school performance, memory problems, intrusive visual images
Emotional reactions	Crying, emotional outbursts, excessive clinginess, irritability, sadness, separation or stranger anxiety, disaster-related or generalized fears	Anger, denial, guilt, helplessness, loss of interest in pleasurable activities, low moods, self-blame, disaster-related and generalized fears	Anxiety, denial, fears of growing up, grief, survivor guilt, shame, humiliation, depression, resentment, suicidal thoughts, revengeful wishes, impulsivity, rage, hopelessness, despair
Behavioral reactions	Anxious behaviors, reenactment play, regressive behaviors, temper tantrums, hyperactivity	Hyperarousal, hypervigilance, aggressive behaviors, hyperactivity, peer problems, repeated telling of the disaster and disaster-related play, social withdrawal	Hyperarousal, acting out behaviors, peer problems, premature entrance into adulthood, social withdrawal, isolation, deviance, delinquency, school refusal, lack of responsibility, loss of interest in pleasurable activities, alcohol and drug use

Source. Adapted from Dogan-Ates 2010.

close to home, and asking to sleep with parents. Sleep disturbances and nightmares (e.g., dreams of imaginary creatures such as witches and monsters) are common reactions seen in preschoolers. Additionally, young children who lack the emotional vocabulary to express their feelings may engage in reenactment through traumatic play by playing the same scene over and over again (Davis and Siegel 2000). This population is vulnerable to dissociation, particularly when there is a component of victimization with interpersonal trauma (Hagan et al. 2015).

In summary, preschoolers who have been exposed to disasters have higher incidences of heightened trauma-specific and fear reactions, developmentally regressive behaviors, and traumatic reenactment of the disaster experience seen within their play. There is evidence for an increase in behavioral problems such as whining and temper tantrums.

Postdisaster Reactions of School-Age Children

School-age children may show a decline in school performance in the aftermath of a disaster. With natural disasters, living conditions and schooling may be disrupted or destroyed. Following a wildfire, children were found to have a decrease in their school performance and an increase in their school absenteeism (McFarlane et al. 1987). Three months after Hurricane Hugo, children with more severe posttraumatic stress disorder (PTSD) symptoms had a greater decline in school performance than those who had fewer symptoms (Shannon et al. 1994).

A study of the aftermath of a 1984 sniper attack on a crowded elementary school playground in South Central Los Angeles where 1 child and a passerby were killed and 13 children were injured showed varying degrees of exposure in the 159 children interviewed. As the degree of exposure increased, the number of PTSD symptoms reported similarly increased. Of the children on the playground, 77% had moderate to severe PTSD symptoms compared with 67% who were at school and <26% who were at home at the time of the attack (Pynoos et al. 1987).

Dollinger et al. (1984) found that both children and their parents had heightened levels of specific fears following a lightning strike disaster than did a nontraumatized control group. These children showed fears of storms, animals, noises, death, enclosed spaces, and separation from their parents. They also had sleep disturbances and somatic complaints that were associated with their fears of storm and death. Galante and Foa (1986) showed that children who were exposed to an earthquake disaster exhibited trauma-specific fears that reoccurred around the anniversary of the disaster.

In summary, school-age children show heightened specific fears, separation anxiety, and PTSD symptoms after exposure to a disaster. They may have a decline in school performance; increased refusal to attend school; and cognitive problems, including poor concentration and/or problems with reading and comprehension. As a result of a disaster, children may lose their social supports and may be less likely to continue to engage in pleasurable activities (e.g., sports, theater, art).

Postdisaster Reactions of Adolescents

Adolescents can be viewed as more adult-like than child-like on the basis of their cognitive functioning and understanding what the trauma means to them. In contrast to school-age children, adolescents tend to exhibit a sense of foreshortened future, negative expectations, and altered attitudes about their career goals and romantic relationships. Some adolescents may not engage in long-term planning because they have lost hope and trust in their future. Postdisaster rates of risk-taking behaviors—including alcohol and other drug use—are higher among adolescents than younger children and may be curbed with an "interdisciplinary, school-based health care center approach" (Schiff and Fang 2016, p. 4).

Studies have suggested that adolescents may show signs of depression, belligerence, and anxiety following a disaster. In a study following the 1972 Buffalo Creek Dam collapse, Gleser et al. (1981) found that adolescents exhibited more depression and belligerence than younger children, with 39% having moderate to severe depression compared with their school-age (32%) and preschool (14%) counterparts. Higher rates of comorbidity with PTSD, depression, and anxiety were noted with adolescents. Najarian et al. (1996) found that 2.5 years after a 1988 earthquake in Armenia there were higher rates of PTSD, depression, and behavioral problems in adolescents affected by the disaster than in the control group. Similar to school-age children, adolescents who are closer to the exposure source (the most affected area) have higher rates of PTSD than those adolescents who are farther away from the source (moderately or less affected areas).

In summary, adolescents may exhibit confrontational behaviors, lack of affect, and defiant or disruptive behaviors such as truancy, drug and alcohol use, and premature sexual activity. The involvement in these risk-taking behaviors can be life threatening and life changing to adolescents' social lives, education, and interpersonal relationships. Peer relationships, which can serve as a source of support, can be negatively impacted. In adolescence, lack of peer relationships can lead to isolation and decreased engagement in daily activities.

Assessments

Emergency Care Systems

The first lines of care for children are usually out-of-hospital providers or disaster medical assistance teams (DMATs) who arrive on the scene of the disaster. There have been deficiencies demonstrated with the preparedness of DMAT and emergency medical services (EMS) agencies in caring for children. A survey of DMATs (Shirm et al. 2007) has shown that they are lacking in pediatric equipment and training and protocols for assessment and management. EMS agencies do not fare much better for the pediatric population: although 73% had written protocols, only 13% of those protocols were specific to children. Almost 70% did not have any specific plan for a mass casualty at a school, and more than 60% did not include any provision for children or adults with special needs (Shirm et al. 2007). Efforts have been made on a federal level to improve the planning and preparedness for children. In 2009, the National Commission on Children and Disasters was formed to conduct a comprehensive study on children in relation to preparedness, response, and recovery for all major disasters and emergencies. In 2010, the commission released its recommendations to the U.S. President and Congress, including establishing a dedicated federal grant for prehospital EMS disaster preparedness, requiring first responders and EMS vehicles to stock pediatric equipment according to national guidelines for basic life support and advanced life support, and developing a national strategy for pediatric emergency transport and patient care during disasters (National Center for Disaster Preparedness 2010).

Currently, overcrowded emergency departments are not prepared to handle the additional surge of patients in the face of large disasters. Pediatric patients are particularly vulnerable on the basis of both the general difficulties involved in emergency departments being able to quickly respond to the urgent needs of children in disaster situations and factors unique to this population.

In 2009, the American Academy of Pediatrics partnered with the American College of Emergency Physicians and published a revised joint policy on the guidelines for care of children in the emergency department (American Academy of Pediatrics et al. 2009). Within these guidelines are recommendations for administration, staffing, equipment, supplies, medications, and quality improvement. Even with this information widely available, only 6% of emergency departments had all the equipment outlined in the joint policy (Gausche-Hill 2009). Most of the equipment that was missing consisted of smaller-size items for infants and children such as pediatric Magill forceps for removal of foreign bodies, oral and nasal cannulas, and vascular access catheters. Only half of emergency departments had quality improvement measures, and some were not even aware that national guidelines existed for emergency departments.

Screening and Triaging Postdisaster

After community disasters, it is vitally important to consider the level of trauma exposure in order to direct people to the most appropriate services and level of care. Pfefferbaum et al. (2013) outlined a service approach based on exposure for both the community and society at large. Those children and families directly exposed who are at risk for developing psychiatric disorders such as PTSD are treated under the medical model. Those who are directly exposed but do not develop a psychiatric disorder and those children and families who are indirectly affected may still suffer distress and challenges from the disruption in their lives. Referral for social support would be more appropriate for these two latter groups, as illustrated in Figure 2–1.

Screening can be used to help identify children in large groups who are at a heightened risk of developing psychiatric disorders (e.g., emergency shelters, faith assistance centers, medical and pediatric health centers, day care centers, schools, faith-based organizations, volunteer organizations, community facilities). Saylor and Deroma (2002) recommended that screenings should occur periodically to obtain a baseline and provide surveillance moving forward. An assessment framework can be used as a model for screening children who were directly exposed or indirectly affected by the disaster (Figure 2–1). If the population is small or the disaster is particularly severe, screening can be omitted in favor of comprehensive clinical evaluations for all children and family members or close associates who were directly exposed.

A comprehensive clinical evaluation includes a full diagnostic assessment with the goal of identifying any psychopathology in order to guide treatment and appropriate referrals. (See Table 2–2 for a list of appropriate screening instruments.) When there is a history of psychopathology or prior trauma, a clinical evaluation should be certified even in the absence of an acute presentation. Clinical evaluations can be done in hospitals or clinics, evacuation centers, schools, or shelters. When establishing a psychiatric diagnosis, the clinician should not rely solely on symptom checklists or questionnaires but rather should focus on assessing the child for all diagnostic criteria of a psychiatric disorder during the course of clinical interviewing in corroboration with parental or caregiver reports (Pfefferbaum et al. 2013). Parents can provide important information regarding

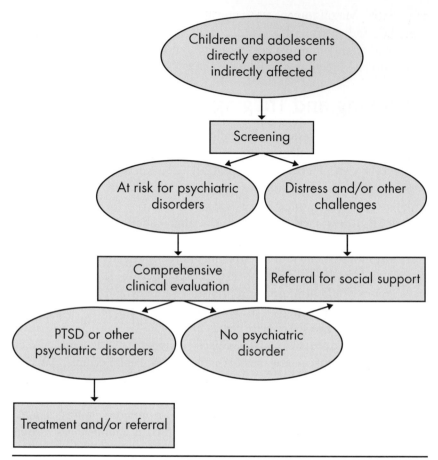

FIGURE 2–1.   Assessment of children and adolescents postdisaster.
PTSD=posttraumatic stress disorder.
Source.   Adapted from Pfefferbaum and North 2013.

the child's history, experiences, behaviors, and functioning, but it must be noted that parents may underestimate clinical symptoms in this population (Scheeringa et al. 2012). Children are the best at recounting their own personal experiences, perceptions, and internal reactions following a disaster. Additional sources of information may include school personnel, family members or close associates familiar with the child, daycare workers, and mental health providers.

Predisaster disorders and preexisting conditions should be noted because these disorders can place children at a higher risk for adverse outcomes following a disaster. Clinicians should not assume that all psychopathology is directly caused by the disaster. Ultimately, clinical

TABLE 2–2. Screening instruments for youth and young adults

Measure or questionnaire	Reference	Age range	Time to complete
Beck Anxiety Inventory (BAI)	Hagan et al. 2015	17 years and older	5–10 minutes
Beck Depression Inventory-II (BDI-II)	Thakar et al. 2013	13 years and older	5–10 minutes
Child Behavior Checklist (CBCL)	Scheeringa et al. 2012	6–18 years	15–20 minutes
Child Revised Impact of Events Scale (CRIES)	Fayyad et al. 2017	8–18 years	<5 minutes
Childhood Trauma Questionnaire (CTQ)	Bernstein and Fink 1998	12 years and older	5 minutes
DISC Predictive Scales (DPS)	Pfefferbaum and North 2016	9–17 years	20 minutes
Strengths and Difficulties Questionnaire (SDQ)	Fayyad et al. 2017	3–16 years	5 minutes
Trauma Symptom Checklist for Children (TSCC)	Hagan et al. 2015	8–16 years	15–20 minutes
Trauma Symptom Checklist for Young Children (TSYC)	Hagan et al. 2015	3–12 years	15–20 minutes
Traumatic Events Screening Inventory-Parent Report Form Revised (TESI-PR)	Hagan et al. 2016	0–6 years	20–30 minutes
UCLA Child/Adolescent PTSD Reaction Index for DSM-5 (PTSD-RI)	Pynoos and Steinberg 2013	7–17 years	20–30 minutes

judgment must be used to determine what the symptoms represent, the level of severity, and whether or not the symptoms fit current diagnostic criteria.

International Psychiatry

Some complex disasters, such as international wars and civil conflicts, are not just a single circumscribed event but may occur over years. These disasters can displace large groups and result in subsequent traumatic events. Genocide, terrorism, and mass refugee immigration may further impact those affected by war. As infrastructure and native supports collapse, there is a greater challenge to meet the mental health needs of the surviving people. International psychiatry seeks to understand global mental health disparities and recognizes the need for international collaboration when it comes to assessing large groups, delivering services, and conducting research necessary for developing policy and evidence-based interventions.

For example, Cambodia was ravaged by war and genocide under the Khmer Rouge in the 1970s, causing the population to fall by 20%–40% and triggering a consequent mass global diaspora. The only two psychiatrists in the country were killed during this time, and the only psychiatric hospital was converted into a "retraining facility." A number of international studies in the decades that followed looked at mental health outcomes in this population. These studies have included more than 6,600 individuals in publications spanning 1986 to 2014. Assessing such large groups requires international collaboration, ability to work across pluralistic health care systems, and an understanding of cultural concepts of distress (e.g., *baksbat* or "broken courage") (Chhim 2013). Rates of PTSD and major depressive disorder vary widely depending on which study is considered (Ritter 2014). Of note, the rates of PTSD were highest in groups outside of Cambodia and Thailand. Youth affected by the Khmer Rouge genocide and refugee immigration were less likely to have a diagnosable psychiatric disorder if they were living with their nuclear family following relocation to the United States.

Sociocultural and Policy Implications

Public Health Systems and Agencies

The role of the public during the three phases of the disaster cycle—prevention, response, and recovery—is crucial in order for health systems and agencies to be able to support and sustain community efficacy and resiliency. Shaw (2007) referred to these three phases as the pre-impact, impact, and post-impact phases. Public health systems and agencies can be very instrumental in preserving, promoting, and sustaining the resilience of children and families. Clinicians working within these systems "should assess and monitor risk and protective factors across all phases of a disaster" (Pfefferbaum et al. 2013, p. 1230). Table 2–3 highlights some of the empirical biopsychosocial risk and protective factors that may be considered when assessing large groups of youth.

TABLE 2–3. Risk and protective factors that can influence the postdisaster developmental trajectory in youth

	Risk factors	Protective factors

Biological factors	• Prior trauma exposure (priming)
	• Family psychopathology
	   – Maternal symptoms of PTSD or depression
	   – Parental psychopathology and poor mental health
	   – Mothers with highly punitive discipline styles
	   – Parents who manifest symptoms
	   – Number of maternal disorders
	   – Negative family emotional tone
	   – Parental overprotectiveness
	   – Self-reported maternal escape or avoidance coping
	• Problematic substance use since the disaster
	• Physical adversity
	   – Physical injury from traumatic event
	   – Chronic and complex traumatic stress
	   – Physical illness or injury caused or exacerbated by a storm
	• Pretrauma psychiatric problems
		• Neurobiological integrity
		   – Intelligence
		   – Cognitive ability
		   – Communication skills
		   – Higher scores on cognitive tests
		   – Cognitive flexibility
		   – Social skills
		• Familial/hereditary factors
		   – Parental responses to trauma
		   – Positive parenting attitudes
		   – Parental competence
		   – Warm and caring parents
		   – Parental harmony
		   – Effective parenting
		• Ability to elicit caretaking behaviors

TABLE 2–3. Risk and protective factors that can influence the postdisaster developmental trajectory in youth *(continued)*

Risk factors	Protective factors
Psychological factors	

Risk factors

- Degree of traumatic exposure
- Functional impairment
- Degree of fear
- Reversal of the dependency role
- Witnessing a threat to a caregiver
- Self-report emotional sensitivity
- Excessive prohibition of regressive behaviors
- Perceptions of the events
- Severity of the trauma
- Attachment status
- Serious risk of death
- Death of family member or close friend
- Victimization resulting from lawlessness after a storm
- Victimization of a loved one
- Victimization
- Psychological adversity
- Avoidance symptoms
- Anxiety before the storm
- Traumatic reminders
- Traumatic loss

Protective factors

- Adaptive coping and problem-solving skills
- Humor
- Tendency to express opinions even if different from others
- Positive self-concept and image of self
- Intact self-regulation
- Social competence
- Adaptability to new situations
- Ease with transitions
- Empathy
- Resilience
- Feeling of safety and security
- Positive emotions
- Internal locus of control
- Self-esteem
- Hope
- Optimism

TABLE 2–3. **Risk and protective factors that can influence the postdisaster developmental trajectory in youth** *(continued)*

	Risk factors	Protective factors

Social factors	• Living in areas that are continually exposed to disasters
	• Exposure to media coverage of the disaster
	• Financial strain
	  – Unemployment
	  – Income loss
	  – Lower family income
	  – Culture of poverty
	  – Urban poverty
	  – Difficulty meeting children's basic needs
	• Distressed family environment
	  – Children experiencing family violence during war
	  – Decreased parental supervision
	  – Ongoing difficulties associated with housing
	  – Parent-child dysfunction
	  – Child maltreatment
	  – Incarceration
	  – Parenting stress
	  – Challenges in parenting
	  – Family violence
		• Higher social support
		  – Perceived high instrumental support
		  – School support
		  – Support through other social and community-based institutions
		  – Valued school affiliation
		• Religion and spirituality
		  – Religious affiliation
		  – Engagement in religious activities
		  – Limited exposure to quarrels about religion and politics
		• Family support
		  – High family socioeconomic status
		  – Parental education
		  – Having parents who spend time with their children and support them with school work
		  – Strength and continuity of familial relationships and parental monitoring of their children's behavior
		  – Using nonviolent means of communication and discipline

TABLE 2–3.   Risk and protective factors that can influence the postdisaster developmental trajectory in youth (*continued*)

Risk factors	Protective factors
Social factors (*continued*)	
• School	• Family support (*continued*)
– Perceiving teachers as not kind	– Positive family environment
– Failing school	– Family cohesion
• Property loss	– Affectional ties with the family
– Having toys lost during war	– Caring positive parent-child relationships
• Anxiety at the neighborhood level	– Extended family
• Access to substance use	• Having leisure activities
• Gang violence	• Avoidance of television time
• School and community violence	• Maintaining routines
• Personal victimization in the school and/or community	
• Relationship to victims and survivors	
• Physical proximity	

Note.   PTSD=posttraumatic stress disorder.

Prevention Phase

During the prevention phase, the goals of public health are the following: optimize and enhance preparedness within systems serving families and children, promote community efficacy and resilience, and identify available resources. In order to effectively respond to a disaster, public health workers need to have specialized skills, capabilities, and knowledge. Many organizations, such as the American Red Cross, provide disaster mental and behavioral health training, such as psychological first aid for first responders and providers. Disaster mental and behavioral health training should include program and intervention evaluation, research, phase of emergency planning, and attention to crisis risk communication cycles. It is important to integrate mental and behavioral health resources into a disaster response.

Promoting community resilience is a critical goal during the prevention phase of a disaster. *Community* can consist of a group of people living in an identifiable locality or sharing common interests. Norris and colleagues (2008, p. 131) define community resilience as "a process linking a set of adaptive capacities to a projective positive trajectory of functioning and adaption after a disturbance." They found that high levels of personal resilience and wellness can ground community resilience. Community resilience focuses on collective action and outcomes. Public health agencies can work within communities to build and foster resilience. Public health systems should also identify available resources by updating contact information of agencies, clarifying their respective roles and responsibilities during disaster events, and linking potential resources.

Disaster Response Phase

The goals of this phase are the following: assess the impact of the disaster event, inform and educate the public, and facilitate referral to clinicians for timely evaluation and treatment and other services. Mental and behavioral health surveillance, needs assessment, and screening serve several purposes when assessing the impact of a disaster. Screening and triage focus on identifying the appropriate clinical intervention, level of care needed, and urgency with which the services are provided.

During the disaster response phase, public health agencies can provide the public with timely risk communication and health education. With the rapid spread of information through television and radio news, the Internet, and social media, individuals can be affected remotely (e.g., teens living outside the affected area learn about a school shooting through vivid pictures on Instagram), and they may want to know more details about the extent of the disaster. Disasters may involve both objective and subjective risk; generate great concern; and evoke fear, hypervigilance, anxiety, apathy, outrage, distrust, anger, helplessness, depression, frustration, and a decreased sense of control, which may negatively impact behavior and function. Public health agencies may provide developmentally appropriate mental and behavioral health education to children and parents on the expected and normative psychological reactions to disasters, explain certain problems that might require further help from mental health professionals, and provide instructions on how to access mental and behavioral health services within the community.

The last goal during the disaster response focuses on facilitating referral to treatment and other services provided by shelters, medical facilities, religious organizations, community centers, child care facilities, and schools. Assisting with finding employment opportunities for parents who have lost their jobs as a result of the disaster is another valuable part of helping families recover.

Disaster Recovery Phase

The goals of the disaster recovery phase include the following: identify unmet needs, reduce the impact of primary and secondary events, reestablish normalcy, investigate longer-term event effects, and formulate policy. Interventions aimed at mitigating or preventing the effect of secondary events of trauma will help improve health outcomes for subsequent trauma exposures. Public health agencies should find ways to reduce any unnecessary or preventable psychological trauma associated with the recovery phase (e.g., decrease separation time between a lost child and parents or caregiver). Public health workers need to be trained to recognize adverse mental and behavioral health outcomes in children and families following a disaster to be able to make appropriate and timely referrals. These workers may benefit from additional training in basic crisis counseling techniques such as psychological first aid.

As a result of a disaster, there can be initial observations of heroism, altruism, and hopefulness during the response phase, which can be replaced with disillusionment and realization of the harsh realities of loss, grief, hardship, and community destruction. Many families experience losses of various types and have subsequent unmet needs that warrant identification. The death of loved ones, insufficient food and clothing, and temporary or permanent termination of parent employment can be distressing. Public health activities can be undertaken to help minimize the extent of these secondary stressors. Return to normalcy involves understanding of an adaptation to losses rather than a return to a predisaster state. Public health agencies should focus on assisting schools, families, and child care agencies to return to predictable and supportive routines.

The disaster recovery phase has been the least studied phase and remains poorly defined because there are no clear temporal boundaries delineating when the recovery phase starts and ends. Public health should support large-scale, longitudinal, population-based epidemiological studies to fill in any gaps in the understanding of the postdisaster effects on children and families. Outcome and long-term intervention research should be conducted to determine best practices for helping children and families affected by disasters. Once best practices are known, public health policy and advocacy work should support preventative and remedial interventions for children and adolescents who are at risk.

Conclusion

In this chapter, we discussed how children and adolescents are a vulnerable population and provided a framework on how to assess groups of children and adolescents from a developmental perspective. We provided some background information on the challenges faced by practitioners within public health systems as they attempt to ensure rapid triage and emergency management and described the challenges of screening large groups and the role of international psychiatry. Last, we discussed the roles of public health systems and agencies during the disaster cycle and how we need to evaluate our strategies, policies, and procedures at each phase while considering biopsychosocial risk and protective factors.

There is greater need for recognizing and promoting international research and opportunities for establishing "international interdisciplinary working teams" (Schiff and Fang 2016). War, refugee immigration, community violence and victimization, terrorism, and natural disasters are some of the traumatic events that affect large groups and that can have a global impact. International collaboration among trauma experts, clinicians, and first responders holds promise for addressing the challenges faced when assessing large groups of traumatized youth.

KEY CONCEPTS

- Children are a particularly vulnerable population compared with adults because of their developmental differences and disparities in accessing mental health services.
- Children and adolescents should be assessed on the basis of their developmental level and unique biopsychosocial risk and protective factors.

- Although screening is appropriate for large groups of children following disaster situations, children directly exposed to severe disasters may need to proceed straight to a comprehensive clinical evaluation.
- For large-scale disasters, international psychiatry holds promise for collaborative approaches to assessing large groups and addressing mental health needs in a culturally sensitive manner.

Discussion Questions

1. Given the widespread use of social media, what types of psychosocial supports can we use online to help those who might be remotely affected by disasters?

2. Considering the variable rates of PTSD following a potentially traumatizing event, how can we assess resilience versus psychopathology in children and adolescents?

3. Focusing on the prevention phase, how can we improve our current systems to promote community and personal resilience?

Suggested Readings

Byron BH, Ruzek JI, Wong M, et al: Disaster mental health training: guidelines, considerations, and recommendations, in Interventions Following Mass Violence and Disasters: Strategies for Mental Health Practice. Edited by Ritchie EC, Watson PJ, Friedman MJ. New York, Guilford, 2006, pp 54–79
Pfefferbaum B, North CS: Assessing children's disaster reactions and mental health needs: screening and clinical evaluation. Can J Psychiatry 58(3):135–142, 2013
Shaw JA, Espinel Z, Shultz JM: Care of Children Exposed to the Traumatic Effects of Disaster. Arlington, VA, American Psychiatric Publishing, 2012

References

American Academy of Pediatrics; Committee on Pediatric Emergency Medicine; American College of Emergency Physicians; et al: Joint policy statement-guidelines for care of children in the emergency department. Pediatrics 124(4):1233–1243, 2009 19770172
Bernstein DP, Fink L: Childhood Trauma Questionnaire: A Retrospective Self-Report. San Antonio, TX, Pearson, 1998

Chhim S: Baksbat (broken courage): a trauma-based cultural syndrome in Cambodia. Med Anthropol 32(2):160–173, 2013 23406066

Davis L, Siegel LJ: Posttraumatic stress disorder in children and adolescents: a review and analysis. Clin Child Fam Psychol Rev 3(3):135–154, 2000 11225750

Dogan-Ates A: Developmental differences in children's and adolescents' post-disaster reactions. Issues Ment Health Nurs 31(7):470–476, 2010 20521917

Dollinger SJ, O'Donnell JP, Staley AA: Lightning-strike disaster: effects on children's fears and worries. J Consult Clin Psychol 52(6):1028–1038, 1984 6520273

Fayyad J, Cordahi-Tabet C, Yeretzian J, et al: Resilience-promoting factors in war-exposed adolescents: an epidemiologic study. Eur Child Adolesc Psychiatry 26(2):191–200, 2017 27312537

Galante R, Foa D: An epidemiological study of psychic trauma and treatment effectiveness for children after a natural disaster. J Am Acad Child Adolesc Psychiatry 25(3):357–363, 1986

Gausche-Hill, M: Pediatric disaster preparedness: are we really prepared? J Trauma 67(2 suppl):S73–S76, 2009 19667856

Gleser GC, Green BL, Winget C: Prolonged Psychosocial Effects of Disaster: A Study of Buffalo Creek. New York, Academic Press, 1981

Hagan MJ, Hulette AC, Lieberman AF: Symptoms of dissociation in a high-risk sample of young children exposed to interpersonal trauma: Prevalence, correlates, and contributors. J Trauma Stress 28(3):258–261, 2015 26062136

Hagan MJ, Sulik MJ, Lieberman AF: Traumatic life events and psychopathology in a high risk, ethnically diverse sample of young children: a person-centered approach. J Abnorm Child Psychol 44(5):833–844, 2016 26354023

McFarlane AC, Policansky SK, Irwin C: A longitudinal study of the psychological morbidity in children due to a natural disaster. Psychol Med 17(3):727–738, 1987 3628633

Najarian LM, Goenjian AK, Pelcovitz D, et al: Relocation after a disaster: posttraumatic stress disorder in Armenia after the earthquake. J Am Acad Child Adolesc Psychiatry 35(3):374–383, 1996 8714327

National Center for Disaster Preparedness: Children and Disasters. New York, Earth Institute, Columbia University, 2010. Available at: https://ncdp.columbia.edu/policy/policy-portfolio/children-disasters/. Accessed June 29, 2018.

Norris FH, Stevens SP, Pfefferbaum B, et al: Community resilience as a metaphor, theory, set of capacities, and strategy for disaster readiness. Am J Community Psychol 41(1–2):127–150, 2008 18157631

Pfefferbaum B, North CS: Assessing children's disaster reactions and mental health needs: screening and clinical evaluation. Can J Psychiatry 58(3):135–142, 2013

Pfefferbaum B, North CS: Child disaster mental health services: a review of the system of care, assessment approaches, and evidence base for intervention. Curr Psychiatry Rep 18(1):5, 2016 26719308

Pfefferbaum B, Shaw JA; American Academy of Child and Adolescent Psychiatry (AACAP) Committee on Quality Issues (CQI): Practice parameter on disaster preparedness. J Am Acad Child Adolesc Psychiatry 52(11):1224–1238, 2013 24157398

Pynoos RS, Steinberg AM: The UCLA PTSD Reaction Index for DSM-5. Los Angeles, CA, Behavioral Health Innovations, 2013

Pynoos RS, Frederick C, Nader K, et al: Life threat and posttraumatic stress in school-age children. Arch Gen Psychiatry 44(12):1057–1063, 1987 3689093

Ritter JT: International psychiatry: Cambodia as a case study—Part II. Grand rounds presentation at the University of Hawaii John A. Burns School of Medicine, Honolulu, HI, June 2014

Saylor C, Deroma V: Assessment of children and adolescents exposed to disaster, in Helping Children Cope With Disasters and Terrorism. Edited by La Greca AM, Silverman WK, Vernberg EM, et al. Washington, DC, American Psychological Association, 2002, pp 35–53

Saylor CF, Swenson CC, Powell P: Hurricane Hugo blows down the broccoli: preschoolers' post-disaster play and adjustment. Child Psychiatry Hum Dev 22(3):139–149, 1992 1555486

Scheeringa MS, Myers L, Putnam FW, et al: Diagnosing PTSD in early childhood: an empirical assessment of four approaches. J Trauma Stress 25(4):359–367, 2012 22806831

Schiff M, Fang L: Adolescents' exposure to disasters and substance use. Curr Psychiatry Rep 18(6):57, 2016 27087347

Shannon MP, Lonigan CJ, Finch AJ Jr, et al: Children exposed to disaster: I. Epidemiology of post-traumatic symptoms and symptom profiles. J Am Acad Child Adolesc Psychiatry 33(1):80–93, 1994 8138525

Shaw JA: Children: Stress, Trauma, and Disasters. Miami, FL, Disaster Life Support Publishing, 2007

Shirm S, Liggin R, Dick R, et al: Prehospital preparedness for pediatric mass-casualty events. Pediatrics 120(4):e756–e761, 2007 17908733

Swenson CC, Saylor CF, Powell MP, et al: Impact of a natural disaster on preschool children: adjustment 14 months after a hurricane. Am J Orthopsychiatry 66(1):122–130, 1996 8720649

Thakar D, Coffino B, Lieberman AF: Maternal symptomatology and parent-child relationship functioning in a diverse sample of young children exposed to trauma. J Trauma Stress 26(2):217–224, 2013 23529875

3

Assessment of Individuals

Chad Shenk, Ph.D.
Heather Bensman, Psy.D.
Brian Allen, Psy.D.

PEDIATRIC TRAUMA—environmental events involving actual or threatened death, serious injury, or sexual violence—affects up to two-thirds of all children younger than 18 years in the United States (Copeland et al. 2007). Trauma-exposed youth experience a range of adverse effects, including the onset of psychiatric disorders across different diagnostic domains, as well as a host of physical health outcomes. Moreover, the majority of children exposed to one trauma experience multiple traumas and adversities that can sustain the risk for adverse health outcomes even into adulthood (Felitti et al. 1998). Assessing pediatric trauma exposure at the points of clinical care where families receive health services can promote detection of a trauma history, more accurately inform clinical decision making and differential diagnosis, and guide more effective courses of therapy to address patient complaints. In this chapter, we review the state-of-the art methods for assessing pediatric trauma in childhood and adolescence so that the practicing clinician can better detect, diagnose, treat, and refer patients they serve. Emphasis is placed on pediatric trauma measures that meet the following criteria: they are available across different developmental stages and different assessment structures (e.g., interview, self-report); they include caregiver reports of trauma exposure history; they include an assessment of posttraumatic stress disorder (PTSD) as conceptualized in the fifth edition of the *Diagnostic and Statistical Manual of Mental Disorders* (DSM-5; American Psychiatric Association 2013); and they provide information on the sociocultural value, financial cost, administration time, and potential challenges of the measure. Information on how to access each instrument is also provided. Currently available assessment instruments are listed in Table 3–1.

Developmental Approaches

Preschool and School-Age Children

Assessing pediatric trauma in infants and young children often requires the clinician to interview primary caregivers who have an established relationship with the child so that changes in mood and functioning as a result of the trauma can be determined most accurately. This necessitates that the clinician has a firm understanding of typical infant and child development so that deviations from normative patterns and milestones can be readily identified. For example, in addition to the symptoms included in the criteria for PTSD, young children may demonstrate changes in sleep and appetite, vague somatic complaints, regressive behaviors, toileting difficulties, and increased clinginess to caregivers. In addition, caregivers can often experience sadness and guilt about their young child having been exposed to a trauma. In our experience, it is important for clinicians to recognize and normalize this reaction in caregivers during the interview so that the accuracy of information gained during the interview is enhanced and the transition to clinical services is most appropriate.

Diagnostic Infant and Preschool Assessment

The Diagnostic Infant and Preschool Assessment (DIPA; Scheeringa and Haslett 2010) is a semistructured clinician interview administered with the child's caregiver that assesses 16 different psychiatric conditions that may exist in children from birth to age 6 years. The DIPA begins with a standardized assessment of 11 traumatic life events common for children in this age range, including exposure to vehicle accidents, animal attacks,

TABLE 3–1. Summary of instruments for the assessment of pediatric trauma

	Age range	Respondent(s)	What is assessed	Administration	Cost	Source
Diagnostic Infant and Preschool Assessment (DIPA)	Birth to 6 years	Caregiver	Trauma and symptoms	Clinician-administered interview	Free	https://medicine.tulane.edu/sites/g/files/rdw761/f/DIPA-2017-2-14.pdf
Traumatic Events Screening Inventory for Children (TESI-C)	Birth to 18 years	Youth and caregiver options	Trauma	Clinician-administered interview	Free	www.ptsd.va.gov/professional/assessment/child/tesi.asp
UCLA PTSD Reaction Index for DSM-5 (UCLA PTSD-RI-DSM-5)	Birth to 18 years	Youth and caregiver	Trauma and symptoms	Self-report, caregiver report, or clinician interview	Varies (contact publisher)	www.reactionindex.com/index.php/
Kiddie Schedule for Affective Disorders and Schizophrenia (K-SADS-PL)	3–18 years	Youth and caregiver	Trauma and symptoms	Clinician-administered interview	Free	www.kennedykrieger.org/patient-care/faculty-staff/joan-kaufman
Comprehensive Trauma Interview (CTI)	12 years and older	Youth	Trauma and symptoms	Self-report and clinician-administered interview	Free	Contact jgn3@psu.edu

TABLE 3–1. Summary of instruments for the assessment of pediatric trauma *(continued)*

	Age range	Respondent(s)	What is assessed	Administration	Cost	Source
Childhood Trauma Questionnaire (CTQ)	12 years and older	Youth	Trauma	Self-report	$177.15 for kit (manual and 25 questionnaires); $71.45 for 25 questionnaires	www.pearsonclinical.com/psychology/products/100000446/Youthhood-trauma-questionnaire-a-retrospective-self-report-ctq.html

physical abuse, natural disasters, and drowning. Items endorsed in this section of the assessment are then followed by a clinical interview of the caregiver to assess developmentally appropriate symptoms of PTSD, such as nightmares, increased frequency or severity of temper tantrums, avoidance of adults, reluctance to discuss the trauma, new troubles in school, and reenacting the trauma in play situations, consistent with recent modifications to DSM-5 for children younger than age 7 years.

Other psychiatric disorders assessed with the DIPA include major depressive disorder, attention-deficit/hyperactivity disorder, separation anxiety disorder, and generalized anxiety disorder. The DIPA can be completed in 30–60 minutes depending on the total number of symptoms endorsed. Earlier versions of the DIPA have shown acceptable levels of reliability and validity, although psychometric testing of the recent update to DSM-5 is needed. The DIPA is available to clinicians free of charge at https://medicine.tulane.edu/sites/g/files/rdw761/f/DIPA-2017-2-14.pdf.

Traumatic Events Screening Inventory for Children (TESI-C)

The Traumatic Events Screening Inventory for Children (TESI-C; Ribbe 1996) was originally developed as a 15-item clinician-administered interview conducted with a child or adolescent age 4–18 years to determine whether he or she has ever experienced a traumatic event and if so, the total number of traumas to which he or she was exposed. Traumatic events assessed with the TESI-C include exposure to domestic violence, community violence, natural disasters, accidents, physical injuries, physical abuse, and sexual abuse. The TESI-C has moderate to good interrater reliability across different traumatic events, with noted criterion and convergent validity.

The TESI-C has since been revised into a developmentally sensitive 24-item clinical interview (TESI-CRF-R; Ghosh-Ippen et al. 2002) that assesses the presence of additional types of trauma exposure common to this age range, such as an animal attack or kidnapping. Like the TESI-C, the TESI-CRF-R is administered by the clinician with the child and takes approximately 10 minutes to complete depending on the severity of trauma exposure. There is also a 24-item clinical interview that can be administered with the child's caregiver, the Traumatic Events Screening Inventory–Parent Report Revised (TESI-PRR; Ghosh-Ippen et al. 2002), that allows for an assessment of trauma exposure in children age 0–6 years. The TESI-CRF-R and TESI-PRR are available to clinicians free of charge at www.ptsd.va.gov/professional/assessment/child/tesi.asp.

School-Age Children and Adolescents

As children age and cognitive abilities advance, the number of available assessment strategies for pediatric trauma exposure increases and diversifies. Namely, school-age children and adolescents are generally able to participate directly in clinical interviews as well as complete child report versions of a variety of instruments. This can greatly enhance assessment in terms of efficiency, comprehensiveness, and accuracy by recruiting both caregivers and children as reporters of trauma exposure and any resulting symptoms. Direct assessment with school-age children and adolescents can also begin the process of having the child recognize and discuss his or her trauma history as a means of preparing him or her for a subsequent course of treatment in which communication about trauma exposure is expected.

Within these age groups, there can be highly diverse presentations of posttraumatic symptoms. Within school-age children, it is common to see behaviors that could be confused with attention-deficit/hyperactivity disorder. For example, when children have reexperiencing symptoms of intrusive memories and flashbacks, they may have significant difficulty attending to educational activities, remaining focused on homework, and following tasks through to completion. Additionally, children may attempt to distract themselves from these intrusive symptoms by engaging in off-task, attention-seeking, and disruptive behaviors. Alternatively, some children and adolescents may demonstrate presentations that mimic agoraphobia, generalized anxiety disorder, or depressive disorders, with increased isolation or reluctance to engage in previously enjoyed activities and decreased motivation across various areas of life.

UCLA Child/Adolescent PTSD Reaction Index for DSM-5

The UCLA Child/Adolescent PTSD Reaction Index for DSM-5 (UCLA PTSD-RI; Pynoos and Steinberg 2013) is a widely used measure of both pediatric trauma exposure and posttraumatic stress symptoms that is appropriate for youth ages 7–18 years. Youth self-report and caregiver report versions are available, including the assessment of trauma exposure via caregiver report for children age 6 and younger. Additionally, the measure is commonly implemented in a clinician-administered interview format.

A previous version, the UCLA PTSD-RI for DSM-IV, included a brief trauma screen assessing the youth's exposure to 12 discrete types of trauma, including war, natural disaster, sexual abuse, and painful medical procedures, recorded in a yes/no format. The current iteration expanded this brief screen into a detailed and comprehensive Trauma History Profile (THP). The THP is a clinician-administered tool for aggregating information across youth self-report, caregiver report, obtained records, and other sources. Scores are recorded for 22 discrete forms of trauma and other adverse events, such as neglect, bullying, community violence, and forced displacement (e.g., refugee status), as well as details of the traumatic event, the youth's role in the event (e.g., victim, witness, learned about later), and the age at which the event was experienced. The THQ can also be administered directly to children as a self-report assessment of pediatric trauma exposure should the child have the cognitive abilities to do so accurately. A PTSD symptom severity scale measuring intrusive thoughts, avoidance of trauma reminders, changes in mood and cognitive attributions, and hypervigilance maps directly onto DSM-5 PTSD criteria, including an assessment of the dissociative subtype. The DSM-5 PTSD diagnostic algorithm is included in the scoring of the UCLA PTSD-RI for DSM-5 to aid in making a formal psychiatric diagnosis.

Available psychometric analyses used the previous version for DSM-IV and generally found acceptable reliability and validity estimates as well as a factor structure resembling the DSM-IV structure for PTSD (Elhai et al. 2013; Steinberg et al. 2013). Psychometric analyses of the revised version of the UCLA PTSD RI for DSM-5 are under way. The current version of the UCLA PTSD RI is now a licensed and copyrighted instrument available for purchase at www.reactionindex.com/index.php/.

Kiddie Schedule for Affective Disorders and Schizophrenia—Present and Lifetime Version for DSM-5

The Kiddie Schedule for Affective Disorders and Schizophrenia—Present and Lifetime Version (K-SADS-PL) for DSM-5 (Kaufman et al. 2016) is a multicomponent interview that assesses a variety of disorders described in DSM-5. It is appropriate for use with children between ages 3 and 18 years (Birmaher et al. 2009) and is typically used in research settings. It is a semistructured interview that includes the DSM-5 Cross-Cutting Symptoms Measures, an unstructured introductory interview, a diagnostic screening interview, a supplementary completion checklist, appropriate diagnostic supplements, and the Summary Lifetime Diagnostic Checklist.

Assessment of exposure to traumatic events occurs during the diagnostic screening interview. The clinician uses a probe indicating that he or she will ask about a number of "bad things that sometimes happen to children your age" (Kaufman et al. 2016, p. 46) and requesting information about whether they have ever happened to the child. The K-SADS-PL assesses 12 different types of trauma, including being involved in car accidents, being involved in other types of accidents, experiencing a fire, witnessing a disaster, witnessing a violent crime, being the victim of a violent crime, being confronted with traumatic news, experiencing terrorism, living in a war zone or experiencing war-related events, witnessing domestic violence, experiencing physical abuse, and experiencing sexual abuse. Additionally, there is a final question that evaluates for anything else "really bad" or "scary" that the child experienced or witnessed. There is a prompt associated with the final question to be used to obtain additional information about possible traumatic incidents if there is concern about parental substance abuse and/or neglect. In response to questions regarding each type of trauma, the clinician assigns a score of 0–2 for the individual responses of the child and of the parent. A score of 0 signifies that there is no information, 1 indicates that the trauma was not experienced, and 2 indicates that the trauma was experienced. If any of the items is endorsed, then the clinician continues with the PTSD portion of the diagnostic screening interview to assess for the presence of PTSD symptoms.

There is limited research regarding the K-SADS-PL DSM-5 since the 2013 update of DSM, but there is much information regarding the prior version of this tool, the K-SADS-PL, which assessed for psychopathology as defined in DSM-IV (Birmaher et al. 2009; Kaufman et al. 1997). Traditional paper administration of the K-SADS-PL for DSM-5, as well as web-based administration via adolescent self-report, caregiver report, or clinician-administered interviews, are available at www.kennedykrieger.org/patient-care/faculty-staff/joan-kaufman.

Adolescents and Transitional-Age Youth

As adolescents continue to develop and approach adulthood, assessment of pediatric trauma exposure relies almost exclusively on youth interviews and self-report instruments. Establishing rapport and asking questions in a standardized yet developmentally appropriate manner can facilitate the assessment of trauma exposure with the adolescent population. Nonetheless, continuing to obtain caregiver report may be useful, particularly in cases in which the youth displays avoidance about a traumatic event and denies having experienced it when in fact the event did occur.

The Comprehensive Trauma Interview

The Comprehensive Trauma Interview (CTI; Noll et al. 2003) is an interview developed to measure exposure to both DSM-defined traumatic events and co-occurring childhood adversities (e.g., bullying, unwanted sexual advances on the Internet) in both youth age 12 years and older and adults. The CTI is a multicomponent instrument assessing exposure to pediatric trauma and adversity as well as subsequent PTSD symptoms. First, respondents complete a 30-item self-administered screening component, the CTI Screen, which assesses exposure to pediatric trauma and adversity. Second, using responses from the CTI Screen and with the assistance of the clinical interviewer, participants identify the most distressing event (MDE) they have ever experienced in their lifetime and then rate their subjective distress in response to the MDE. Details about the MDE and all other items endorsed on the CTI Screen are then gathered in a semistructured interview to gain information about these events, including age at onset, duration, and relationship to a potential perpetrator. Prior research on the CTI (Barnes et al. 2009) demonstrated moderate to substantial reliability in individual recall of adverse events and with information on exposure to child maltreatment using data collected from child protective services.

After information about exposure to adverse events is obtained, the CTI-PTSD Symptoms scale is administered as a fully structured interview in which all respondents are asked the same questions in the same format to assess the presence, onset, and duration of PTSD symptoms, along with areas of functional impairment, in response to the MDE regardless of whether or not it was a DSM-defined trauma. The CTI, including the CTI-PTSD Symptoms scale, is a reliable and valid instrument according to the DSM-IV conceptualization (Shenk et al. 2016), and a psychometric evaluation of revisions for DSM-5 is under way. The CTI is available at no charge by contacting the scale's developer (see Table 3–1).

Childhood Trauma Questionnaire

The Childhood Trauma Questionnaire (CTQ; Bernstein and Fink 1998) is a 28-item self-report measure appropriate for youth ages 12 through adult. The measure asks respondents to report how accurately they believe each statement describes their experiences growing up, using a Likert scale ranging from 1 (never true) to 5 (very often true). Items are summed to yield total scores for each of five scales: emotional abuse, physical abuse, sexual abuse, emotional neglect, and physical neglect. As such, the CTQ is more accurately conceptualized as a self-report measure of the respondent's maltreatment experience as opposed to trauma more broadly conceived.

A helpful feature of the CTQ is the inclusion of a three-item minimization/denial scale meant to detect when individuals are potentially not answering questions in a forthright manner. Multiple studies demonstrated that the CTQ is interpreted similarly across various samples (e.g., normative samples, adolescents on inpatient units, adults receiving services for substance use) and that it corresponds well with criterion methods of determining maltreatment history (Bernstein et al. 2003). Replicated studies of the factor structure are available, and reliability estimates appear acceptable (Bernstein and Fink 1998). The CTQ is a licensed and copyrighted instrument available for purchase (minimum of 25 required) at www.pearsonclinical.com/psychology/products/100000446/childhood-trauma-questionnaire-a-retrospective-self-report-ctq.html.

Overcoming Potential Challenges

When assessing traumatic events in the pediatric population, it is important to first establish rapport and demonstrate that a trained professional will be available to provide support in response to an endorsement of a traumatic event. Additionally, it is strongly recommended that clinicians have identified resources in the community (e.g., domestic violence shelters, medical providers) to address any urgent concerns associated with disclosed traumas.

The assessment of pediatric trauma also assumes that children and caregivers are willing to disclose or discuss painful events. There are multiple reasons as to why children and youth may not disclose the traumatic experiences that they have had, including feelings of shame, guilt, embarrassment, anxiety, and fear. In the case of possible child abuse or domestic violence, both parents and children may be anxious about the possible involvement of law enforcement or children's protective agencies and the consequences that may occur as a result. Children may be fearful that they will be blamed for the incidents, that they will be punished, that their relationship with caregivers will be negatively impacted, or that no one will believe them. Both parents and children may be fearful of reporting violence in the home because of concerns that it will become more severe after reports have been made, possibly causing significant injury or death.

Finally, it is generally recommended that information on pediatric trauma exposure be obtained from multiple sources, such as child and caregiver reports. Although ideal, obtaining information in this way will inevitably result in discrepancies regarding whether or not a specific trauma occurred as well as the severity of psychiatric symptoms that resulted. It is often best in these situations to err on the side of a trauma occurring if one is endorsed and on the side of the greatest severity of symptoms reported by any one source for determining trauma exposure and need for clinical intervention.

Children and youth may present with a specific identified trauma, and clinicians may be tempted to proceed with an assessment, assuming this index trauma is the primary event of concern. However, trauma experiences are highly correlated, and it may be the case that 1) multiple trauma exposures are present and 2) the most significant traumatic exposure is not the index trauma. For instance, children with sexual abuse histories are often referred for services precisely because they have a sexual abuse history. It is not uncommon for such children to have also experienced chronic physical abuse or exposure to domestic violence, and the impact of these experiences may be more detrimental than a single sexual abuse experience. As such, clinicians are urged to conduct a thorough trauma screen for each child and not rely solely on the identified index trauma.

Pediatric trauma screening measures and interviews often assess traumas as defined by criterion A of DSM's conceptualization of PTSD. DSM-5 made significant changes to the definition of trauma that will have an impact on pediatric trauma assessment. Most notably, DSM-5 has removed the unexpected or accidental death of a family member or friend due to natural causes as a traumatic event. Pediatric trauma assessments will need to update existing screening measures to conform to this new definition, should the goal ultimately be to assess PTSD symptoms according to the current DSM taxonomy. Moreover, self-report screens assessing exposure to different traumatic events often do not evaluate whether the events endorsed were of significant intensity to cause symptoms of PTSD. Follow-up questions to assess for the severity of trauma involved in the actual or threatened death, serious injury, emotional abuse, or sexual violence described in criterion A should evaluate the frequency, duration, and level of exposure that the child experienced, such as whether he or she was a direct victim or observer or only heard about the event.

In addition, DSM-5 now outlines criteria for PTSD in children younger than age 7 years. This is a new developmental stage for the diagnosis of PTSD. However, reliable and valid measurement of trauma exposure and resulting PTSD in this age range is a newly initiated effort. Assessing trauma exposure with younger children (ages 0–6 years) is similar to the process used with older children and adolescents. However, two considerations are necessary. First, given the child's age, it is likely in most instances that a self-report of exposure is not attainable. The clinician must rely on the reports of caregivers and others to ascertain the type of trauma the child experienced and the extent of exposure. Second, the clinician should be especially cognizant of the impact of "non-trauma" forms of adverse experiences on children, such as loss of a loved one or parental separation due to divorce. Given children's relatively limited ability to cope with external stressors, traumatic events that occur, for instance, during a separation from a caregiver hold the potential for inducing distress to a degree that may not be expected with older children and adolescents exposed to a similar event. As such, assessing the caregiver's ability to respond to the child may be particularly salient with younger children.

Sociocultural and Policy Implications

The decision to use one or more pediatric trauma assessments can depend on the measure's ability to assess a range of traumas across a range of ages and cultures and the cost of using copyrighted measures. The UCLA PTSD-RI is widely used in clinical research both for conducting a screen of traumatic experiences and for the assessment of PTSD symptoms among people of different cultural and ethnic groups. It has proven quite versatile, with effective implementation across a wide range of ethnic groups; numerous different languages; and for various types of index traumas, including an earthquake in Armenia, community violence in Los Angeles, terrorism in Norway, and sexual abuse in various countries. In a national sample of more than 6,000 youth, no cultural or ethnic differences were identified for scores on the UCLA PTSD symptoms scale (Steinberg et al. 2013). Although some guidance is available to describe the manner in which the THP may be used in practice, no psychometric analyses are published yet evaluating the quality of the PTSD symptoms scale in the latest iteration based on DSM-5. The UCLA PTSD-RI is now available only by purchase of a license to administer, which may limit the feasibility of the instrument for wide-scale use in many settings.

The CTQ has been used in multiple settings, including outpatient, inpatient, and clinical research, and has been administered in multiple countries in various translations, including Spanish, Dutch, and German. It can be completed typically in less than 5 minutes, with the added value of a validity scale to assess the accuracy of the respondent's reporting. However, there are several factors to consider. The CTQ focuses exclusively on the assessment of child maltreatment and does not assess other, more common types of pediatric traumas. There is also no symptom assessment available as a component or supplement to the standard CTQ. Finally, at the time of this writing, the cost of the CTQ, a copyrighted assessment, is

$177 for the manual and 25 copies of the instrument, which may limit feasibility.

The K-SADS-PL is available in Spanish and has been evaluated in a number of diverse sociocultural settings. This instrument is freely available to clinicians and can be administered in a variety of methods, which may be beneficial to the clinician depending on the age or reading level of the child respondent. There are official trainings in the K-SADS-PL should this be of interest to the clinician. The K-SADS-PL also has the advantage of including a host of psychiatric disorders common to traumatized children and adolescents. However, administration time can be extensive depending on the number of traumas and psychiatric symptoms endorsed.

In sum, there are many factors to consider when choosing a pediatric trauma exposure instrument. These factors involve the time available to the clinician to conduct an assessment, the age range of the pediatric population served, the financial resources available to pay for licensed instruments, and the desire to conduct a comprehensive psychiatric interview following an assessment of pediatric trauma. Prioritizing these factors will aid clinicians in deciding which instrument to use when assessing trauma exposure with the patients they serve.

Family Evaluation

When a child experiences trauma, it is also important to complete an assessment of family members and their reaction to the trauma given that they will likely be the primary sources of support for the child and can play a key role in promoting resilience. Additionally, family members may have directly undergone the same situation, may have vicariously experienced trauma through their child's account, or may have their own trauma history that affects their ability to cope with the current situation; therefore, they may benefit from their own intervention as well. Ideally, the clinician will be able to meet individually with the child, with the primary caregivers, and with the whole family together in order to evaluate individual reactions as well as family interactions and communication patterns. An initial focus should be assessing for any acute safety concerns within the family, followed by an evaluation of how each person is affected by the traumatic experience and how this may affect their interactions with other family members.

Areas to assess include current and historical exposure to trauma, as well as symptoms associated with any endorsements of trauma. It is also beneficial to evaluate symptoms of other psychiatric conditions and to assess for any factors that may affect parenting abilities. In considering how the family will respond to trauma, it is beneficial to evaluate any family violence and family separations, including those that have resulted from the current trauma. Given that assessments are likely to be used for treatment planning, it is important to identify adaptive family coping skills; strengths within the various family relationships; and factors contributing to resilience, such as caregivers' support for both the child and themselves. All of the areas mentioned can be evaluated through clinical interviews, although there are standardized measures available for many of these domains.

Conclusion

Pediatric trauma exposure is common and can affect not only a child's mental health but also his or her physical health and functioning across domains. Many clinicians may not be aware of the scope and potential effects of trauma exposure on the health of their patients. For instance, pediatric trauma exposure can significantly limit a child's response to well-established interventions for some of the most common psychiatric complaints in this population (Shenk et al. 2014). Failure to routinely screen for pediatric trauma in the health settings most often visited by children and families can limit accurate diagnosis and treatment planning. Therefore, one strategy for increasing awareness of and screening for trauma exposure is to routinely assess for pediatric trauma at well-child visits completed by pediatricians and family medicine physicians. It is also critical that psychiatrists and clinical psychologists screen for a trauma history in the children and families they serve in order to rule in or rule out the relevance of pediatric trauma exposure for an individual patient's presenting complaints. In this chapter, we described several well-established measures assessing pediatric trauma exposure from infancy to adulthood, including important feasibility and cultural considerations. Appropriate assessment of trauma will lead not only to a more informed diagnosis but also to the opportunity to provide appropriate referrals for intervention.

Assessment as a standard practice within medical settings can also potentially destigmatize the experience of trauma because providers can approach the subject by explaining that traumatic experiences occur in all segments of the population. Normalization of symptoms associated with the trauma, including those that are listed as criteria for PTSD (e.g., nightmares, intrusive memories, avoidance of certain people or places, emotional numbing, irritability), as well as those that are not necessarily diagnostic (e.g., increased separation anxiety) can help the patient and family understand that their responses are within the realm of what is expected in response to significant stress. It is strongly recommended that the clinician assessing pediatric trauma provide brief education regarding the prevalence of trauma exposure, the most common posttraumatic symptoms that occur, and the empirically supported treatments that are available to address symptoms of children and youth experiencing trauma so that an accurate sense of hope can be instilled in patients and caregivers. The National Child Traumatic Stress Network (www.nctsn.org) maintains a detailed listing of empirically supported treatments and promising practices to address trauma in the pediatric population.

KEY CONCEPTS

- Pediatric trauma affects up to two-thirds of all children in the United States younger than age 18 years.
- Comprehensive assessment by trained clinicians offers the best opportunity to detect pediatric trauma and resulting psychiatric symptoms while guiding optimal treatment planning.
- Several state-of-the-art instruments are available for assessing pediatric trauma and psychiatric symptoms in a developmentally and culturally sensitive manner.
- Valuable technical information regarding access to and administration of these instruments is given along with extensive clinical insight into how to overcome common barriers.

Discussion Questions

1. How common is pediatric trauma exposure?

2. What are the most effective and efficient means to assess pediatric trauma in your practice?

3. What barriers exist to assessing pediatric trauma?

4. How can we assess trauma exposure in diverse populations?

Suggested Websites for Additional Information

International Society for Traumatic Stress Studies: www.istss.org
National Child Traumatic Stress Network: www.nctsn.org
Substance Abuse and Mental Health Services Administration: www.samhsa.gov

References

American Psychiatric Association: Diagnostic and Statistical Manual of Mental Disorders, 5th Edition. Arlington, VA, American Psychiatric Association, 2013

Barnes JE, Noll JG, Putnam FW, et al: Sexual and physical revictimization among victims of severe childhood sexual abuse. Child Abuse Neglect 33(7), 412–420, 2009 19596434

Bernstein DP, Fink L: Childhood Trauma Questionnaire: A Retrospective Self-Report. San Antonio, TX, Pearson, 1998

Bernstein DP, Stein JA, Newcomb MD, et al: Development and validation of a brief screening version of the Childhood Trauma Questionnaire. Child Abuse Negl 27(2):169–190, 2003 12615092

Birmaher B, Ehmann M, Axelson DA, et al: Schedule for affective disorders and schizophrenia for school-age children (K-SADS-PL) for the assessment of preschool children—a preliminary psychometric study. J Psychiatr Res 43(7):680–686, 2009 19000625

Copeland WE, Keeler G, Angold A, et al: Traumatic events and posttraumatic stress in childhood. Arch Gen Psychiatry 64(5):577–584, 2007 17485609

Elhai JD, Layne CM, Steinberg AM, et al: Psychometric properties of the UCLA PTSD Reaction Index part II: investigating factor structure findings in a national clinic-referred youth sample. J Trauma Stress 26(1):10–18, 2013 23417874

Felitti VJ, Anda RF, Nordenberg D, et al: Relationship of childhood abuse and household dysfunction to many of the leading causes of death in adults: the Adverse Childhood Experiences (ACE) Study. Am J Prev Med 14(4):245–258, 1998 9635069

Ghosh-Ippen C, Ford J, Racusin R, et al: Traumatic Events Screening Inventory–Parent Report Revised. San Francisco, CA, Child Trauma Research Project of the Early Trauma Network and National Center for PTSD Dartmouth Child Trauma Research Group, 2002

Kaufman J, Birmaher B, Brent D, et al: Schedule for Affective Disorders and Schizophrenia for School-Age Children-Present and Lifetime Version (K-SADS-PL): initial reliability and validity data. J Am Acad Child Adolesc Psychiatry 36(7):980–988, 1997 9204677

Kaufman J, Birmaher B, Axelson D, et al: K-SADS-PL DSM-5. November 2016. Available at: www.kennedykrieger.org/sites/default/files/community_files/ksads-dsm-5-screener.pdf. Accessed March 14, 2018.

Noll JG, Horowitz LA, Bonanno GA, et al: Revictimization and self-harm in females who experienced childhood sexual abuse: results from a prospective study. J Interpers Violence 18(12):1452–1471, 2003 14678616

Pynoos RS, Steinberg AM: The UCLA PTSD Reaction Index for DSM-5. Los Angeles, CA, Behavioral Health Innovations, 2013

Ribbe D: Psychometric review of Traumatic Event Screening Instrument for Children (TESI-C), in Measurement of Stress, Trauma, and Adaptation. Edited by Stamm BH. Lutherville, MD, Sidran Press, 1996, pp 386–387

Scheeringa MS, Haslett N: The reliability and criterion validity of the Diagnostic Infant and Preschool Assessment: a new diagnostic instrument for young children. Child Psychiatry Hum Dev 41(3):299–312, 2010 20052532

Shenk CE, Dorn LD, Kolko DJ, et al: Prior exposure to interpersonal violence and long-term treatment response for boys with a disruptive behavior disorder. J Trauma Stress 27(5):585–592, 2014 25270151

Shenk CE, Noll JG, Griffin AM, et al: Psychometric evaluation of the Comprehensive Trauma Interview PTSD Symptoms scale following exposure to child maltreatment. Child Maltreat 21(4):343–352, 2016 27659904

Steinberg AM, Brymer MJ, Kim S, et al: Psychometric properties of the UCLA PTSD reaction index: part I. J Trauma Stress 26(1):1–9, 2013 23417873

Weathers FW, Blake DD, Schnurr PP, et al: The Life Events Checklist for DSM-5 (LEC-5)—Standard, 2013. Washington, DC, National Center for PTSD. Available at: www.ptsd.va.gov/professional/assessment/te-measures/life_events_checklist.asp. Accessed March 14, 2018.

4

The Forensic Evaluation

Michael Kelly, M.D.
Anne B. McBride, M.D.

FORENSIC EXPERTS—evaluators and practitioners who specialize in the overlapping fields of child and adolescent psychiatry and the law—frequently encounter childhood trauma as an overrepresented experience that can have lasting consequences. In this chapter, we first review several important legal concepts and provide a historical context for the evaluation of posttraumatic stress disorder (PTSD) in forensic settings. Next, we review epidemiological data and developmental trajectories associated with different types of childhood trauma. Then, we discuss how an evaluator can conduct a forensic evaluation in a trauma-informed, developmentally sensitive manner and how forensic evaluators quantify the extent of psychological damages as part of their evaluations. Finally, we address several sociocultural and policy implications of forensic evaluations of traumatized youth.

Legal Background

The American legal system is divided into two main categories for handling rule violations or disputes among adults: civil law and criminal law.

and Keeshin 2011). Of note, traumatized youth whose symptoms are subthreshold for PTSD are still known to experience similar levels of functional impairment and psychological distress as youth who meet DSM criteria for PTSD (Carrion et al. 2002).

Among youth in juvenile detention, the frequency of trauma exposure is significantly higher than it is in the general population. In a study of 898 detained youth ages 10–18 years, Abram et al. (2004) found that 92.5% had experienced one or more traumas, and 11.2% of this population met criteria for PTSD within the preceding year. Figure 4–1 illustrates the significant overlap between trauma, PTSD, and youth involved in the juvenile justice system.

The Forensic Evaluation

Developmental Trajectories

Because the age of the child or adolescent who is being evaluated impacts the method of data collection, forensic evaluators should consider developmental differences when gathering information required to diagnose PTSD (for the diagnostic criteria, see Box 1–1 in Chapter 1, "The Clinical Interview"). For example, younger children may have difficulty verbalizing symptoms or emotions associated with PTSD, particularly because their language skills are still developing over time. DSM-5 (American Psychiatric Association 2013) now offers developmentally sensitive PTSD criteria for preschoolers.

Parent or guardian collateral report can be an integral part of the forensic evaluation for youth. However, there is an abundance of literature suggesting that parents often underestimate their children's trauma-related symptoms. Evaluators must also remain cognizant of youth potentially minimizing their difficulties as a means of coping. In addition, children with limited verbal abilities (e.g., from developmental delay) may not be able to articulate their responses to trauma. Thus, it is essential that forensic evaluators have experience in identifying trauma-related symptoms in youth from all developmental levels. Concurrently, in cases in which sustained trauma is documented, evaluators should review available sources of information such as police reports, child protective services records, or related medical or mental health records to better understand the extent of the trauma and its impact on the child.

Forensic evaluators should recognize that although PTSD is the most common diagnosis associated with trauma, trauma-exposed youth can also

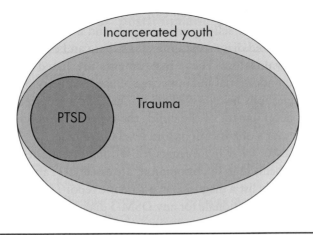

FIGURE 4–1. **Overlap between the juvenile justice system, trauma, and posttraumatic stress disorder (PTSD).**

be diagnosed with various associated comorbid or unrelated premorbid conditions (e.g., depression, anxiety, substance use, behavioral disorders, learning disorders, attention-deficit/hyperactivity disorder). Adequate training in child development and childhood psychopathology is necessary to navigate the challenges in evaluating such youth and their often-complicated overlapping symptoms and impairments.

Evaluation Structure

The forensic evaluation should include an interview with the minor and a collateral interview with the parent(s) or guardian(s) to obtain a full psychosocial history. Forensic evaluators use a developmental approach to interview the minor on the basis of his or her age and developmental level. Electronically recording forensic evaluations is becoming a more common practice. As Corwin and Keeshin (2011, p. 513) noted, electronic recording can serve to protect "subjects in these evaluations from errors in citing their statements and behaviors, and protects the evaluator from allegations of misrepresentation." Record review is an essential part of any forensic evaluation and an important means by which forensic evaluators can identify consistencies and/or inconsistencies in the information obtained through forensic interview and the collateral accounts of others. It is imperative that forensic evaluators look at other available records such as the child's mental health, medical, educational, juvenile court, and/or police records in order to obtain information on his or her functioning before, at the time of, and after a reported trauma.

2006). In civil cases, additional professionals (e.g., vocational specialists, health economists) are often used to assist in determining the long-term financial damages associated with trauma (Corwin and Keeshin 2011).

Other Challenges in the Forensic Evaluation

Challenging aspects of forensic evaluations of youth who are the confirmed and/or suspected victims of childhood trauma include dual agency, malingering, suggestibility, child sexual abuse syndrome and accommodation syndrome, and bias.

Dual Agency

The relationship between forensic evaluators and examinees is distinct from that of the doctor-patient relationship. For example, a treatment provider's first obligation is to that of her or his patient; however, a forensic evaluator's obligation is to provide unbiased consultation to the courts or the retaining party (i.e., the client). Furthermore, the issue of informed consent and the limits of confidentiality are of primary importance in any forensic evaluation. Forensic psychiatrists adhere to ethical principles that include the following (from the American Academy of Psychiatry and the Law's ethical guidelines):

> At the outset of a face-to-face evaluation, notice should be given to the evaluee of the nature and purpose of the evaluation and the limits of its confidentiality. The informed consent of the person undergoing the forensic evaluation should be obtained when necessary and feasible. If the evaluee is not competent to give consent, the evaluator should follow the appropriate laws of the jurisdiction. (American Academy of Psychiatry and the Law 2005)

Forensic evaluators must be cognizant of the potential for a forensic evaluee to forget about the evaluator's role at some point, incorrectly assuming that their communications are to be kept confidential. Evaluators should be vigilant and thoughtful about maintaining appropriate boundaries and roles when conducting forensic assessments versus providing psychiatric or psychological treatment.

Consideration of Malingering

Given the nature of the potential gains involved in civil, juvenile, and criminal matters, one essential aspect of the forensic evaluation in cases of suspected trauma involves the consideration of malingering. DSM-5 describes malingering as "the intentional production of false or grossly exaggerated physical or psychological symptoms, motivated by external incentives such as avoiding military duty, avoiding work, obtaining financial compensation, evading criminal prosecution, or obtaining drugs" (American Psychiatric Association 2013, p. 726). Although discussion of all the methods experienced forensic evaluators sometimes use to assist in the detection of feigned psychiatric symptoms is beyond the scope of this text, it is important to note that malingering must be considered in a forensic evaluation. Forensic evaluators who notice marked inconsistencies between forensic interview, collateral reports, and/or the available records should consider malingering in their differential diagnosis. In addition, the endorsement of symptoms that are highly atypical or that deviate from usual developmental trajectories should raise some concern for feigned and/or exaggerated psychiatric symptoms.

Memory, Suggestibility, and the Forensic Examination

Forensic experts are sometimes asked to evaluate childhood sexual abuse allegations. Following several highly publicized cases involving false accusations of abuse in the 1980s (e.g., the McMartin preschool trial), research involving memory and suggestibility in children and adolescents blossomed after children's false accusations were linked closely to suggestible interview techniques (Ceci et al. 1994; Goodman et al. 2017; Poole and Lindsay 1998). Children's eyewitness testimony is a broad topic; however, there are several key points that can be summarized from the literature. Children cannot testify reliably about events occurring before age 2 years. Although even young children are capable of reporting accurate memories of traumatic events, they tend to have more limitations with memory recall than do older children and adults. In general, children are more suggestible than adults. To minimize interview errors or potential biases when evaluating child abuse, centers specializing in child abuse evaluation (e.g., Children's Advocacy Centers) arose in the 1980s to provide response and prevention services, education, and leadership in the field. Structured interview protocols requiring specialized training have been developed to standardize initial investigations involving child abuse (Brown and Lamb 2015; Lamb et al. 2007; Sternberg et al. 2001). In the next subsection, we briefly discuss the psychiatric literature related to a topic that has received a lot of attention in the press and exemplifies concerns related to evaluations involving suspected child abuse.

tional means of reducing bias and increasing transparency in forensic evaluations.

Sociocultural and Policy Implications

In our view, forensic evaluators should attempt to remain cognizant of their own potential biases; the types of bias that can be associated with forensic evaluations; the potential for bias in the civil, criminal, and juvenile justice systems; and the way that evaluees' cultural, racial, and ethnic identities impact the perception of mental illness, mental health professionals, the legal system, their communities, and themselves. At the same time, child and adolescent forensic psychiatrists have opportunities to be at the forefront of policy change and societal improvement. For example, specialists may weigh in on important issues such as the overprescribing of antipsychotics to foster care youth, evidence-based approaches to treating detained youth, or educating the courts on the developmental impact on delinquency. Moreover, by performing thorough, ethical evaluations and providing excellent care to youth within the various legal systems, child and adolescent forensic psychiatrists can exemplify a high standard that should permeate through communities and society.

Conclusion

Trauma frequently plays a role in forensic evaluations, particularly those involving children and adolescents. The forensic evaluator who specializes in child development is often tasked with examining and opining on the impact of trauma on youth within the legal system, including within both civil and criminal juvenile law. Forensic evaluations are different from clinical evaluations, and the forensic evaluator should understand the complexities involved in this distinct role. It is important for clinicians to know the unique aspects of forensic evaluations in order to avoid problems related to dual agency and to serve their patients' best interests. Forensic evaluators working on cases involving trauma-exposed youth need to have a strong grasp of child development, be knowledgeable about the tools used to help assess psychic trauma in clinical and forensic settings, and possess solid forensic report–writing skills. It is our hope that this chapter informs the burgeoning practice of forensic evaluation and proves useful to clinicians seeking to help their clients navigate criminal, juvenile, and civil court matters; collaborate with forensic evaluators when needed; and have a better understanding when reading forensic reports.

KEY CONCEPTS

- Interpersonal trauma is more likely than noninterpersonal trauma to result in PTSD.
- Detained youth have significantly higher rates of trauma exposure than that of the general population.
- Traumatized children who do not meet full DSM-5 criteria for PTSD are still at risk for experiencing severe and long-term negative consequences from trauma.
- Child sexual abuse syndrome and child sexual abuse accommodation syndrome are ideas based on clinical observation and were not intended to be used as a means of reliably distinguishing between false and accurate reports of child sexual abuse.

Discussion Questions

1. In what ways does the role of a forensic evaluator differ from that of a treatment provider?

2. What steps, if any, can forensic evaluators take in order to minimize bias?

3. What are some important developmental factors to consider when performing a forensic psychiatric evaluation on traumatized youth?

4. What are some of the tools that forensic evaluators use in order to screen for trauma symptoms and perform comprehensive diagnostic evaluations?

Suggested Readings

Buchanan A, Norko MA (eds): The Psychiatric Report: Principles and Practice of Forensic Writing. New York, Cambridge University Press, 2011

Grisso T: Forensic Evaluation of Juveniles. Sarasota, FL, Professional Resource Press/Professional Resource Exchange, 2013

Scott ES, Steinberg LD: Rethinking Juvenile Justice. Cambridge, MA, Harvard University Press, 2009

References

Abram KM, Teplin LA, Charles DR, et al: Posttraumatic stress disorder and trauma in youth in juvenile detention. Arch Gen Psychiatry 61(4):403–410, 2004 15066899

Achenbach TM, Edelbrock C: Child Behavior Checklist. Burlington, VT, University of Vermont, 1991

American Academy of Psychiatry and the Law: Ethics guidelines for the practice of forensic psychiatry. American Academy of Psychiatry and the Law, Bloomfield, CT, May 2005. Available at: www.aapl.org/ethics-guidelines. Accessed March 14, 2018.

American Psychiatric Association: Diagnostic and Statistical Manual of Mental Disorders, 5th Edition. Arlington, VA, American Psychiatric Association, 2013

Bernet W, Corwin D: An evidence-based approach for estimating present and future damages from child sexual abuse. J Am Acad Psychiatry Law 34(2):224–230, 2006 16844803

Briere J: Trauma symptom checklist for children. Odessa, FL, Psychological Assessment Resources, 1996

Bromet E, Sonnega A, Kessler RC: Risk factors for DSM-III-R posttraumatic stress disorder: findings from the National Comorbidity Survey. Am J Epidemiol 147(4):353–361, 1998 9508102

Brown DA, Lamb ME: Can children be useful witnesses? It depends how they are questioned. Child Dev Perspect 9(4):250–255, 2015

Carrion VG, Weems CF, Ray R, et al: Toward an empirical definition of pediatric PTSD: the phenomenology of PTSD symptoms in youth. J Am Acad Child Adolesc Psychiatry 41(2):166–173, 2002 11837406

Ceci SJ, Huffman MLC, Smith E, et al: Repeatedly thinking about a non-event: source misattributions among preschoolers. Conscious Cogn 3(3–4):388–407, 1994

Corwin DL, Keeshin BR: Estimating present and future damages following child maltreatment. Child Adolesc Psychiatr Clin N Am 20(3):505–518, 2011 21683916

Duncan L, Georgiades K, Wang L, et al: Psychometric evaluation of the Mini International Neuropsychiatric Interview for Children and Adolescents (MINI-KID). Psychol Assess 30(7)916–928, 2018 29199837

Everson MD, Sandoval JM: Forensic child sexual abuse evaluations: assessing subjectivity and bias in professional judgements. Child Abuse Negl 35(4):287–298, 2011 21546087

Finkelhor D, Hamby SL, Ormrod R, et al: The Juvenile Victimization Questionnaire: reliability, validity, and national norms. Child Abuse Negl 29(4):383–412, 2005 15917079

Foa EB, Johnson KM, Feeny NC, et al: The Child PTSD Symptom Scale: a preliminary examination of its psychometric properties. J Clin Child Psychol 30(3):376–384, 2001 11501254

Goodman GS, Jones O, McLeod C: Is there consensus about children's memory and suggestibility? J Interpers Violence 32(6):926–939, 2017

Lamb ME, Orbach Y, Hershkowitz I, et al: A structured forensic interview protocol improves the quality and informativeness of investigative interviews with children: a review of research using the NICHD Investigative Interview Protocol. Child Abuse Negl 31(11–12):1201–1231, 2007 18023872

London K, Bruck M, Wright DB, et al: Review of the contemporary literature on how children report sexual abuse to others: findings, methodological issues, and implications for forensic interviewers. Memory 16(1):29–47, 2008 18158687

Luthra R, Abramovitz R, Greenberg R, et al: Relationship between type of trauma exposure and posttraumatic stress disorder among urban children and adolescents. J Interpers Violence 24(11):1919–1927, 2009 18945918

Malloy LC, Lyon TD, Quas JA: Filial dependency and recantation of child sexual abuse allegations. J Am Acad Child Adolesc Psychiatry 46(2):162–170, 2007 17242619

Murrie DC, Boccaccini MT, Guarnera LA, et al: Are forensic experts biased by the side that retained them? Psychol Sci 24(10):1889–1897, 2013 23969777

Poole DA, Lindsay DS: Assessing the accuracy of young children's reports: lessons from the investigation of child sexual abuse. Appl Prev Psychol 7(1):1–26, 1998

Pynoos RS, Steinberg AM: The UCLA PTSD Reaction Index for DSM-5. Los Angeles, CA, Behavioral Health Innovations, 2013

Soykoek S, Mall V, Nehring I, et al: Post-traumatic stress disorder in Syrian children of a German refugee camp. Lancet 389(10072):903–904, 2017 28271834

Sternberg KJ, Lamb ME, Orbach Y, et al: Use of a structured investigative protocol enhances young children's responses to free-recall prompts in the course of forensic interviews. J Appl Psychol 86(5):997–1005, 2001 11596815

Summit RC: The child sexual abuse accommodation syndrome. Child Abuse Negl 7(2):177–193, 1983 6605796

PART II
Treatment

TABLE 5–1.   Core components of trauma intervention

Trauma-focused assessment

Crisis intervention and stabilization; establishing safety, consistency, and predictability

Engagement and relationship building (with providers and/or caregivers)

Psychoeducation about trauma and traumatic stress

Skill development in emotion identification, emotion expression, and emotion regulation

Trauma processing through approach and exposure

Integration of the trauma experience

Building empowerment, optimism, and resilience

Consequently, a wide variety of intervention approaches for child trauma have been successfully developed, implemented, and evaluated. Some interventions are designed to focus on specific types of childhood trauma, such as sexual abuse or community violence, whereas others provide more general intervention to address a variety of trauma types and include interventions that focus on addressing experiences of chronic or complex trauma (see Ford and Courtois 2015). Intervention approaches range from being individually focused, to parent and/or family focused, to systems focused. Similarly, we have seen support for group therapy interventions, as well as interventions that focus on a specific identified patient. It is beyond the scope of this chapter to provide a comprehensive overview of all trauma-focused interventions for youth; for further information about specific interventions approaches, readers are referred to the National Child Traumatic Stress Network, the National Registry of Evidence-Based Programs and Practices, and the California Evidence-Based Clearinghouse for Child Welfare. As our field advances toward a personalized medicine approach, we will learn which interventions work best for which youth (and which trauma types). In the meantime, researchers have identified a number of core components of trauma intervention that cut across all evidence-based practices. A summary of these core components of trauma intervention is presented in Table 5–1.

Although different interventions may interchange the order of delivery of some of these components, the core practices should generally be delivered in the order listed in Table 5–1 so as to first establish a foundation of safety and skill development before engaging in in-depth processing of traumatic experiences (in which distress is often expected to surface). Many of the core components of trauma intervention are covered in more detail in Chapters 6–15, which address specific therapeutic modalities and interventions. In this chapter, we focus on a few of the general principles of psychotherapy that are especially important in any practice approach for addressing traumatic stress in youth.

Engaging With Trauma

Trauma intervention for youth begins with engaging youth and their families around the topic and theme of trauma. Knowing that avoidance is a key element of the trauma response, we can expect many youth and families to demonstrate some reluctance or difficulty (which is often covert if not expressed explicitly) in approaching the topic of trauma. In addition, many youth and caregivers are simply unaware of the connection between their psychopathology and their experiences of trauma and adversity. Therefore, it can be important to be direct and straightforward, yet gentle, about the focus of the therapeutic work. Openly acknowledging that the therapeutic work will involve a focus on traumatic life experiences makes the goals of the intervention clear, helps to prepare the youth and family for the work ahead, and begins the process of countering avoidance through approach.

Language and Terminology

The process for engaging with trauma, including the language we use to discuss and refer to trauma, should vary by patient age, developmental stage, and family readiness. In some cases, youth and families will enter the clinical setting knowing that their difficulties stem from trauma exposure (e.g., "Ever since the accident, I have felt nervous and anxious whenever I am in a car—I think I've been traumatized"). In such cases, the patient has begun the engagement work for the provider. However, it is often not so easy. In many cases, especially for young children, the caregiver will raise the issue of trauma but will express doubt about how to broach the topic with the child. For young children, it can be helpful to talk about "scary" experiences and "the time(s) when I felt very afraid." Young children may need to describe these events (and thereby engage with trauma) through such mediums as art or play because they may still be developing the skills and language to describe such experiences verbally.

In addition, many youth and families may have some level of stigma or preexisting negative conceptions of the term *trauma*. In these cases, the clinician can initiate the conversation using such terms as "stress," "stressful life experiences," or "the time(s) I felt threatened or in danger" to introduce the topic and begin the work of engaging with trauma. However, it is important to move quickly to name "trauma" and to directly reference specific experiences (such as "the shooting at your home," "the sexual assault," or "the arguments between your mom and dad") as being the focus of the treatment; using this terminology and directly referencing the trauma serve to counter the avoidance that youth and families may naturally experience and send a clear message about the nature of the upcoming work. Given that the process of engaging around trauma will vary on the basis of consideration of patient characteristics such as developmental stage and level of readiness, it is important that the provider proceed in a gentle and sensitive fashion, giving careful thought from the outset as to how he or she will go about discussing, describing, and addressing trauma and what language and terminology to use.

Assessment

The engagement process often begins with assessment. The practices of trauma-focused assessment are discussed in more detail in Chapter 2 ("Assessment in Schools or Other Large Groups") and Chapter 3 ("Assessment of Individuals"). Here, we note that the process of conducting a trauma screen, in which the clinician asks about exposure to various specific types of traumas and assesses for trauma-related symptoms and distress, begins the process of engaging with trauma. Initial trauma-focused assessment sends the message that "this is what we are here to talk about and work on together; these are the themes and issues that are relevant for our work." Trauma-focused assessment also provides an early opportunity for psychoeducation. Through assessment, youth and their families learn about the typical types of experiences that can be traumatic, and they explore common responses to trauma, many of which are likely affecting them.

Psychoeducation

Psychoeducation about the impact of trauma is important for normalizing youth responses to trauma and for helping youth and families to understand their trauma-related reactions and distress. Although the specific content and concepts taught can vary across intervention approaches, at its core, psychoeducation involves the presentation of information about the prevalence of trauma exposure and the common psychological, emotional, behavioral, and physiological reactions to trauma. Through these conversations and activities, youth learn that they are not alone in their experience of trauma, that their trauma responses are expected (i.e., the youth is not "crazy"), and that there are pathways to recovery. These lessons can be taught by providing and reviewing informational handouts (e.g., handouts available from the National Child Traumatic Stress Network at www.nctsn.org), describing the neurobiology of stress and trauma, and playing question-and-answer games (e.g., What Do You Know? card game by the CARES Institute, available at www.caresinstitute.org/Products.php), among other approaches.

Motivational Enhancement

Engagement around trauma also often involves building and enhancing motivation to address trauma. Once again, youth and their families may experience trauma-related avoidance that may serve to prevent or deter them from addressing trauma as a core component of the therapeutic effort. It can take extra effort on the part of the clinician to enhance motivation and develop a commitment to address the trauma and tolerate the distress that is inherently involved in trauma processing. Psychoeducation lays the foundation for motivational enhancement by providing an understanding of how trauma experiences are connected to current difficulties and presenting problems.

Motivational interviewing approaches (Miller and Rollnick 2013) are important elements of this engagement process. For example, carefully examining and highlighting the costs and benefits of addressing versus not addressing trauma can enhance motivation for trauma work. Identifying and making explicit the expected barriers to addressing trauma is another element of motivational interviewing approaches that can enhance treatment success. In addition, values-based approaches, such as those from acceptance and commitment therapy (Hayes et al. 1999; Walser and Westrup 2007), that place engagement with trauma within the context of personal life goals and values can serve to enhance motivation for trauma treatment. Enhancing motivation, developing understanding of the rationale for trauma treatment, and building the commitment to therapy early in the process is important for trauma intervention because youth and families will typically have to persevere through challenging content and emotions during the course of the intervention.

Case Conceptualization

Finally, engagement on the part of the clinician or provider entails trauma-focused case conceptualization and treatment planning. Regardless of the specific approach, interventions for youth exposed to trauma and

---

TABLE 5–2.   Reflection questions to guide trauma-focused case conceptualization

---

What has happened to the individual? What stressful or traumatic experiences might be relevant for understanding the presenting problem?

When did the trauma occur, and when did the problems emerge? Is there a connection? Who was involved or associated with the trauma experience?

How might the problem thoughts, feelings, and/or behaviors have been adaptive in the past? How did these cognitive, emotional, and/or behavioral responses previously help the individual to survive or cope with a threat or stressor?

What is the function of the thoughts, feelings, and/or behaviors underlying the problem? What are the antecedents and consequences of the problem? Are the precursors or responses related to, shaped by, or influenced by trauma experiences?

What information is being communicated or expressed by the problem behavior?

Where did the individual experience lost opportunities for skill development due to exposure to trauma and adversity (i.e., what were the child's developmental stage and primary tasks of development at the time of trauma exposure?)?

---

traumatic stress require consideration of the role of trauma experiences in shaping the presenting problems, diagnoses, and primary concerns. Trauma-informed case conceptualization involves using trauma history as the context for understanding emotional, behavioral, and psychological difficulties. Such difficulties, and the related functional impairments stemming from child trauma exposure, can typically be understood as being the result of 1) adaptive efforts to cope with a malevolent or threatening environment, 2) attempts to understand and integrate the trauma experience(s) (often occurring through reenactment), 3) efforts to express or communicate the individual's level of distress or difficulty, and/or 4) missed opportunities to develop and practice a given skill due to the presence of trauma exposure. Specific questions that can inform and guide trauma-informed case conceptualization are presented in Table 5–2.

By conducting trauma-focused case conceptualization, providers and clinicians can develop treatment plans and objectives that directly address the core issues (related to the trauma experience) that underlie the problems presenting at the surface (e.g., difficulties with attention, communication, and emotion and behavior regulation). For example, treatment recommendations for aggressive behaviors often emphasize behavioral reinforcement planning. However, behavior management alone for a child with a history of trauma exposure does not address the underlying need to develop emotion regulation skills. A trauma-informed intervention ap-

Capitalizing on efforts to establish safety, security, and predictability, the therapist can find opportunities in the development of a trusting relationship to help the youth have a sense of agency, control, and empowerment in his or her relationships. Such opportunities may include eliciting the youth's input in developing therapy goals, establishing therapy and household routines and reinforcement plans, and selecting coping practices. In general, efforts to actively involve the youth in the intervention process (versus being a passive recipient) serve to increase the quality of the therapeutic relationship. The therapist and caregiver should seek to offer the appropriate balance of structure and support that will promote the youth's sense of agency and ability to meet stated goals and objectives (Wachtel 2016), thereby increasing the youth's empowerment in the context of his or her relationships. The area and level of agency and autonomy should be developmentally tailored; a preschool or school-age child will need greater levels of structure, guidance, and oversight relative to an adolescent or transition-age youth.

Another important element of a safe, trusting, and responsive relationship is the experience of attunement. Youth (and individuals of all ages) feel safe and have positive relationship experiences when they feel seen, heard, and understood. Providers and caregivers working with youth exposed to trauma should therefore take careful effort to identify, reflect, and demonstrate empathy for youth and their experiences of cognitive, emotional, behavioral, and physiological dysregulation. These efforts are facilitated by the work done in psychoeducation and skill-building components of trauma-focused intervention (e.g., emotion identification, emotion expression). In addition, reflective-listening and perspective-taking skills, practices, and activities play an important role in trauma intervention because they enhance the quality of the relationship through demonstration of attunement to the youth's experience. Every interaction that demonstrates attunement, prioritizes the needs of the child, and helps the child feel safe and secure alters that child's experience and his or her schema of what a relationship should entail. As Bruce Perry states, every positive, attuned interaction with a trustworthy other can help rewire the brain (Perry 2006).

The principles and practices discussed above apply to both the patient-therapist relationship and the youth-caregiver relationships. Providers should institute the practices described above in their individual interactions with youth and also should promote the use of these practices in caregiver interactions with youth. For the latter, guidance and support in these efforts can be accomplished through individual sessions with caregivers, collateral case consultation, or dyadic or family sessions. The ex-

proach might focus on developing physiological regulation skills as a means of addressing the aggressive or disruptive behaviors that stem from emotional hyperarousal occurring in response to trauma reminders.

Establishing Safety

Another essential element of trauma intervention involves establishing a sense of safety within both the context of the therapy intervention and the context of the patient's broader life. Trauma inherently involves an experience of real and/or perceived threat to an individual's (or loved one's) well-being. Fully addressing and processing trauma and traumatic stress first requires that a baseline level of stability and security be established. Although many youth and families experience ongoing adversity and trauma that can make the task of establishing safety challenging, there are numerous measures that can be taken to increase the sense of readiness and preparedness to establish a stable grounding foundation (see Cohen et al. 2012). For example, providers can help youth and families develop safety plans and identify resources to access in the case of future trauma exposure (e.g., identifying family and social supports, crisis and emergency hotlines, and local shelters). Developing goals and skills for coping also helps to establish a sense of safety because patients and families feel increasingly empowered in managing their own emotional, cognitive, and behavioral responses.

Establishing safety also involves developing and advancing predictability and consistency across multiple settings. At the core of the traumatic stress response is the inherent loss of control or agency over what is happening to the individual (or what is happening around him or her), resulting in experiences of dysregulation and disorganization. Therefore, it is important that the youth (and family) have a sense of control over their environment, that they identify areas where they are able to exert control, and that they experience a sense of consistency and organization in their activities. Trauma intervention involves work to establish predictable routines (e.g., in therapy, at home, at school) and consistent responses from caregivers and caregiving environments (e.g., see Blaustein and Kinniburgh 2010). Psychoeducation and coaching should be provided to ensure that care is taken to prepare for or address major transitions or changes in routine. By establishing a sense of safety and predictability for youth and families affected by trauma, clinicians and providers can offer a new experience in operating within a grounding foundation that provides stability and security as youth and families move through trauma treatment and generalize skills and practices into their everyday lives. The safe foundation contributes to the quality of familial, social, and therapeutic relationships, which are discussed next.

Relationship Development and Care

Trauma intervention leans heavily on relationship quality and relationship resources. Although the importance of the therapeutic relationship and therapeutic alliance is a key element of all mental health interventions (Karver et al. 2006), it is especially important for youth exposed to trauma. Childhood trauma (and especially interpersonal trauma such as assault, abuse, neglect, and violence exposure) inherently involves the violation of trust and security within the individual's relationships: either someone did something to harm me or someone I love, or someone failed to protect me from harm or adversity. Histories of trauma involving disrupted attachment, interpersonal violation, and/or failure of the caregiver or system to uphold the "protective shield" can present immediate challenges to the goal of establishing a trusting relationship. It will be natural for many youth (and their families) to experience some doubt or insecurity about the quality and reliability of both new and established relationships. Therefore, clinicians and providers should anticipate that extra effort may be required to establish trust and security in both the patient-therapist and the youth-caregiver relationships. Although this task may be challenging, it is important to keep in mind that the results can be transformative. The development of a single trusting relationship can alter the trajectory of a child who may not have had such a relationship in his or her prior experiences.

In order to develop a trusting relationship, the provider might begin by making explicit the patient's history of relationship violations and providing context for difficulties in current relationships. The provider can align with the youth and family by acknowledging the difficulty of not feeling able to trust others or feel safe in relationships. In this effort, it will be important to distinguish harmful or unsafe relationships (in which a trauma or violation occurred) from other experiences of positive and trustworthy relationships so as to avoid overgeneralization and globalizing of negative experiences. These efforts overlap with elements of cognitive restructuring and trauma processing that are key in many trauma-focused interventions discussed in subsequent chapters in this book.

tent and exact nature of the involvement of caregivers and other supportive relationships in the therapeutic work will vary by the youth's age and developmental stage, caregiver availability, and treatment modality. However, given that trauma always occurs within the context of a relationship, it is important that the provider address this context and work with the relationship in some form, whether it be directly or indirectly. An essential byproduct of trauma-focused intervention is increased youth-caregiver and family communication about trauma in general and about specific trauma experiences and outcomes; providers should make efforts to ensure progress toward this outcome.

Finally, care for the therapeutic relationship with youth and their families includes open acknowledgment of the limitations and boundaries of the relationship. Although the specifics of these limitations and boundaries will vary across providers, clinics, and agencies, it is essential that these relationship expectations are made clear throughout the course of the intervention. What is the extent of provider availability to the youth and family? What role(s) will the provider fill in the life of the youth and family? How long is the therapeutic relationship expected to last?

This last question begins to touch on the topic of termination. Termination and case closure can be particularly challenging for youth and families who have experienced trauma because traumatic experiences often involve unexpected or uncontrollable loss. Therefore, it is important that therapists addressing trauma take special care in preparing for termination and closure, setting appropriate expectations for how and when termination will take place, providing opportunities for youth agency in the termination process, and ensuring opportunities to prepare for and process reactions to termination. Some providers say that "it is never too early to talk about termination." Careful attention to this process will ensure that the youth maintains a positive association with the therapeutic relationship and that safety and stability in ongoing relationships is bolstered. A revisiting of psychoeducation, youth skill building, and youth and family goals and resources is often required as part of the termination and closure process.

Addressing Shame and Self-Blame

Experiences of shame and self-blame are common for youth (and all individuals) exposed to trauma, especially interpersonal traumas. In an effort to make sense of the occurrence of trauma and victimization in their life, youth often attribute culpability to themselves, arriving at conclusions such as "trauma happened to me because I am a bad person and I deserve it," "my mom and dad fought so much because I caused them so much trouble," "I didn't do enough to stop what was happening," or "it was my fault for not being smarter and protecting myself." These experiences of shame and self-blame are often the drivers of trauma-related psychopathology, and they are either core components or strong associates of symptoms of depression, anxiety, and posttraumatic stress disorder.

Shame and self-blame often emerge in the metacognitive processes involved in an individual's interpretation of his or her reactions and responses to traumatic events. Given the important role of metacognition, clinicians need to assess, evaluate, and treat the cognitive, emotional, and behavioral manifestations of shame and self-blame in the course of their work with patients. Experiences of shame and self-blame may emerge through direct assessment (including use of validated questionnaires), review of the trauma narrative, and/or interpretation of themes in a child's play or relational interactions. Approaches for addressing shame and self-blame will vary according to patient characteristics and treatment modality, with approaches including (but not limited to) narrative processing, cognitive restructuring, play, and mindfulness or acceptance practices. Addressing shame and self-blame often results in a shift in a youth's self-perception and identity: by highlighting the context for the trauma experience, the youth's efforts to protect himself or herself and others, and the responsibility of perpetrators for their actions, youth often move from seeing themselves as victims to seeing themselves as resilient survivors. This powerful shift is commonly associated with reductions in trauma-related psychopathology.

Overcoming Potential Challenges
Maintaining Confidentiality

Challenges related to maintaining confidentiality are common in trauma treatment. As with any therapeutic or clinical service, confidentiality policies and limitations to confidentiality should be presented and reviewed at the outset of services as part of the consent process. This procedure is especially important for trauma intervention for youth because there is greater likelihood that a need for reporting will emerge during the course of therapy (e.g., because of disclosure of child abuse or the presence of suicidal ideation or self-harm). Given the histories of violation of trust

should also expect to provide some level of flexibility to accommodate family needs—establishing stability and regularity can be an ongoing process in which optimal routines develop over time.

In addition, many youth and families exposed to trauma face adversity due to limited resources and low socioeconomic status. Stressors related to insecurity with food, housing or shelter, employment, education, and finances are destabilizing and can serve as barriers to treatment. In many cases, providers will need to first assist families in identifying resources to meet these basic needs before progressing into trauma therapy. In addition, challenges related to transportation, caregiver (or youth) work schedules, and caregiving responsibilities (e.g., for younger family members) will require collaborative problem solving between the therapist, youth, and family. Providers will need to consider optimal locations of service delivery (e.g., in clinic, school based, home based) based on a given family's needs and limitations as well as achievable levels and means of caregiver involvement.

Different trauma treatment approaches recommend and require different levels of caregiver involvement; therefore, providers may wish to select their approach in part on the basis of caregiver availability and may also need to consider modifications to modes of caregiver involvement (e.g., telephone). In addition, provider efforts devoted to establishing safety and enhancing motivation for treatment (as discussed earlier) will also help to address the barriers that many youth and families commonly face while seeking trauma services.

Sociocultural and Policy Implications

Individual responses to trauma, as well as the work done in psychotherapy to address these responses, occur within a larger context of family, community, school, political, and sociocultural systems (Bronfenbrenner 1979). These systems impact individual trauma experiences and responses. Therefore, it is important that we as providers attend to these systems, acknowledge their impact, and effect change where possible as part of the therapy process. That is, in addition to attending to the youth patient, we must also consider, process, and address the needs of the families, communities, and cultures that contextualize the youth's experience. This often involves addressing multigenerational legacies of exposure to trauma and adversity by bringing these historical and cultural traumas into the therapy work. This may be done by directly processing historical traumas with the patient and/or caregiver, by incorporating this information into case conceptualization, by working to address basic family and systems needs (e.g., due to resource shortage), and/or by ensuring appropriate services for previous generations (e.g., parents, grandparents) to address their own experiences of traumatic stress.

Caregiving systems, such as schools, foster homes, and juvenile justice systems, can become organized around trauma in such a way that the systems demonstrate the same trauma symptoms of hypervigilance, avoidance, arousal or reactivity, and hopelessness or numbing that we see in individuals (Bloom and Farragher 2013). Youth existing within traumatized and trauma-organized systems may experience exacerbation of their own symptoms and distress because the dynamics of the system have the potential to be triggering or retraumatizing. Clinicians and providers have an opportunity to influence these systems through intervention and advocacy at multiple levels—individual, systems, and policy—as discussed in the following subsection.

Advocacy for Youth Exposed to Traumatic Stress

Part of the role of therapists and mental health professionals supporting youth exposed to trauma is to serve as an advocate. Therapists frequently interact with providers within school, juvenile justice, foster care, employment, and primary care systems. Each of these interactions offers an opportunity to provide psychoeducation about trauma and to advance a trauma-informed system of care, both in general and in relation to specific patients. These interactions lead to shifts in perspective and approach as a given provider enters his or her work with youth exposed to trauma and as therapists encourage outside providers to use trauma as context for their interactions with youth. The result is that youth experience improved relationships and interactions with providers and systems, feel safe in their service setting, and ultimately experience improved outcomes related to their traumatic stress.

As advocates, we can strive to make connections across systems, and, even if just little by little, we can help to build a consistency of knowledge, language, and responses when addressing themes of trauma. On large scales, we can advocate for policy changes that 1) advance trauma-informed services and systems and 2) promote public health messaging that normalizes responses to trauma and emphasizes the importance of addressing traumatic stress. With these efforts, therapists have an oppor-

Ford JD, Courtois CA: Treating Complex Traumatic Stress Disorders in Children and Adolescents: Scientific Foundations and Therapeutic Models. New York, Guilford, 2015

Hayes SC, Strosahl KD, Wilson KG: Acceptance and Commitment Therapy: An Experiential Approach to Behavior Change. New York, Guilford, 1999

Karver MS, Handelsman JB, Fields S, et al: Meta-analysis of therapeutic relationship variables in youth and family therapy: the evidence for different relationship variables in the child and adolescent treatment outcome literature. Clin Psychol Rev 26(1):50–65, 2006 16271815

Miller WR, Rollnick S: Motivational Interviewing: Helping People Change, 3rd Edition. New York, Guilford, 2013

Perry BD: The neurosequential model of therapeutics: applying principles of neuroscience to clinical work with traumatized and maltreated children, in Working With Traumatized Youth in Child Welfare. Edited by Webb NB. New York, Guilford, 2006, pp 27–52

van Dernoot Lipsky L: Trauma Stewardship: An Everyday Guide to Caring for Self While Caring for Others. Oakland, CA, Berrett-Koehler, 2009

Wachtel T: Defining Restorative. Bethlehem, PA, International Institute of Restorative Practices, 2016. Available at: www.iirp.edu/images/pdf/Defining-Restorative_Nov-2016.pdf. Accessed March 16, 2018.

Walser RD, Westrup D: Acceptance and Commitment Therapy for the Treatment of Posttraumatic Stress Disorder and Trauma-Related Problems. Oakland, CA, New Harbinger, 2007

6

Play Therapy

Julia LaMotte, M.S.
Karen Smith, Ph.D.

PLAY IS IMPORTANT. The realm of imagination, where emotions can be explored, illustrated, enacted, and transformed, is fertile ground for growth. Children's play is essential for the healthy mastery of developmental skills across cognitive, social, physical, and emotional domains of functioning. It enhances executive functioning (e.g., planning, organization, behavior regulation) and facilitates the attainment of appropriate social skills (turn-taking), emotional expression/regulation, and physical activity levels.

Play is fun—it challenges and entertains and delights—and the self-perpetuating pleasure that it induces compels the child to keep playing. With repetition, the function of the play evolves to serve a variety of purposes related to brain adaptation. Burghardt (2005) suggested that these processes follow a sequential arc, evolving from very simple to novel and creative behavior. Initially, play operates as a primary process, depleting excess metabolic energy and building a child's behavioral repertoire. Secondary-process play facilitates behavioral flexibility, neural processing, and motor coordination. As the child matures, play transforms from being mostly physical to an exploration of cognitive or mental territory. Tertiaryprocess play aids further behavioral and neural development that promotes social competence, innovation, and creativity.

In this way, a child's play can be understood as an effort to make sense of the world around him or her in a developmentally appropriate manner. Play creates a context for self-exploration and emotional expression while providing a space for dealing with unpredictable events and the sense of loss of control (Pellis et al. 2005). It is no surprise that mental health providers have identified and used play as a powerful modality for the delivery of therapeutic interventions with children.

The Association of Play Therapy defines play therapy as

> the systematic use of a theoretical model to establish an interpersonal process wherein trained play therapists use the therapeutic powers of play to help patients prevent or resolve psychosocial difficulties and achieve optimal growth and development. (Ray and McCullough 2015, p. 2)

But what does that mean in practice? Play therapy is the play therapist's ability to quickly analyze and skillfully direct the patient's play that separates play therapy from play. (A description of developmentally appropriate activities will be provided later in the section "Developmental Approaches.") Play therapy has unique theoretical roots; however, in its implementation it is flexible enough to allow the therapist to adapt and use this treatment modality as an effective augmentation of multiple evidence-based child therapies. In the last several years, contemporary play therapy has made notable gains within the field of evidence-based treatments for children through rigorous research; see Bratton et al. (2005) for a comprehensive meta-analysis of the efficacy of play therapy.

Play and Trauma

Early work by Bessel van der Kolk (2003) emphasized the importance of play in brain development, particularly for children who have experienced trauma. The encoding of a traumatic event or series of events involves many brain structures that rely on nonverbal communication, such as the amygdala (emotions and behavior), thalamus (sensory and motor signals), hippocampus (emotion and memory), and brain stem (central nervous system regulation). Other areas of the brain (frontal lobes) are responsible for encoding and later meaning making of these events. Play therapy allows children to represent the traumatic event nonverbally, a process similar to that by which the event was encoded, thereby accessing emotions that cannot necessarily be described in words. Furthermore, with the assistance of a skilled play therapist, children may be able to create a cohesive narrative for the event that was previously nonexistent. In the words of Haim G. Ginott (1960, p. 243), "toys are the child's words and play is the child's language." We would argue that the dynamic process of play therapy teaches the child to become "bilingual," using the language of play to build a meaningful narrative about the event that can be communicated to others and using language to then re-encode the trauma narrative into his or her brain circuitry. Play becomes a therapeutic bridge between the inexpressible and the spoken, which then opens the possibility of using other forms of evidence-based treatments that require and rely on verbal communication.

Trauma-Focused Play Therapy

After a traumatic event has occurred, it is common for children to express their internal turmoil through play. Posttraumatic play is often repetitive, highly structured, and sometimes literal and may involve reenactment of the traumatic event through the use of dolls, figurines, and other toys. It is not surprising, then, that trauma-focused play therapy has emerged as an efficacious and developmentally appropriate intervention for young children through adolescence.

Similarly, Gil (2017) describes the model of trauma-focused integrative play therapy (TFIPT) as having three reparative strategies for improving the child's social-emotional well-being: following the child's pace, considering the therapeutic relationship as context, and facilitating or processing the child's posttraumatic play. TFIPT emphasizes the integration of strategies to address the child's trauma using a balance between the child's receptivity, pacing, and clinical judgment.

In practice, play therapists must develop a skill set that is in tune with the idiosyncrasies of play. It is important to distinguish whether the child's play behaviors are helping to resolve the traumatic memories (dynamic play) or are potentially contributing to further trauma by reinforcing unresolved feelings of hopelessness (stagnant play). When implementing trauma-focused play therapy, the clinician must carefully observe the child's play behavior to determine whether it is dynamic or stagnant in nature. Although play may begin as stagnant, subtle shifts—such as the presence of previously nonexistent characters or objects, changes in the outcome of the play scenario, or the child assuming a more active role as an agent of change in the play narrative—may signal that the play is becoming dynamic, serving to resolve the trauma. Availability of appropriate affect, variability in play, decreased rigidity, and physical fluidity are additional signs of dynamic play. Of course, caregivers may also observe these changes in the child's play at home or at school, along with other positive changes in the child's social-emotional and behavioral functioning; therefore, collaboration between the therapist and the family is essential as therapy progresses.

Unfortunately, there are no formal guidelines or benchmarks to help determine the pace of posttraumatic play therapy. Decisions regarding when a therapist should intervene in the child's play and become more directive in shaping the trauma narrative are left to clinical judgment and, sometimes, intuition. Early intervention in the play may inhibit overall effectiveness, whereas waiting too long may prolong and reinforce feelings of hopelessness. A gradual, watchful approach wherein the therapist starts slowly with subtle involvement in the play (e.g., providing a verbal narrative as the play unfolds) and over time introduces more challenging interventions (e.g., asking questions, redirecting a segment of play, suggesting an alternative outcome) can be a trial-by-error endeavor. Posttraumatic play is repetitive in nature; therefore, the therapist has many opportunities to note and encourage change. It can be helpful to videotape sessions to facilitate objective observation of the child's play, track progress over the course of therapy, and anticipate opportunities for direct intervention.

Developmental Approaches

This section was written with the attainment of normative developmental milestones in mind. It is imperative that the therapist have a clear developmental framework prior to treatment onset in order to adequately assess the patient's progress and the overall therapeutic effectiveness. When planning for play activities, the clinician is strongly encouraged to consider the child's developmental abilities and level of social-emotional maturity in addition to his or her chronological age. Given the impact of trauma on brain development, there will likely be discrepancies between the child's competencies in various developmental domains. Do not hesitate to offer a range of materials, some of which may seem "too young" for the child's age. Let the child choose where to start: he or she will know.

We have compiled a list of play materials that can facilitate the play therapy process (Table 6–1), but these suggestions are only a starting point. For additional creative resources, see Lowenstein's (2011) publicly available e-book and the suggested readings at the end of this chapter.

TABLE 6–1. Suggested play materials

Art materials (crayons, markers, finger paints, paper, cartoon paper, clay, Play-Doh, magazines)

Stuffed animals and puppets

Soap bubbles

Dolls

Playhouse

Cars, trains, and rescue vehicles (ambulance, police)

Legos and blocks

Figurines (animal, family members, superheroes)

Stress balls or squishy balls

Dry erase board and markers

Board games and card games (chess, checkers, Uno, Guess Who)

Sand tray

Blank storybooks

Music CDs and blank CDs

Video recorder

Note. Assessment of the patient's developmental stage will help inform appropriateness of play materials. Although we have provided an array of suggested materials with ascending age in mind, these are merely suggestions.

Preschoolers

Psychological intervention with young children may be difficult given that cognitive abilities are limited at this age, which might pose a potential barrier to traditional talk therapy interventions. For example, it would be developmentally inappropriate to ask a preschooler to make connections between thoughts, feelings, and actions because at this age, children are still honing their cause-and-effect abilities. Therefore, play therapy may be of particular interest for young children because it deemphasizes verbal abilities and uses the natural language of play. This is consistent with the results from a recent meta-analysis, which yielded an average effect size of 0.53 for the use of play therapy in children 7 years and younger (Lin and Bratton 2015).

Although advances in child intervention are significant, many evidence-based treatments have not been proven to be effective for young children. Additionally, many early childhood interventions focus on behavioral and environmental changes that caregivers must implement. However, some children who have experienced trauma may have limited involvement with their pre–traumatic event caregivers, so play therapy is unique in that therapeutic intervention can occur without caregiver participation. Clinicians should expect the play of preschoolers to be egocentric, symbolic, and imaginative and should not focus too heavily on whether the child is factually correct in the expression and representation of real-life events. Ryan et al. (2017) provide a promising multidisciplinary model based in neurobiology that capitalizes on regulatory activities targeted at specific brain regions known to be impacted by trauma in children.

School-Age Children

As children transition into school age, a shift from imagination to concrete thinking begins to arise. Increased awareness of social norms and emphasis on objective rules may begin to shape play behaviors. Creative play allows children to reenact events while identifying with a character in the narrative rather than directly expressing their own thoughts and feelings. In this same manner, the therapist can guide the child through the reexperiencing of emotions in the play while suggesting additional coping skills to assist with any fear or anxiety related to the trauma. For example, the clinician may ask whether the character in the narrative would like to practice deep breathing rather than directing this suggestion to the child. The clinician's understanding of developmentally appropriate behaviors will aid him or her in assessing whether progress is being made or whether additional or more direct intervention is appropriate.

Adolescents and Transitional-Age Youth

It is a common misperception that play therapy is not an appropriate treatment model for adolescents because play is often characterized as "juvenile" and deemed inappropriate for teenagers. However, adolescence serves as a transitional period between childhood and adulthood when verbal expression of internal dialogue is developing and the representation of inner emotions may best be captured through modalities other than direct talk therapy.

Whereas adolescent play behaviors serve a more complex purpose (e.g., task-oriented instead of free play), teenagers may vacillate between their current abilities and previously acquired skills during a play session. An adolescent may find play therapy and other interventions that emphasize creative expression (e.g., drawing or art, poetry, games) easier to engage in than traditional therapeutic techniques that rely heavily on verbal expression. Building an alliance with a self-conscious, emotionally wary teenager can be difficult; therefore, inclusion of play therapy activities may decrease initial resistance to the therapeutic process by providing an indirect method of emotional expression. After developing trust and positive rapport with the therapist indirectly, the adolescent may be willing to engage in more direct discussion of the traumatic event. The therapist may decide to incorporate other appropriate trauma interventions at this juncture given the solid framework already built between the teenager and the therapist.

In contrast to traditional manualized treatment approaches, TFIPT can look very different from case to case. For this reason, we have provided a list of issues to consider when deciding when or how to use this modality (Table 6–2). For example, in a case where a young child has experienced a traumatic motor vehicle collision with the loss of a family member, TFIPT can be used to target the psychological effects of the traumatic event as well as feelings of loss and bereavement. Of course, in the case of a medical trauma, it is also important to have an understanding of the child's current cognitive functioning as it relates to possible traumatic brain injury. This may also be a relevant consideration in other types of trauma.

Overcoming Potential Challenges

With the implementation of any therapeutic intervention, it is likely that the clinician will face a variety of challenges, each unique to the individual case. Although we cannot provide a step-by-step guide for every potential challenge, we have included some areas of further consideration specific to trauma-focused play therapy. First, it is crucial that the therapist continually assess progress to differentiate between what is deemed *toxic* or *stagnant play* versus *dynamic play*. Gil (2017) has developed a checklist to assist with assessment of behaviors relevant to this differentiation. Of course, it is ultimately the clinician's judgment to determine when further intervention is warranted. The absence of adequate positive change may be indicative of the need to incorporate other empirically based interventions into the treatment.

One challenge unique to trauma-focused play therapy is monitoring the level of involvement of caregivers. We have emphasized the importance of assessment to determine developmental competencies; however, this information may be unavailable or unreliable depending on the child's history with the caregiver. Ultimately, the onus is placed on the therapist to adequately assess the child's developmental status both to in-

---

TABLE 6–2. Recognizing opportunities for decision making in the course of play therapy

---

Recognizing the opportunity to use play therapy

- Consider the characteristics of the trauma that has been experienced.
- Assess the child's behavioral and emotional symptoms.
- Take note of whether there are medical consequences that necessitate a nonverbal approach.

Getting started

Indirect techniques

- Create a safe, nurturing therapeutic environment that deemphasizes verbal communication.
- Provide a range of developmentally appropriate materials for play.
- Observe play behavior without interference.

Direct techniques

- Describe the child's play.
- Become an active participant in play.
- Ask questions about the play.
- Ask for guidance from the child before you participate.

Assessing progress

- Record changes in play or narrative from stagnant to dynamic.
- Use caregivers as informants for behavior change outside of session.

Recognizing opportunities to integrate other treatment

- As play becomes more directive, weave in alternative approaches as part of the play scenario.
- Consider play as an exposure technique.

---

form decisions about appropriate play materials and to direct treatment goals. Additionally, it is at the discretion of the clinician to decide when it is appropriate to involve caregivers or relevant adults in the therapeutic play activities. This is a difficult balance because too much parental involvement may jeopardize rapport with the therapist, but caregivers may become frustrated if they are excluded and may stop bringing their child to treatment. In some instances, the caregiver may have experienced the traumatic event as well, which might present additional challenges to the treatment. Preparation with caregivers prior to involvement in sessions, including discussion of the caregiver's potential trigger behaviors, is critical.

More broadly, the very nature of play therapy poses difficulty for manualization of this type of treatment. Although fantastic resources are available (see the Suggested Readings section for additional information), the shift in empirically based treatments has seen a rise in the use of treatment manuals that provide a week-by-week guide for providing therapy. Known resources may serve as a foundation for understanding the tenets of play therapy; however, given the personalized nature of the trauma narratives being enacted, it is likely that treatment will differ from clinician to clinician and from patient to patient. As play therapy gains acceptance as an empirically sound form of intervention, perhaps researchers will be able to develop more specific protocol manuals.

Sociocultural and Policy Implications

As mentioned in the subsection "Preschoolers," results of a meta-analytic review of empirical research demonstrated robust efficacy of play therapy across diverse populations of children (Lin and Bratton 2015). Because the language of play is universal, it is not surprising that this therapeutic technique can benefit individuals from a range of sociodemographic backgrounds. However, although all children play, there are many cultural differences in what play looks like and what its purpose is perceived to be.

Awareness of the cultural background of one's patient may help inform the family's receptiveness to treatment as well as engagement throughout. Shen (2016) described the potential influence of parental views of play on children's level of engagement in play therapy: Whereas Hispanic caregivers have a tendency to value play, Asian parents may become more restrictive around early school age. Cultural diversity may explain differences in children's responsiveness to therapy across ethnicity; most groups of children (African American, Hispanic, and Native American, as well as children who were biracial or multiracial) were more responsive to play therapy than talk therapy alone, with the exception of Asian ethnicities. Broad statements about differences between ethnic groups are often unhelpful; therefore, clinicians are encouraged to develop cultural competence because the unique cultural and familial context of the children who come to therapy may vary.

Furthermore, the focus of cultural implications should be directed at the inclusion of culturally relevant play materials (e.g., dolls or figures of diverse skin tones and cultural attire, ethnically diverse play foods). In a survey of play therapy counselors, the majority said they used culturally appropriate adaptations of play techniques and materials; however, de-

Ginott HG: A rationale for selecting toys in play therapy. J Consult Psychol 24(3):243–246, 1960 13850211

Lambert SF, LeBlanc M, Mullen JA, et al: Learning more about those who play in session: the National Play Therapy in Counseling Practices Project (phase I). J Couns Dev 85(1):42–46, 2007

Lin YW, Bratton SC: A meta-analytic review of child-centered play therapy approaches. J Couns Dev 93(1):45–58, 2015

Lowenstein L: Favorite Therapeutic Activities for Children, Adolescents, and Families: Practitioners Share Their Most Effective Interventions. Toronto, ON, Canada, Champion Press, 2011. Available at: www.lianalowenstein.com/e-booklet.pdf. Accessed March 16, 2018.

Pellis SM, Pellis VC, Foroud A: Play fighting: aggression, affiliation, and the development of nuanced social skills, in Developmental Origins of Aggression. Edited by Trembley R, Hartup WW, Archer J. New York, Guilford, 2005, pp 47–62

Ray DC, McCullough R: Evidence-Based Practice Statement: Play Therapy (research report). Clovis, CA, Association for Play Therapy, 2015 (revised 2016). Available at: https://cdn.ymaws.com/a4pt.site-ym.com/resource/resmgr/About_APT/APT_Evidence_Based_Statement.pdf. Accessed March 16, 2018.

Ryan K, Lane SJ, Powers D: A multidisciplinary model for treating complex trauma in early childhood. Int J Play Ther 26(2):111–123, 2017

Shen Y: A descriptive study of school counselors' play therapy experiences with the culturally diverse. Int J Play Ther 25(2):54–63, 2016

van der Kolk BA: The neurobiology of childhood trauma and abuse. Child Adolesc Psychiatr Clin N Am 12(2):293–317, 2003 12725013

7

School-Based Interventions

Sheryl H. Kataoka, M.D., M.S.H.S.
Pamela Vona, M.P.H., M.A.
Bradley D. Stein, M.D., Ph.D.

THERE ARE NEARLY 15,000 school districts and more than 100,000 schools in diverse communities across the United States. Within the walls of a school, some of the nation's most vulnerable youth can be found: students with preexisting mental health disorders, students with histories of trauma and neglect, and students who are at risk because they live in poverty or are experiencing discrimination due to their ethnic or racial background or their sexual orientation or identity. A national survey of youth found that 61% had experienced a form of trauma, crime, or abuse in the prior year, with some experiencing multiple traumas (Finkelhor et al. 2009).

Childhood trauma can affect key developmental and functional outcomes critical to school performance (Pat-Horenczyk et al. 2009). Exposure to violence is associated with lower grade point average and decreased rates of high school graduation; decreased IQ; and significant deficits in attention, abstract reasoning, long-term memory for verbal information, and reading ability (Delaney-Black et al. 2002). Students with

schoolwide or in classroom settings and include programs such as bullying and substance use prevention and whole-school approaches such as Positive Behavioral Interventions and Supports. Targeted trauma prevention interventions (tier 2), the focus of this chapter, can then be made available for those students who continue to be at risk for trauma-related mental health disorders despite tier 1 services. Tier 2 services, which include early identification and targeted intervention for students, play a critical role in schools to prevent serious functional impairment in students. Often, these tier 2 interventions can reach large numbers of students because they are commonly delivered in groups. Several tier 2 school-based interventions have been designed to intervene early with students who present with posttraumatic stress symptoms. Finally, those few students needing more intensive treatments can be referred for tier 3 services, such as individual or family therapy.

Evidence-Based Targeted Trauma Interventions Across Developmental Levels

A growing number of targeted trauma interventions have been implemented and evaluated in school settings worldwide. These include international programs that intervened with children exposed to war and terror-related trauma (Gelkopf and Berger 2009) as well as programs delivered in U.S. schools to both groups and individuals (Langley et al. 2015; Stein et al. 2003). The most common evidence-based trauma interventions employ components of cognitive-behavioral therapy (CBT) such as psychoeducation, relaxation skills, cognitive restructuring, trauma narrative, safety planning, affect modulation, and in vivo mastery of trauma reminders. However, issues of engagement, identification of traumatic stress symptoms, and parent involvement are important in delivering trauma interventions across developmental levels in schools. In the next section, we present three examples of evidence-based targeted prevention interventions designed for delivery in primary and secondary schools for general types of trauma (see Table 7–1 for a summary).

Bounce Back

Few trauma interventions evaluated for use in schools exist for younger elementary school–age students. Bounce Back was developed to address this need (Langley et al. 2015). Uniquely, Bounce Back blends the evidence-based practices of CBT and a developmentally appropriate approach for young children. This intervention is designed with elements and engage-

TABLE 7–1. **Comparison of targeted trauma-informed prevention programs in schools**

	Bounce Back	Cognitive Behavioral Intervention for Trauma in Schools	Support for Students Exposed to Trauma
Age range	5–11 years	10–15 years	10–16 years
Method of delivery	Mental health clinician	Mental health clinician	Nonclinical school staff
Number of group sessions	10	10	10
Number of individual sessions	2–3	1–3	NA
Parent involvement	Introductory meeting and sharing of trauma narrative	Introductory meeting	NA

Note. NA=not applicable.

ment activities to be developmentally appropriate for 5- to 11-year-olds and activities to engage parents because parental involvement is a crucial component in working with young children. The process of identifying students who are appropriate for Bounce Back also takes into account the developmental level of these students. Each student meets individually with a therapist to review possible traumatic exposures and symptoms, and therapists obtain feedback from parents about areas of functional impairment to focus on during treatment.

Bounce Back consists of 10 weekly 1-hour sessions delivered in groups of four to six students, 2–3 individual sessions with each student lasting 30–50 minutes, and 1–3 educational sessions with groups of parents. This intervention is designed to decrease child posttraumatic stress and anxious and depressive symptoms and improve functioning in school for students who have experienced one or more traumatic events. Bounce Back includes sessions with psychoeducation about trauma, relaxation training, cognitive restructuring, social problem solving, positive activities, and trauma-focused intervention strategies such as the trauma narrative and gradual approach to anxiety-provoking situations.

Bounce Back has incorporated several treatment elements to engage and teach young children skills for coping with traumatic stress. Even before presenting the core components of coping skills and strategies, therapists lay the foundation for identifying and naming feelings and providing simple language for communicating those feelings. Once that foundation is laid, therapists provide concrete examples of topics to be covered, often using familiar "story time" activities that use children's books to illustrate a concept. Concepts in each lesson are presented in a straightforward and concrete manner, with trauma narratives conveyed through the creation of a storybook with pictures created by students.

Another example in Bounce Back of helping students remember and draw on the skills that have been taught in group sessions is through such tools as courage cards that students design themselves as part of the group activity. Younger students are also engaged in treatment through creative games and other experiential activities to engage them in the skills and strategies being taught. In addition, parents of students in Bounce Back are invited to a one-on-one session with the child and the group leader so that the child can share his or her trauma narrative.

Bounce Back has been found to be effective when delivered by school counselors. In a randomized controlled trial comparing students in Bounce Back with students on a waitlist, Bounce Back students had greater improvements in child- and parent-reported posttraumatic stress disorder symptoms, parent-reported emotion regulation, and child-reported anxiety and social adjustment (Langley et al. 2015).

Cognitive Behavioral Intervention for Trauma in Schools

The Cognitive Behavioral Intervention for Trauma in Schools (CBITS) program was created using a community-partnered approach, with shared program and evaluation development between clinician researchers and school staff and administration. This collaboration formed when Los Angeles Unified School District leaders identified mental health effects of violence exposure among their students that needed to be addressed. In partnership with researchers, the district surveyed more than 28,000 sixth graders and found that 94% had been exposed to violence in the past year and 40% had experienced knife or gun violence.

During the development of CBITS, school district leaders indicated that they wanted a trauma intervention that could be delivered by the district's psychiatric school social workers and evaluated in the naturalistic setting of these clinicians delivering the intervention. In order to accommodate the vast numbers of students in need of CBITS and the limited number of clinical staff available to deliver this targeted prevention program, a time-limited, brief group modality instead of intensive individual therapy was suggested. To fit within the context of the school schedule, the CBITS groups also needed to be delivered "bell-to-bell" during a single class period and during the school day when counseling was available.

To start, middle- and high-school students independently complete a screening questionnaire, although some students benefit from having the questions read aloud to them in a large-group classroom setting. After eligibility is determined on the basis of trauma exposure and symptoms, students are placed in groups of six to eight. The groups meet for 1-hour weekly sessions over the course of about 10 weeks, and each student receives one to three individual sessions to work with a therapist on his or her trauma narrative. In addition, parents are invited and encouraged to attend one or two optional psychoeducational sessions, and a similar optional psychoeducational session is also delivered to teachers.

Students learn the core components of cognitive-behavioral skills across the 10 group sessions. In sessions 1 and 2, students are introduced to the group; receive psychoeducation about common reactions to trauma; learn about the connection between thoughts, feelings, and actions; and are introduced to relaxation skills. In sessions 3 and 4, students focus on understanding the link between thoughts and feelings and learn skills for disrupting negative or dysfunctional thoughts. In session 5, students begin to build a behavioral hierarchy that involves approaching anxiety-provoking situations that they want or need to be able to do in a gradual way with use of alternative coping strategies. In addition to the group sessions, students meet individually with the group leader to further process the memory of their traumatic experience by verbalizing a trauma narrative. Sessions 6 and 7 involve exposure to the memory of the traumatic event after completing the individual sessions through imagination, writing, drawing, and sharing with group members. Sessions 8 and 9 focus on building social problem-solving skills, and session 10 includes a review, relapse prevention planning, and a celebration of progress.

CBITS has been shown to improve posttraumatic stress disorder and depressive symptoms among students exposed to violence compared with students on a waitlist (Stein et al. 2003). Findings also suggest that CBITS may benefit students' school performance, with youth who receive CBITS early in the school year achieving higher math and language arts grades than do students who receive the intervention later that same academic year (Kataoka et al. 2011). In addition to improving symptoms following general and multiple exposures to violence, CBITS has also been shown to improve symptoms following a natural disaster (Jaycox et al. 2010).

Support for Students Exposed to Trauma

Support for Students Exposed to Trauma (SSET) is an adaptation of the CBITS intervention, developed in recognition of the scarcity of mental health clinicians in many schools. The intervention is a series of 10 lessons designed to be delivered by nonclinicians such as teachers or school counselors to reduce students' trauma-related distress. SSET includes a wide variety of CBT-based skill-building techniques geared toward changing maladaptive thoughts and promoting positive behaviors.

SSET teaches core cognitive-behavioral skills similar to those found in CBITS. However, each of the 10 SSET sessions is presented as a "lesson plan" to align with a format familiar to teachers. Lesson plans include didactic presentation of materials, practice activities to promote mastery of the skill, and independent practice prior to the next lesson. Like CBITS, each session is designed to be completed within a class period (about 45 minutes per session). SSET does not include the individual trauma narrative sessions or parent sessions. In a preliminary study of students, SSET was found to reduce trauma-related mental health symptoms in preadolescent sixth- and seventh-grade students (Jaycox et al. 2009).

Strategies for Overcoming Common Implementation Challenges in Schools

As interventions that are designed for school settings, Bounce Back, CBITS, and SSET have a relative advantage over usual care, are compatible with other behaviorally oriented practices in schools, and minimize complexity through clearly presented lessons developed in collaboration with school-based clinicians. Despite these advantages, implementing group-based trauma interventions in schools can be challenging. In the next subsection, we address common implementation issues and strategies for overcoming these situations.

School Engagement

One main challenge in delivering a targeted trauma prevention program in schools can be school engagement. Despite the availability of school-based evidence-based treatments (EBTs) that can effectively address students' traumatic stress symptoms, schools often must balance multiple competing demands with limited resources and time and may not see the relevance of a trauma intervention to their educational mission. Typically, a school's primary focus is the academic development of students, with mental health interventions viewed by some school stakeholders as tangential to the primary mission of schools. Therefore, buy-in and communication are particularly important aspects of delivering trauma interventions in school settings. One critical aspect of fostering school buy-in is mission-policy alignment. For schools, this alignment can include linking students' mental health to academic achievement and presenting to school administrators data regarding the links between trauma exposure and school performance and the positive ways that targeted prevention programs can impact academics.

In addition, teachers may have concerns about students missing class time to attend targeted prevention programs when interventions are delivered as "pull-out" sessions. Flexible implementation strategies that take a collaborative approach with each school and partner with administrators and teachers on best times to deliver the program (e.g., during noncore academic classes or during a different class each week) can help to address some concerns about missed educational time. Studies reveal that in-service programs and other opportunities to communicate with teachers and staff are useful in aligning the mission of schools with delivery of preventative trauma programs (Langley et al. 2010).

Identification of Students for Targeted Prevention in Schools

Another key challenge in implementation of trauma-informed targeted school-based prevention is in identifying students who might benefit from the program. One common way this is accomplished is through universal screening because trauma-related symptoms often go unobserved by parents and teachers. However, school providers must be cautious to screen only the number of students that they would have the capacity to treat. In addition, it is highly recommended, and often required by school districts, to obtain parental consent for administering mental health screening, especially regarding sensitive subjects such as traumatic stress and exposure to trauma. Despite efforts to streamline the screening process, it requires additional personnel time and resources that differ from the typical duties of school-based clinicians and includes logistics of both obtaining parent permission and administering the screening itself. Some schools and districts have developed a routine screening of all students as part of the structure of the routine school practice, and others have

context can include historical trauma, racism and microaggressions, trauma exposure during immigration, and community fears of deportation, as well as cultural expressions of distress, communication styles, and family values. The trauma-informed school system framework (see Figure 7–1) illustrates some of these factors, with particular attention paid to the culture of the school and of the community being served.

One approach in balancing both the implementation of an evidence-based targeted prevention intervention and the cultural context and priorities of the community is through a community-partnered approach (Minkler and Wallerstein 2011). Community-partnered participatory research is built on the principles of community-based participatory research, which was developed in under-resourced communities of color to promote collaboration between the community, providers, and academic partners through trust building and two-way knowledge exchange (Jones and Wells 2007). In this model, community members identify the priorities for research, and cultural and community knowledge are integrated into intervention development, implementation, and dissemination. Interventions that have relied on community partnerships for engagement in and implementation of services have been able to maintain the core components of effective interventions while integrating culturally relevant examples and context throughout the delivery of the intervention, as in Bounce Back, CBITS, and SSET.

Policy Implications

Given the growing recognition that trauma exposure negatively impacts academic achievement and that schools provide an optimal setting in which to provide trauma-informed mental health services for children, many federal and state education and health care policy initiatives are calling for wider use of evidence-based trauma-informed services in schools. At the federal level, the U.S. Department of Education supports a number of initiatives that call for the use of trauma-informed interventions. The Every Student Succeeds Act (2015) makes explicit provisions for trauma-informed approaches in student support and academic enrichment. Project School Emergency Response to Violence (SERV) provides funds to helps schools and/or districts recover from a violent and/or traumatic event. Project Prevent awards grants to local education agencies to aid their ability to identify, assess, and serve students who have been exposed to chronic violence. This mechanism explicitly funds mental health services for trauma and anxiety. Similarly, School Climate Transformation grants award resources to local education agencies to facilitate their development of an evidence-based multi-tiered framework to support students' behavioral health needs. Finally, the Promoting Student Resilience program funds mental health services in school districts recovering from acts of civil unrest.

In addition to the Department of Education initiatives, a number of federal health policies and programs expand access to trauma-informed behavioral health services. In December 2014, the "free care rule" was reversed. Before this change, the rule prevented states from receiving Medicaid funds for services that ordinarily are provided for free. This change allows schools to bill for health and mental health services as long as Medicaid requirements are met. The Affordable Care Act (2010) enhances access to behavioral health services by middle- and low-income children. Additionally, the revision to the free care rule enhances schools' ability to receive Medicaid funding to provide such services. The Safe Schools/ Healthy Students and National Child Traumatic Stress Network initiatives, administered by the U.S. Department of Health and Human Services through the Substance Abuse and Mental Health Services Administration, aim to enhance the provision of trauma-informed interventions to students in the school setting.

State health initiatives have also been launched to enhance the provision of trauma-informed services in schools. For example, California's Mental Health Services Act includes a Prevention and Early Intervention initiative that explicitly allocates resources for the provision of trauma-informed services in schools. Additionally, Massachusetts, Pennsylvania, Washington, and Oregon have each passed legislation that allocates funding to enhance trauma-informed approaches in schools. Given the extent of these federal and state policies, schools likely need guidance on how to identify students eligible for services, select appropriate trauma-informed interventions, and train their mental health workforce in evidence-based trauma practices.

Conclusion

At a time of increased recognition of the deleterious, life-long effects to youth of untreated exposure to traumatic events (Felitti et al. 1998), a combination of events and progress has created opportunities for schools to more effectively meet the needs of many traumatized students through targeted prevention interventions. Recent years have seen not only the development of school-based targeted prevention programs demonstrated to be effective in helping trauma-exposed children but also development of other elements that can enhance the successful delivery of such interventions (Kletter et al. 2013). These elements include approaches to engaging school decision-makers and obtaining their support for trauma-informed targeted prevention, identifying students likely to benefit from such services, and ensuring that school personnel delivering the interventions have received necessary training and implementation support. It is critical that personnel consider the sociocultural environments of the school and community in any effort to deliver school-based trauma services (or services of any kind). Federal and state initiatives can provide financial support to schools seeking to deliver school-based targeted prevention for traumatic stress.

Schools' primary mission is educating students, not meeting their mental health needs, but schools can play a critical role in reducing the unmet need for children's mental health services that exists in our current mental health care delivery system, and such services provide individual, family, and social benefits for the children, families, and schools involved. These benefits are likely to be most profound for children in socioeconomically disadvantaged communities because these children are more likely to be exposed to a range of traumatic events and to have greater difficulties accessing effective mental health services. This chapter helps to provide a road map for mental health clinicians, educators, and other stakeholders desiring to use school-based targeted prevention services to better meet the needs of children exposed to traumatic events.

KEY CONCEPTS

- Clinicians need to understand the impact of trauma exposure on students' school functioning.
- It is important to recognize the key components of successful school-based interventions for students exposed to trauma.
- Several state and federal policy initiatives exist that help to foster the implementation of trauma services in schools.

Discussion Questions

1. How can targeted trauma-informed prevention interventions be integrated into other forms of support services in a school?

2. With limited resources, what are some strategies schools can use in implementing targeted trauma prevention programs?

3. How can core components of targeted trauma-informed programs based on cognitive-behavioral therapy be implemented across primary and secondary schools?

Suggested Readings

Chafouleas SM, Johnson AH, Overstreet S, et al: Toward a blueprint for trauma-informed service delivery in schools. School Ment Health 8(1):144–162, 2016

Kataoka S, Langley AK, Wong M, et al: Responding to students with posttraumatic stress disorder in schools. Child Adolesc Psychiatr Clin N Am 21(1):119–133, x, 2012 22137816

Nadeem E, Jaycox LH, Langley AK, et al: Effects of trauma on students: early intervention through the cognitive behavioral intervention for trauma in schools, in Handbook of School Mental Health. Edited by Weist MD, Lever NA, Bradshaw CP, et al. New York, Springer, 2014, pp 145–157

References

Delaney-Black V, Covington C, Ondersma SJ, et al: Violence exposure, trauma, and IQ and/or reading deficits among urban children. Arch Pediatr Adolesc Med 156(3):280–285, 2002 11876674

Felitti VJ, Anda RF, Nordenberg D, et al: Relationship of childhood abuse and household dysfunction to many of the leading causes of death in adults: the Adverse Childhood Experiences (ACE) study. Am J Prev Med 14(4):245–258, 1998 9635069

Finkelhor D, Turner H, Ormrod R, et al: Violence, abuse, and crime exposure in a national sample of children and youth. Pediatrics 124(5):1411–1423, 2009 19805459

Gelkopf M, Berger R: A school-based, teacher-mediated prevention program (ERASE-Stress) for reducing terror-related traumatic reactions in Israeli youth: a quasi-randomized controlled trial. J Child Psychol Psychiatry 50(8):962–971, 2009 19207621

Jaycox LH, Langley AK, Stein BD, et al: Support for students exposed to trauma: a pilot study. School Ment Health 1(2):49–60, 2009 20811511

Jaycox LH, Cohen JA, Mannarino AP, et al: Children's mental health care following Hurricane Katrina: a field trial of trauma-focused psychotherapies. J Trauma Stress 23(2):223–231, 2010 20419730

Jones L, Wells K: Strategies for academic and clinician engagement in community-participatory partnered research. JAMA 297(4):407–410, 2007 17244838

Kataoka S, Jaycox LH, Wong M, et al: Effects on school outcomes in low-income minority youth: preliminary findings from a community-partnered study of a school trauma intervention. Ethn Dis 21(3 Suppl 1):S1–71–77, 2011 22352083

Kletter H, Rialon RA, Laor N, et al: Helping children exposed to war and violence: perspectives from an international work group on interventions for youth and families. Child and Youth Care Forum 42(4):371–388, 2013

Langley AK, Nadeem E, Kataoka SH, et al: Evidence-based mental health programs in schools: barriers and facilitators of successful implementation. School Ment Health 2(3):105–113, 2010 20694034

Langley AK, Gonzalez A, Sugar CA, et al: Bounce back: effectiveness of an elementary school-based intervention for multicultural children exposed to traumatic events. J Consult Clin Psychol 83(5):853–865, 2015 26302251

Minkler M, Wallerstein N: Community-Based Participatory Research for Health: From Process to Outcomes. New York, Wiley, 2011

Pat-Horenczyk R, Qasrawi R, Lesack R, et al: Posttraumatic symptoms, functional impairment, and coping among adolescents on both sides of the Israeli-Palestinian conflict: a cross-cultural approach. Appl Psychol 58(4):688–708, 2009

Ramirez M, Wu Y, Kataoka S, et al: Youth violence across multiple dimensions: a study of violence, absenteeism and suspensions among middle school children. J Pediatr 161(3); 542-546, 2012 22521110

Stein BD, Jaycox LH, Kataoka SH, et al: A mental health intervention for schoolchildren exposed to violence: a randomized controlled trial. JAMA 290(5):603–611, 2003 12902363

Substance Abuse and Mental Health Services Administration: SAMHSA's Concept of Trauma and Guidance for a Trauma-Informed Approach (HHS Publ No SMA-14-4884). Rockville, MD, Substance Abuse and Mental Health Services Administration, July 2014. Available at: https://store.samhsa.gov/shin/content/SMA14-4884/SMA14-4884.pdf. Accessed March 16, 2018.

Vona P, Wilmoth P, Jaycox LH, et al: A web-based platform to support an evidence-based mental health intervention: lessons from the CBITS web site. Psychiatr Serv 65(11):1381–1384, 2014 25124275

Vona P, Baweja S, Santiago CD, et al: A cross-site partnership to examine implementation and sustainability of a school-based trauma program. Ethn Dis (in press)

UCSF Healthy Environments and Response to Trauma in Schools (HEARTS)

Joyce Dorado, Ph.D.
Martha Merchant, Psy.D.

UCSF HEARTS: Key Elements of an Approach to Addressing Trauma in Schools

The University of California, San Francisco Healthy Environments and Response to Trauma in Schools (UCSF HEARTS) program is a multilevel, whole-school approach that aims to promote school success and resilience for trauma-impacted children and youth by creating trauma-informed, safe, supportive, equitable, and engaging learning and teaching environments that benefit everyone in the school community. The program works in partnership with schools and school districts, using a trauma-informed approach to build the capacity of school personnel to increase teaching and learning time in classrooms and reduce time spent on disciplining

TABLE 8–1.   UCSF HEARTS core guiding principles for creating trauma-informed schools

Principle	Trauma-informed lens rationale	Description of principle
Understanding trauma and stress	When we do not understand trauma, we are more likely to misinterpret trauma-related behaviors as "willful," "sick," or "crazy," which can lead to ineffective, stigmatizing, and/or punitive reactions to people impacted by trauma.	Understanding how trauma and stress can affect individuals, relationships, and organizations helps to reframe otherwise confusing or aggravating behavior. This assists us in recognizing trauma's effects more accurately, which leads to more compassionate, strength-based, and effective responses to trauma-impacted people that promote healing rather than reactions that inadvertently retraumatize and cause harm.
Cultural humility and responsiveness	We come from diverse cultural groups that may experience different traumas and stressors, react to these adversities differently, and experience differences in how others respond to our traumatic experiences.	When we are open to understanding the trauma and adversity caused by historical, institutionalized, and societal oppression and respond to them with cultural humility, we can work together to mitigate these harms, and equity is enhanced.
Safety and predictability	Trauma unpredictably violates our physical, relational, and emotional safety, resulting in a sense of threat and a need to focus resources on managing risks.	Establishing physical, relational, and emotional safety, as well as predictability in the environment, enables us to focus resources on healthy development, wellness, learning, and teaching.

TABLE 8–1. UCSF HEARTS core guiding principles for creating trauma-informed schools *(continued)*

Principle	Trauma-informed lens rationale	Description of principle
Compassion and dependability	Trauma can leave us feeling isolated or betrayed, which may make it difficult to trust others and receive support.	By fostering relationships that are compassionate and attuned, as well as dependable and trustworthy, we re-establish trusting connections with others that foster healing and well-being.
Resilience and social-emotional learning	Trauma can derail the development of healthy skills in regulating emotions, cognitions, and behaviors, as well as healthy interpersonal skills, which may then compound trauma's negative effects.	Promoting wellness practices and building social-emotional learning competencies of self-management, self-awareness, social awareness, relationship skills, and responsible decision making (www.CASEL.org) help us to be resilient and more successful in school and at work.
Empowerment and collaboration	Trauma involves a loss of power and control that can make us feel helpless and hopeless.	When we are given meaningful opportunities to have voice and choice and our strengths are acknowledged and built on, we feel empowered to advance growth and well-being for ourselves and others and can work together to forward the cause of social justice.

Source. Modified from Dorado JS, Martinez M, McArthur LE, et al.: "Healthy Environments and Response to Trauma in Schools (HEARTS): A whole-school, multi-level, prevention and intervention program for creating trauma-informed, safe, and supportive schools." *School Mental Health* 8:163–176, 2016, Table 1: UCSF HEARTS Core Guiding Principles for Creating Trauma Informed Schools, p. 167. With permission of Springer Science+Business Media New York 2016.

(with repeated incidents) eventual expulsion. These reactions, however, are not an effective method for creating positive change for students like Ryan, nor are they effective for a school community. Further, unnecessarily punitive discipline procedures such as these add to the risk of such students dropping out or being pushed out of school (Public Counsel 2015).

One simple, profound change we can make in order to create more trauma-informed schools is a shift in perspective. In the face of confusing, undesirable behaviors, we tend to ask, "What is wrong with you?" If instead we ask, "What has happened to you?" we allow the opportunity to see beyond the surface behaviors to the underlying causes driving the behavior (Bloom 1995). Note that we are not suggesting that these questions are being or should be asked out loud, particularly in the middle of a heated situation. However, asking these questions internally can shift the way we understand, feel, and react to or respond to the situation. This shift is in accord with broader initiatives for creating more trauma informed-systems (Substance Abuse and Mental Health Services Administration 2014) and can facilitate a more effective and compassionate response that can help students succeed in school rather than engendering a punitive reaction that can ultimately lead to students' disengagement from school. Shifting our perspective, along with an understanding of the effects of chronic stress and trauma, can help schools recognize students like Ryan as needing support as opposed to simply requiring discipline.

Consider the vignette again, this time including the underlying chronic stress and traumatic events (i.e., what has happened?) and the resulting experiences of the student, teacher, classroom, and school (inserted in italics):

> Ryan is an *African American* fifth-grade boy *from a very low-income neighborhood where community violence is a frequent occurrence. He has been witnessing severe domestic violence between his parents since he was a baby. One night, in front of Ryan, his father beat up and injured his mother so badly that a neighbor called 911. His father was handcuffed and taken away by the police, and his mother was taken in an ambulance to the hospital. Ryan slept little that night, terrified by the events and anxious about what would become of his mother and father. In the morning, Ryan asked his neighbor to take him to school. Ryan attends a chronically under-resourced public school that serves children largely from Ryan's neighborhood. The school has experienced two lockdowns due to community violence in the past several months. Ryan's teacher has been overwhelmed by the large number of high-needs children in her classroom as well as the fact that there have been several physical fights between her students in recent weeks. As a relatively new teacher, she has been putting in many extra hours to try to prepare her lessons and manage student difficulties, and she is exhausted.* This morning, when Ryan arrived at school, his teacher, Ms. Lang, *who did not know about his traumatic ex-*

periences, asked him for his homework, but Ryan did not have it. She expressed frustration at him and took away his recess as a consequence. *Ryan was upset and triggered by being in trouble with his teacher.* A short time later, his deskmate accidentally bumped Ryan. *Ryan was already to some degree triggered into a heightened state of vigilance and preparation for defense against threat (i.e., survival mode), and this physical contact fully triggered him into a fight/flight/freeze reaction.* As a result, Ryan punched his deskmate in the stomach. Ms. Lang, naturally upset by this outburst, began to yell at Ryan to stop, *which further escalated him.* Ryan began screaming, kicked over a chair, and hid under his desk. After 10 minutes of trying to extract Ryan from the classroom *(during which time Ms. Lang felt frightened, helpless, and defeated and the other children in the classroom could only look on in fear and frustration),* Ryan was brought to the principal's office. Ryan was then suspended for 5 days for his behavior, *inadvertently exposing Ryan not only to a major loss of instructional time but also to a period of time during which he would have no refuge from the trauma and suffering in his home life* (Dorado 2012b).

When we ask, "What has happened to Ryan?" we can see that he has been impacted by chronic trauma and that his escalated behavior is a trauma-related reaction triggered by his interactions with his teacher and classmate. Similarly, when we ask, "What has happened to Ms. Lang?" we see that she is also experiencing a number of overwhelming stressors and is in a sensitized state that has made her vulnerable to being triggered by Ryan's behavior. Shifting our perspective and looking beyond the surface behaviors through a trauma-informed lens can help us to better understand behaviors and guides a formulation of what is needed to meet the needs behind these behaviors and to prevent escalations from occurring in the future. We can see that what is underlying the interactional escalation between Ryan and Ms. Lang is a triggered fear response, and thus what is needed above all else is to address the underlying fear and do what is necessary to help both Ryan and Ms. Lang feel safe. Asking "What has happened?" also allows us to see Ryan and Ms. Lang's strengths despite the adversities they are facing, such as Ryan's desire to come to school and Ms. Lang's dedication and diligence, and we can build on these strengths to promote resilience and school success.

As illustrated by the approach above, when we bring a trauma-informed lens to challenging situations, we advocate asking "What has happened to you?" not only for the student but also for the staff member, the classroom, and the school as an organization. Taking this wider approach has been crucial. This shift in perspective creates an opportunity to address burnout and secondary traumatic stress in teachers and other school staff. When staff begin to understand that they too are affected by chronic stress and trauma and experience attempts to alleviate these effects, their capacity to recognize the importance of addressing the needs of their trauma-impacted student increases, and they can engage in this work with renewed empathy and hope. Working to counteract an "us versus them" mentality, in which there are traumatized students on one side and adults who have to deal with them on the other, HEARTS strives to foster a mentality of "we are all in this together," advancing the understanding that each and every person can play a role in creating a safer and more supportive school that benefits everyone in the school community.

The traditional mental health approach to addressing trauma in schools is to identify students and refer them to mental health services. However, even on-site, trauma-specific treatment is not enough to create meaningful change for trauma-impacted students and communities if psychotherapy is provided within the context of a negative, unsupportive learning and teaching environment. Although Ryan may be able to build coping skills in the therapy room, too often he will return to his classroom only to be inadvertently triggered into survival ("fight/flight/freeze") mode by trauma reminders in the school environment such as a sudden change in classroom routine, a challenging interaction with another student, or a disciplinary practice that he perceives as a threat. In a school where a student like Ryan is seen as a problem to be fixed, there is a risk that his learning and development might be set aside as the school system tries to find a way to "manage" Ryan and his behaviors. Thus, much of HEARTS aims at improving school climate—the norms, goals, values, interpersonal relationships, and organizational structures of a school. A safe and supportive school climate fosters learning and development and allows everyone at the school to experience growth and satisfaction.

A commonly used educational system approach that can promote supportive school cultures and climates as well as provide more intensive supports as needed is multi-tiered systems of supports (MTSS), a comprehensive framework for integrating and aligning academic and behavioral instruction and support. MTSS is often represented by the same triangular graphic as the one used in public health. Tier 1 indicates the bottom of the triangle and identifies universal supports for all students that are meant to be sufficient to serve the needs of most students. Tier 2 indicates the middle of the triangle, comprising selected interventions for students for whom the universal supports are not sufficient. Tier 3 indicates the smallest, top part of the triangle, which includes targeted and intensive interventions for students for whom both tier 1 and tier 2 supports are not sufficient.

The HEARTS program offers supports and interventions across all three MTSS tiers. Further, for each of the tiers, UCSF HEARTS attends to three levels of the school community: students, adults in the caregiving system (i.e., staff and caregivers), and the school system as a whole. (See Figure 8–1 for a sample of HEARTS supports across the three MTSS tiers that could help to support a student like Ryan.) The six trauma-informed principles are applied in all three tiers across all three levels, guiding development and implementation of practices, strategies, supports, and interventions. Because other chapters in this book cover tier 2 and 3 supports, the bulk of descriptions in the following sections will focus on an application of these principles to tier 1 aspects of HEARTS that are fundamental to making school cultures more safe, supportive, equitable, and trauma informed for the entire school community.

Tier 1: Universal Supports

Understanding Trauma and Stress

Since we began implementing HEARTS in 2009, we have recognized the importance of establishing baseline knowledge on how trauma affects individuals, relationships, and organizations as a whole. Therefore, as part of HEARTS, we have facilitated half-day professional development (PD) trainings before the school year begins. These PDs establish common language and understanding of how chronic stress and complex trauma can affect neurobiology, learning readiness, and behavior in individuals and systems. We also offer strategies for addressing these effects that can be used by all members of the school staff. These initial trainings are then augmented through a series of follow-up trainings and consultation, including a concentration on addressing staff burnout and secondary trauma and increasing staff coping resources and wellness via self-care and organizational strategies.

HEARTS training uses metaphors to make the concepts salient and easy to recall. The first metaphor is that of a vinyl record. Because of use-dependent alterations to the brain, chronic trauma "wears a groove in the brain" the same way that when a song is played repeatedly on a record, the needle on the record player eventually wears a deeper groove on that song's track (Dorado 2012a). A different song can be playing, but if the record player is bumped, the needle will skip across the record and land in the record's deepest groove. Indeed, that groove can become so deep that the needle gets stuck in this groove rather than going on to the next song. Consider Ryan's response to his teacher's reaction. Although the event may not seem traumatic from the outside, Ryan's brain may have been "bumped" into his deep "trauma groove" by Ms. Lang's raised voice

nessed severe domestic violence may have learned to hide or run if someone looks like he or she might be angry. This behavior may be adaptive at home with Ryan's family because it helps to protect him from getting hurt, but at school it is less adaptive because without an understanding of the traumatic context of the behavior, school staff generally consider it unacceptable for students to run away from them and hide. We also highlight the fact that the brain can be rewired throughout the lifespan, instilling hope and encouraging teachers and adults who work with children and youth to continue to provide these young people with new experiences to change the wiring of their brains toward healthier ways of being.

Importantly, HEARTS centers on a systems approach to understanding how trauma affects not only individuals but also relationships, groups, and organizations. A system filled with people impacted by chronic stress and trauma can begin to act like a trauma-impacted organism, in which the organization experiences such symptoms as fragmentation, lack of cohesiveness and integration, extreme reactivity, numbness and lack of empathy, decontextualized decision making by those in authority, and an overly intense focus on threat reduction such that order, control, and rigid rules are prioritized at the expense of creativity, development, and innovation (Bloom and Farragher 2013). When staff are having these negative experiences in their schools, rather than asking, "What is wrong with our organization?" it is more helpful to ask, "What has happened to our organization?" This shift in perspective can help to reduce blame and finger-pointing and can help the organization to concentrate their efforts on healing the underlying chronic stress and trauma on an organizational level instead.

Cultural Humility and Responsiveness

Along with understanding trauma and stress, the principle of *cultural humility and responsiveness* is foundational to creating trauma-informed schools. Racism, sexism, heterosexism, xenophobia, and other forms of societal and institutionalized oppression can be experienced as a form of trauma, termed *insidious trauma* by Maria Root (cited by Brown 2008). Insidious trauma can be caused by the looming threat that one's safety and well-being are not as important as another person's safety and well-being because of the lottery of birth (e.g., the color of one's skin, how one talks, whom one loves, where one was born). When shifting the perspective from "What is wrong with you?" to "What has happened to you?" we advocate that schools consider the possibility that one of the things that may have happened to a student (or adult) with challenging behavioral or emotional presentations could be the chronic experience of insidious trauma.

Furthermore, although most forms of trauma occur across class lines, the trauma of community violence disproportionately affects highly stressed, low-income urban neighborhoods, which, because of historical and institutional racism, are largely inhabited by communities of color (Buka et al. 2001). The negative impact of community violence and other types of trauma on school behavior and learning, combined with insidious trauma and the pernicious effects of implicit and explicit bias in individuals and institutionalized policies and procedures, can have a synergistically adverse effect on students from marginalized communities and can contribute to inequity in suspensions, expulsions, and dropout (Soto-Vigil Koon 2013), feeding what is known as the school-to-prison pipeline. The *school-to-prison pipeline* refers to the way that these inequitably administered punitive and exclusionary disciplinary measures result in students of color and students with disabilities being disproportionately pushed out of school and into the juvenile justice and prison population (e.g., Losen et al. 2012). Because Ryan is an African American student from a low-income community, implicit and institutionalized biases are likely factors that contribute to his school-related difficulties.

Because trauma feeds the school-to-prison pipeline, addressing trauma in schools is a crucial component of stemming this harmful pipeline's flow. Additionally, given that stress and time pressure exacerbate implicit bias (Casey et al. 2012), addressing chronic stress in educators and other school staff can also help to mitigate disproportionality. On the whole, educators are highly motivated to teach all children well and to eliminate the achievement gap. An understanding of how chronic stress and insidious trauma are related to the achievement gap and the school-to-prison pipeline can serve to propel schools toward seeking additional training on addressing the effects of implicit and institutional bias in educational and disciplinary practices. This can be a gateway for creating space to discuss cultural humility issues.

Safety and Predictability

Trauma understanding also helps to bolster practices that align with establishing *safety and predictability*. Because students, teachers, and people in general cannot upshift into learning/thinking brain if they do not feel safe (Cole et al. 2005; Ford 2009), it is critical that schools prioritize establishing physical, relational, and emotional safety for everyone in the school community. Furthermore, creating predictability in the environ-

skills (e.g., emotion management) can help educators to enhance social-emotional learning curricula as needed.

We encourage periodic affect regulation activities, or *brain breaks*, emphasizing that practicing affect regulation on a regular basis can help to strengthen students' emotion management skills. When students are feeling stress or fatigue, such breaks can help to decrease stress arousal, reset the brain and body, and get students' energy level to where it is needed for the classroom task at hand.

Many of our HEARTS schools' classrooms also supplement whole class brain breaks with opportunities for individual students to use calming affect modulation tools when they need them. The materials are contained in a mobile "cool-down kit" or are placed in a space in the classroom (e.g., a "peace corner") where students can go for a few minutes when they are becoming dysregulated (Cole et al. 2005). We recommend that teachers establish routines and structure around the use of these tools, model appropriate usage, and refrain from using the space or kit as a consequence. We also underscore that although these trauma-informed practices can prevent disruptive behavior by providing an opportunity for self-regulation, they should augment, not replace, existing classroom management systems and practices.

In addition to boosting students' resilience, we also work to support resilience in school staff, providing training and consultation in science-based wellness strategies drawn from such sources as the Greater Good Science Center at the University of California, Berkeley. We advocate that schools build into the work day regular opportunities for staff to engage in activities that allow them to take better care of themselves and one another.

Empowerment and Collaboration

Because trauma by its nature can leave people feeling helpless, when youth experience chronic trauma, it can be difficult for them to believe that they can have agency in the world and rise up to challenges, which can hinder school success. Further, unnecessarily taking away a person's power or control around personally important issues can be particularly triggering to someone impacted by trauma. By creating opportunities wherein students and staff can exercise their voice and choice, we can begin to mitigate these negative effects. Knowing that one's voice is heard and that one's choices are valued contributes toward healing from trauma.

Inviting students to participate in team meetings centered on increasing their success in the classroom is one way that educators can facilitate voice and choice. For example, when a student like Ryan is given the opportunity to *collaborate* with the staff support team to build a plan around coping with triggering situations, he feels *empowered* and is better able to use the resulting plan. Further, as students practice asserting their voices for their own personal needs, they may be more likely to seek out opportunities to use their voices to empower and benefit others. One trauma-impacted student in a HEARTS elementary school created a petition and rallied his classmates to speak up about a change in a school procedure that was important to them. This, in turn, further encouraged him to be more engaged in his own classroom learning.

Facilitating empowerment and collaboration by incorporating youth voices in the development and implementation of school-wide social-emotional support systems (e.g., PBIS) can make supports more relevant and practical for the young people we serve and can be an important component in the recovery process for youth impacted by trauma. Furthermore, we empower youth by providing them with knowledge about how their own brains and bodies react to stress and what they can do to self-regulate. Inviting youth to be peer educators and to share these concepts and strategies with classmates helps to engage them in promoting the health, resilience, and well-being of themselves and others.

Tier 2: Selected Interventions

The HEARTS core guiding principles are embedded in tier 2 interventions as well. In one main tier 2 intervention, the HEARTS consultant participates as part of a school's weekly coordinated care team, which typically consists of administrators and mental health, special education, and other support staff who meet regularly to discuss students and school-wide concerns. *Trauma understanding* guides the development of behavioral supports that are less punitive and more resilience building. For example, behavioral contracts are a commonly used tier 2 intervention for students demonstrating a pattern of inappropriate behavior. The behavior contract relies on a system of rewards and consequences designed to motivate the student to engage in more appropriate behavior. PBIS asserts that such contracts are effective for "won't do kids" who are choosing not to do what they are supposed to do in a given situation, but such contracts are not helpful for "can't do kids" who lack the skills to do what is being asked of them. In formulating behavioral contracts, it is important to understand that when triggered into survival brain, a student can temporarily change from a won't do kid to a can't do kid because his or her thinking

study, they indicate that HEARTS is a promising program deemed feasible, acceptable, and useful by educators.

Developmental Considerations

Elementary School–Age Children

Working with elementary school–age children can help prevent future behavioral and academic difficulties that can lead to school failure and dropout. Once children reach the age when they are spending most of their waking hours in school, schools with a safe and supportive climate can be an important protective factor that helps mitigate the effects of trauma and adversity. Caregivers' involvement in their child's schooling is another protective factor (Scales and Leffert 2014). Younger children are particularly dependent on adults for their safety and well-being. Thus, when a school-age child is having difficulty in school, it is crucial that professionals providing academic, behavioral, and/or mental health support to students work collaboratively with the child's caregivers. However, when caregivers do not have a positive working relationship with the school and/or they are themselves struggling with multiple stressors, adversity, and trauma, it can be difficult to engage them in their children's academic and social-emotional supports. HEARTS clinicians and consultants attempt to serve as a relational bridge between caregivers and the school, using a trauma-informed lens to create understanding about what may be getting in the way of caregiver involvement, as well as using trauma-informed principles to guide engagement strategies and approaches (e.g., fostering compassionate, dependable relationships with caregivers and empowering them to take an active part in developing and implementing their child's supports).

High School–Age Youth

HEARTS provides tier 1 professional development training as well as consultation around tier 2 and tier 3 interventions using trauma-informed RP in Oakland Unified School District high schools. When engaging high school educators, it is important to acknowledge and account for ways that high schools are structured differently from elementary and middle schools. For example, trainers must attend to the fact that high school teachers work with many more students than do their elementary school counterparts (often between 100 and 200 students), and thus they need different (e.g., less time-intensive) strategies for developing caring and trustworthy relationships with their students.

In our work with high schools, it has been helpful to review normal adolescent brain development to illuminate why emotionally intense situations can lead to impulsive behaviors in typical adolescents. We explain that although an adolescent may have the physical stature and appearance of an adult, his or her brain is still "under construction," with the more fully developed survival/emotional brain (e.g., the limbic system) more likely to overtake the less developed learning/thinking brain (e.g., prefrontal cortex) when the youth is feeling strong emotions. Thus, adolescents commonly need compassionate, dependable adult allies to provide coregulation and thought partnering when navigating emotionally challenging situations. Moreover, experiencing complex trauma can exacerbate normal adolescent affect regulation challenges, so supportive relationships with trusted adults are all the more crucial.

Unfortunately, because adolescents can at times be perceived as threatening in a way that smaller children may not be, some of our most vulnerable youth may lose support from adults when they need it most (e.g., when youth are triggered into a fear response). Racial bias may make this worse for African American boys as young as 10 years old, who tend to be perceived as older and more culpable for their actions than their same-age peers (Goff et al. 2014). Perhaps because of this, we have experienced a relatively high demand for training around how to deescalate out-of-control, dysregulated students (e.g., students who hit or throw things), especially in middle and high schools. Reframing adolescent behavior in terms of normal brain development and adding a trauma-informed lens to this understanding can help adults keep in mind adolescents' potential vulnerability and need for help. In addition, using requests for deescalation training as an entry point for providing professional development around trauma-informed escalation prevention, deescalation, and postescalation repair has been an effective way to engage educators about the use of trauma-informed practices.

Challenges and Overcoming Them: Lessons Learned

One frequently encountered challenge has been educators' concern about not having the time or energy to add more to their heavy load of programs and initiatives to be implemented (e.g., PBIS, Common Core, RP). In order to create time for professional development trainings, we have worked with school districts to secure funding for stipends to pay for staff time outside the normal work day when needed, as well as to offer continuing education credits when possible. Perhaps more importantly, we have underscored that a trauma-informed approach is not meant to be a stand-alone program to be added to educators' already full plate but instead can integrate with and augment a school's existing programs and practices so that they work more effectively for all students, including the students who otherwise tend to fall through the cracks. A trauma-informed lens can help a school community understand the reasons why investing time and energy in PBIS and RP practices is important, and conversely, these practices, when implemented in a trauma-informed manner, provide well-elaborated strategies and procedures for creating a more trauma-informed, safe, and supportive school.

Turnover in school leadership has also sometimes led to difficulties in program implementation. Because engagement with a school's leadership is essential for success, when school leaders change, we prioritize investing the time to establish a positive working relationship with the new leaders. We empathize with them about the difficulty of inheriting programs put in place by previous leadership. We provide a comprehensive overview of the values, principles, and strategies of HEARTS, discussing these points with the new principal to ensure that HEARTS is aligned with the principal's values and vision for the school. Further, buy-in from the majority of the school's staff about working with HEARTS has tended to help new leadership become more invested in program implementation. We also support the wellness and resilience of new school leaders by 1) developing a compassionate and dependable relationship with them that can provide coregulation in times of stress and 2) providing them with safe and predictable time and space to reflect with us about what they need to feel supported themselves, what they can do to provide trauma-informed leadership for their school, and what they believe is needed for their school community to succeed.

Implications for Social Justice and Policy

School reform efforts to improve school performance; close the achievement gap; and eliminate disproportionality in the meting out of punitive, exclusionary disciplinary measures have ranged from a push for more rigorous standardized testing and curricula (e.g., No Child Left Behind) to major, disruptive structural change via administrative and staff replacements and school restructuring (e.g., U.S. Department of Education School Improvement Grants). However, without a trauma-informed lens that includes a cultural humility approach, even the most well-intentioned efforts can be derailed, and school failure and disproportionality can potentially be made worse. For example, when teachers experience intense stress and anxiety caused by the pressure to obtain high achievement test scores without sufficient support, this stress is passed on to students and can dysregulate students enough to interfere with their ability to access their learning brain and perform their best on these tests. Further, when policies compel replacement of principals and school staff (as was required at schools awarded School Improvement Grant funding), students lose educators with whom they have had caring, trusting relationships. These losses work at cross purposes with the goal of increasing school success for low-achieving students because they echo with the histories of traumatic loss experienced by trauma-impacted students, triggering dysregulation and hindering students' ability to learn. In this way, when attempts to improve school systems are not trauma informed, they can be trauma inducing as opposed to trauma reducing, harming many of the at-risk students whom these efforts are ostensibly aimed at helping.

In addition, we have come to realize the centrality of cultural humility and responsiveness as one of our foundational principles. In fact, it is clear that if an approach or intervention is not socially just (e.g., does not promote racial justice), then it is not trauma informed. Without a cultural humility lens, there is a risk that trauma concepts could be used to pathologize communities of color rather underscoring their resilience in the face of an inequitable sociopolitical environment and institutionalized oppression and the sociocultural trauma that can result.

Moreover, we believe that cultural humility and responsiveness are critical in our work to create safer, more supportive, and equitable school climates. For example, in looking at the demographics of staff at schools serving underresourced communities, we have often observed staff communities where credentialed teachers are largely white, whereas classified staff (e.g., paraprofessionals, school security guards, administrative assistants) are largely people of color, often from the same low socioeconomic status communities where most of the students live. Although classified staff do not have teaching credentials, in addition to their professional experience and training, they often bring tremendous assets to the table, including long-standing relationships with students and their families, invaluable lived experience, and an understanding of the strengths and challenges of communities served by the school. Yet classified staff have frequently expressed to us that they feel disempowered, relatively unvalued, and left out of important decisions concerning the school community. Bringing a cultural humility approach to addressing this challenge is an important step in repairing ruptured staff relationships and knitting together a stronger, healthier school staff community.

Conclusion

UCSF HEARTS is a principle-driven, multi-tiered, whole-school approach for ensuring that all students are afforded the opportunity for both resilience and school success, despite the impact of trauma on some students' lives. Our aim is to use training and consultation to create school communities that promote safety, support, and equity and that make engagement and learning readiness possible. We offer the key components of HEARTS for school communities and professionals to consider when addressing chronic stress and trauma in their schools. Further, HEARTS core guiding principles can be used as a road map to guide the development and implementation of trauma-informed supports and interventions for creating learning and teaching environments where everyone in the school community—students and adults alike—can develop and thrive.

KEY CONCEPTS

- A trauma-informed schools approach applies the science of trauma, resilience, neurobiology, and systems theory to the goal of creating safe, supportive, equitable, and engaging learning and teaching environments that benefit everyone in the school community.

- A trauma-informed approach that involves whole-school culture change, as opposed to the traditional approach of identifying and referring symptomatic students to support services, is needed to create meaningful change for trauma-impacted students and school communities.

- The six HEARTS core guiding principles for creating trauma-informed schools (promoting understanding of trauma and stress, cultural humility and responsiveness, safety and predictability, compassion and dependability, resilience and social-emotional learning, and empowerment and collaboration) can be used as a road map for developing and implementing strategies for mitigating the effects of trauma and chronic stress in schools.

• These core guiding principles should be applied not only to students but to all members of the school community, including teachers, paraprofessionals, support staff, administrators, and parents or caregivers.

• Integrating a trauma-informed approach with existing programs and initiatives (e.g., Positive Behavioral Interventions and Supports, restorative practices, social-emotional learning curricula), as opposed to implementing stand-alone trauma-informed programs, is key to feasibility, effectiveness, and sustainability of trauma-informed practices.

Discussion Questions

1. How might you apply HEARTS key elements and core-guiding principles for creating trauma-informed schools to your work in healing trauma given your role (e.g., as a clinician)?

2. Do your practices and interventions promote each of the six core guiding principles?

3. Do any of your practices or interventions inadvertently thwart any of the six core guiding principles?

4. In your work in healing trauma, do you consider the effects of family, school, neighborhood, culture, and societal context on your patient, and do you include these contextual factors in the interventions you provide?

Suggested Readings

Craig SE: Reaching and Teaching Children Who Hurt: Strategies for Your Classroom. Baltimore, MD, Paul H Brookes, 2008

Hammond Z: Culturally Responsive Teaching and the Brain: Promoting Authentic Engagement and Rigor Among Culturally and Linguistically Diverse Students. Thousand Oaks, CA, Corwin, 2015

Souers K, Hall PA: Fostering Resilient Learners: Strategies for Creating a Trauma-Sensitive Classroom Book. Alexandria, VA, ACSD, 2016

Trauma-Focused Cognitive-Behavioral Therapy

Jessica L. Griffin, Psy.D.
Jessica Wozniak, Psy.D.

Overview of the Trauma-Focused Cognitive-Behavioral Therapy Model

Trauma-focused cognitive-behavioral therapy (TF-CBT) is a time-limited, components-based, phase-based trauma treatment for children ages 3–18 who have experienced single or multiple traumas, including youth with complex trauma experiences and outcomes (Bartlett et al. 2018; Cohen et al. 2017). A hybrid treatment model, TF-CBT integrates several therapies, theories, and interventions, including trauma-sensitive practices, cognitive-behavioral principles, child development, attachment theory, neurobiology, family therapy interventions, empowerment therapy, and humanistic therapy, making it appealing to a variety of practitioners regardless of their stated theoretical orientation(s).

TABLE 9–1.   TF-CBT practice components: goals *(continued)*

TF-CBT component	Goals for treatment	Techniques
Affective regulation	Increase the youth's feelings vocabulary and appropriate expression of feelings and decrease avoidant or other maladaptive symptoms by increasing the youth's language regarding feeling expression	Teach feelings vocabulary and feelings expression: list of feelings, feelings charts and feelings faces, feelings charades, feelings Jenga (Berger and Gehart-Brooks 2000), Color-Your-Life technique (O'Connor 1983), feelings color wheel, emotions thermometer, feelings selfies with adolescents, identifying feelings in pop culture
Cognitive coping	Improve ability to connect thoughts, feelings, and behaviors and assist the youth in identifying alternative thoughts	Teach the cognitive triangle, thought checking (accurate/ inaccurate, helpful/unhelpful thoughts), what are you thinking? team, best friend scenarios, you be the therapist, Socratic questioning and progressive logical questioning
Trauma narrative	Generate an active trauma narration to assist the youth in processing his or her trauma experiences, decrease physiological arousal to trauma reminders, and make meaning of trauma experiences	Create a chapter book regarding the youth's trauma experiences, create a life "timeline," use music or artwork to tell his or her story
In vivo exposure	Develop a hierarchy of feared stimuli in order to assist the youth in decreasing fear response to specific feared situations (e.g., school avoidance, sleeping in his or her own bed)	Develop a hierarchy of feared stimuli (e.g., "baby steps") in order to help the youth master feared situation (e.g., fear of sleeping in own bed, fear of going to school, fear of public restroom)

TABLE 9–1.   **TF-CBT practice components: goals** *(continued)*

TF-CBT component	Goals for treatment	Techniques
Conjoint sessions	Allow the youth to share his or her trauma narrative with caregiver(s) in a supportive way, improve parent-child communication, and strengthen the parent-child relationship	Use parent-child sessions to share child's trauma narrative and facilitate healthy parent-child interaction
Enhancing safety and future development	Teach personal safety skills, including physical and psychological safety; assist family in planning for the future, including future trauma reminders or adversity; and celebrate completion of TF-CBT	Teach body safety, healthy sexuality, planning for the future, and the three *P*s of TF-CBT (predict, plan, permit); prepare for trauma reminders, hold a graduation, and prepare for termination

Note.   TF-CBT=trauma-focused cognitive-behavioral therapy.

search studies, see Cohen et al. 2017; de Arellano et al. 2014; Griffin et al., in press.) TF-CBT has since been used with children and adolescents exposed to multiple traumas, and treatment effects have been shown to persist after accounting for type of trauma experienced (Scheeringa et al. 2011). In addition, RCTs have shown TF-CBT to be effective with both complex trauma and single-incident trauma, even with youth exposed to ongoing trauma (Cohen et al. 2011, 2012b; Murray et al. 2015). (For a review of studies, see Cohen et al. 2017; Griffin et al. in press.) It is also important to note that even though the early studies focused on childhood sexual abuse (de Arellano et al. 2014), the average number of trauma types *in addition to sexual abuse* was 2.6 (Cohen et al. 2004), highlighting that even in those earlier studies, TF-CBT was serving youth with multiple traumatic experiences.

A wealth of studies support the model's efficacy in reducing reexperiencing, hyperarousal, and avoidance PTSD symptoms, with effect sizes ranging from medium to large in most studies. (For a review, see de Arellano et al. 2014.) Empirical research consistently demonstrates the effectiveness of TF-CBT in reducing symptoms of PTSD and behavioral and depressive symptoms in youth and improving positive outcomes since the original multisite RCT (Cohen et al. 2004). (For a review of other studies, see Cohen et al. 2017.)

The family system also benefits from the use of TF-CBT (Cohen et al. 2004, 2017; de Arellano et al. 2014; King et al. 2000). Research has reliably documented parental gains, including decreased parental depression and parental PTSD, increased sense of parental competence and parental support, and reduced emotional distress associated with the child's traumatic experience. Follow-up studies have demonstrated sustainability of these gains over time. The parent/caregiver component is used with the assumption that the caregiver is competent and child focused. However, TF-CBT can be effectively provided *without* the caregiver component. Additionally, TF-CBT can be used with individuals other than biological parents in the caregiver role, such as foster parents, grandparents, and other supportive adults. Of note, TF-CBT is not appropriate for use with offending parents or caregivers.

There are very few limitations to TF-CBT. In recent years, multiple applications of the treatment for special populations or special circumstances (e.g., young children, youth with developmental disabilities, commercially sexually exploited children, court-involved youth) have been developed or are currently in development. Exclusion criteria include children who are in the midst of *active, current* psychosis and children who are *actively* suicidal or homicidal because evidence of effectiveness is limited in this area (de Arellano et al. 2014). Children who have a prior history of psychotic symptoms or prior history of suicidality and/or homicidality are eligible to receive TF-CBT, although monitoring of safety is of utmost priority. Additionally, in a review of 10 TF-CBT RCTs, de Arellano et al. (2014) suggested that more research is necessary to determine effectiveness in treating children and caregivers with substance use disorders and youth with developmental disabilities and the ability to include caregivers with significant mental illness in treatment; more rigorous studies are under way.

TF-CBT continues to be the most rigorously tested and most widely disseminated treatment for traumatized youth, with more RCTs than any other trauma-focused child treatment to date. However, systematic reviews of interventions including TF-CBT (de Arellano et al. 2014; Fraser et al. 2013) have highlighted limitations of the current state of the available research, such as short-term outcomes and the use of wait list control groups or treatment as usual comparisons rather than head-to-head comparison studies.

Although TF-CBT initially grew out of traditional outpatient settings, it is now widely implemented across a variety of therapeutic and community-based settings, including outpatient, residential, inpatient, home-based, school-based, group therapy, and other milieus (Cohen et al. 2016; Konanur et al. 2015). There are a variety of resources to assist clinicians in implementation of TF-CBT, including a manual (Cohen et al. 2017), an applications book (Cohen et al. 2012a), free Web-based training (www.musc.edu/tfcbt2) and consultation services (www.musc.edu/tf-cbt-consult) through the Medical University of South Carolina, a national certification program with a national database of nationally certified TF-CBT clinicians (http://tfcbt.org), and numerous additional resources available through the National Child Traumatic Stress Network (www.nctsn.org), including an implementation guide.

TF-CBT PRACTICE Components

As mentioned earlier, the PRACTICE components of the TF-CBT model (Cohen et al. 2017) are structured in a progressive way to help youth learn the skills necessary to process their trauma history (see Table 9–1). However, gradual exposure begins in the first session and is integrated into all treatment components to help children gain mastery in how to use the skills when trauma reminders or cues occur. TF-CBT is a time-limited treatment model, with a beginning, middle, and an end that emphasizes proportionality across treatment phases (Figure 9–1). In the first phase of treatment, utmost care is paid to safety and stabilization as youth learn coping skills. After youth build skills through the first four PRACTICE components (PRAC), they move on to phase two of treatment and begin trauma narration. Finally, in phase three of treatment, the youth complete the last components of treatment, including in vivo work (as needed), conjoint sessions, and learning how to enhance safety and development. In this final phase, the focus of treatment is on integration and consolidation and ultimately assisting youth in making meaning of their experiences and focusing on their future.

Typically, TF-CBT is implemented in 12–18 sessions but can be done in as few as 8 sessions. Some youth experiencing complex trauma experiences and outcomes may require up to 25 sessions (Cohen et al. 2012b). For youth with complex trauma, the initial phase is longer and includes a larger emphasis on safety (see Figure 9–1 for an overview of TF-CBT and TF-CBT with complex trauma). Each session consists of both individual treatment with the child and an individual session with the parent or caregiver; the content of the caregiver sessions typically parallels the components and information reviewed during the child sessions.

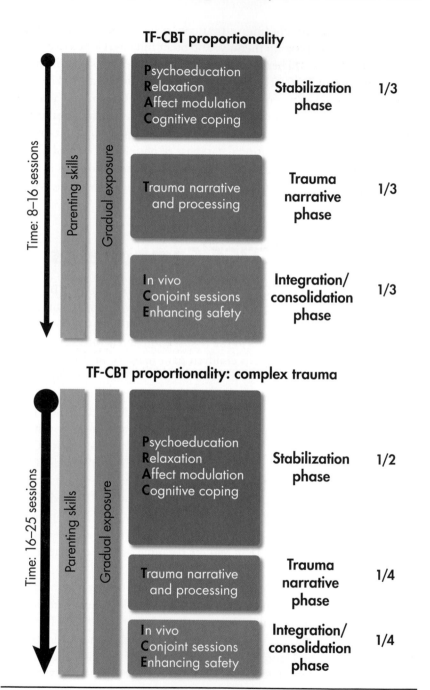

FIGURE 9–1.   TF-CBT components and phases.

TF-CBT typically begins with an initial assessment phase during which the clinician conducts individual interviews of the caregiver and youth and uses clinical assessment tools to carefully assess for both traumatic experiences and trauma-related symptoms. In addition to comprehensive clinical information, the clinician gathers information about the child's functioning prior to the traumatic experience. Information gathered during the assessment can provide a natural segue into the psychoeducation component of TF-CBT, underscoring why a trauma-focused treatment is needed.

Psychoeducation

The psychoeducation component of TF-CBT begins at the first session of treatment, when the child and the caregiver are each provided information about the child's trauma experience(s) and trauma reaction(s) with the goals of normalizing the child and parent's reactions to trauma and helping the youth understand that he or she is not alone and that traumatic experiences are common. Information about typical psychological and physiological responses to trauma is provided both to the youth and to the caregiver. A tone of hopefulness is set for the child and the family with the theme that healing is possible. Although psychoeducation begins at the start of treatment (and ideally at the first phone call), it may continue throughout treatment.

Parenting Skills

The parenting skills component is an essential element of the TF-CBT model. Even the most highly functioning competent parents may struggle with parenting effectively when their child has been through a traumatic experience. The trauma may have directly impacted the parents or their functioning, making it difficult to fulfill responsibilities of daily living, parenting routines, or household responsibilities. A lack of predictability or consistency is problematic for the traumatized child, who benefits from structure in the face of chaos. Thus, the parenting skills component is introduced immediately in the TF-CBT model and is attended to throughout treatment.

Children with a history of trauma are at greater risk of developing behavioral and emotional difficulties, so it is recommended that all parents receive guidance and support in improving their positive parenting practices. The parenting skills component uses several techniques, such as praise, selective attention (e.g., active ignoring, catching a child being good), time-out, behavior management and reward systems, and functional behavioral analysis (determining the function of a particular behavior and where to intervene effectively by exploring the antecedents of the behavior, what happens during the behavior, and the consequences of the behavior). Within TF-CBT, role-playing and modeling techniques are an essential part of treatment, allowing parents to practice the skills with the clinician before applying them at home with their child. Also, because it is clear that parents who do better have children who do better, caregiver self-care strategies are emphasized throughout treatment, and parents are encouraged to practice coping skills and self-care. Caregivers in the TF-CBT model could also include foster parents, grandparents, or other supportive persons in the child's life who serve in a caregiving role. However, as stated in the section "Efficacy and Effectiveness of TF-CBT," TF-CBT may be done without the parent/caregiver component.

Relaxation

The relaxation component of TF-CBT teaches youth valuable skills to assist them in turning down the heightened physiological response to stress and trauma by using a series of techniques. Children who have gone through traumatic experiences are prone to a physiological manifestation of stress (e.g., faster heart rate, agitation, sleep disturbance, restlessness, irritability); youth who have experienced complex trauma experience this hyperarousal chronically, with long-term physical and developmental impact. Relaxation strategies may include deep breathing, progressive muscle relaxation, guided imagery, and mindfulness as well as other self-care strategies such as yoga, meditation, exercise, art, and listening to music.

Affective Regulation

The affective regulation component of TF-CBT allows youth to improve their feelings identification and increase their feelings vocabulary and also to express feelings more effectively. If youth are able to express their feelings more effectively and have the language to express their emotional pain, they are less likely to use maladaptive or avoidant coping strategies (Cohen and Mannarino 2015). Within the affective regulation component, the clinician uses a series of strategies to teach this skill as well as gradual exposure related to the youth's trauma experiences.

Cognitive Coping

Children are particularly prone to inaccurate or dysfunctional thoughts about traumatic experiences (Cohen et al. 2017). These thoughts (e.g.,

"It's all my fault I was sexually abused," "The world is a dangerous place") can negatively impact children's belief systems. The cognitive coping component refers to a variety of techniques that are used in TF-CBT to encourage youth and their caregivers to explore their thoughts in order to challenge those thoughts that are distorted, maladaptive, or inaccurate and/or unhelpful to them and generate newer, healthier thoughts. Within the cognitive coping component, the clinician uses a series of techniques, including the cognitive triangle, to assist youth (and their caregivers) in recognizing how thoughts are related to feelings and behaviors and that changing how they think about a situation can have an impact on how they feel and, subsequently, on their behavior. The cognitive triangle can be used in a variety of circumstances from crises of the week to trauma-specific thought patterns as a means to assist youth in identifying alternative, healthier thoughts and learning the connection between their thoughts and their emotional experiences and behavioral outcomes. Gradual exposure work is also interwoven into the cognitive coping component.

Trauma Narration and Cognitive Processing of Trauma

In the trauma narration component of treatment, the child is desensitized to trauma reminders. As a result, the child experiences decreased physical and psychological hyperarousal at exposure to trauma cues or traumatic memories, which thereby decreases his or her avoidance and trauma-related symptoms. The trauma narration assists youth in undoing the connection between thoughts, reminders, and/or discussion of the traumatic experiences and helps him or her learn how to not be overwhelmed by negative emotions. In addition, trauma narratives assist youth in making meaning of their experiences.

The trauma narration process is done gradually so that each step is only slightly more difficult than the previous one. The emphasis is not on the final trauma narrative product but on the interactive process between the child and the therapist. The trauma narrative can take many forms, such as a chapter book, a poem, a series of drawings, or another modality of the youth's choosing. Over the course of several sessions, the youth is encouraged to describe more details of what happened during (and before and after) the traumatic experience(s) as well as his or her thoughts and feelings during the experience(s). After the child has created a full draft of the trauma narrative, the clinician will then identify, explore, and challenge any inaccurate or unhelpful cognitions in the child's narrative using a series of techniques previously introduced in the cognitive coping component.

In Vivo Mastery of Trauma Reminders

The in vivo component of TF-CBT is the only component of treatment that is optional; it is applied only to overgeneralized fears of innocuous situations, something most children ultimately do not develop. For youth who develop fears of innocuous situations (e.g., fear of sleeping in their own bed, fear of driving in cars, fear of going to school), a stepwise in vivo desensitization plan can be enacted. Therapists are encouraged to desensitize the child not to reality-based fears or actual trauma cues that serve a protective function but to those situations in which feared trauma cues are innocuous reminders.

Conjoint Parent-Child Sessions

The TF-CBT model includes conjoint parent-child sessions at multiple points in treatment whereby the clinician shares information with the child and caregiver such as psychoeducational material and/or practices regarding coping and safety skills. The content of the parent sessions typically parallels the content of the child sessions. That is, if the child is learning affective regulation skills, the clinician also reviews the affective regulation component with the caregiver so that the caregiver is able to practice these skills to reinforce the concepts at home with the child. Later in treatment, in sessions facilitated by the clinician (and after a period of preparation for the youth and caregiver), the child shares his or her trauma narrative with the caregiver. Additional conjoint sessions may address parent-child relationship issues, seek to improve parent-child communication, and increase the child's (and the caregiver's) comfort in talking about difficult topics, including the trauma experience(s). Conjoint sessions are not enacted until the clinician determines that it is clinically appropriate to do so.

Enhancing Safety and Future Development

The final component of TF-CBT addresses physical and psychological safety concerns, healthy sexuality when appropriate, and assertiveness training. Although reviewing body safety is typically reserved for the final component in TF-CBT, in cases of ongoing trauma or complex trauma, this component is moved up earlier in treatment. Throughout treatment, as in any good practice, clinicians should be checking in with the youth regarding his or her safety. Whenever possible, safety planning actively includes the caregiver. To the extent possible, safety planning should include a review of body safety, trauma triggers and reminders, identifying safe sources of support in the child's life, and practicing and/or role-playing the initiation of a safety plan. When appropriate, healthy sexuality and healthy relationships as well as assertiveness training, social skills training, and conflict resolution may be reviewed. Clinicians are encouraged to use a variety of materials, including handouts, body safety books, fact sheets, videos, and even smartphone apps to assist them in safety planning. The final session(s) of treatment include moving toward termination and review of treatment; planning for the future, including future trauma reminders and identifying sources of support; a graduation that celebrates the child's successful completion of treatment; and bringing treatment to a close.

Developmental Approaches in TF-CBT

TF-CBT is implemented from early childhood through adolescence, without major modifications to the core components for each age group. However, the following suggestions are made regarding applications with preschool, school-age, and adolescent and transition-age groups.

Preschool-Age Children

TF-CBT can be used with children as young as 3 years (Scheeringa et al. 2011). Some preliminary data from evaluation studies indicated that TF-CBT results in effective outcomes for young children who experience complex trauma, whereas other models specifically designed for young children (e.g., child-parent psychotherapy) do not demonstrate significant positive findings for this age group (Bartlett et al. 2018). However, certain adjustments need to be made in applying TF-CBT to preschool-age children (Drewes and Cavett 2012). As with therapy with any young child, patience and simplicity are key elements throughout treatment. The clinician will need to adjust the timing and pacing of sessions. For example, a preschool-age child may not be able to tolerate an hour-long session but might benefit from two shorter 30-minute sessions and/or more frequent breaks. Concepts should be explained concretely using examples that are relevant to a young child's life. TF-CBT clinicians are encouraged to use a structured playful approach in order to develop the therapeutic relationship with patients; thus, using play-based techniques is consistent with the core value of TF-CBT being flexible to meet a patient's individual needs. Directive play therapy strategies can be used within the TF-CBT components. Incorporating puppets, dollhouses, or other play materials can help, not only with engagement but to ease the processing of trauma-laden material. Young children may benefit from incorporating more visual activities as well as more movement into the PRAC components. Clinicians should anticipate that preschoolers' trauma narratives may not be as lengthy, but even young children are fully capable of engaging in the trauma narration process. They may wish to create their trauma narratives through a series of drawings or a puppet show or by writing a story together with their therapist. Working closely with caregivers throughout the TF-CBT model is essential when working with preschool-age children.

School-Age Children

When working with school-age children, it is necessary to ask about and incorporate a child's interests into the clinical work. Clinicians are encouraged to be creative in incorporating a child's hobbies or interests, whether they be music, art, video games, pop culture, or sports, into the TF-CBT components in order to increase youth engagement. Simply put, if TF-CBT is not enjoyable, at least to some extent, youth will not want to engage in treatment.

Adolescents and Transitional-Age Youth

TF-CBT can be provided successfully with adolescents in a similar manner to which it is applied to school-age children, again with emphasis on integrating adolescents' interests into treatment components. Additionally, themes appropriate to developmental stages of adolescence may be applied across components. For example, psychoeducation could include education regarding life skills, and the parenting component might consist of helping parents identify appropriate expectations for their adolescent. The parenting component may also include supporting caregivers' abilities to balance autonomy and dependence in their children. No studies to date have examined TF-CBT with transitional-age youth (ages 16–24 years), although efforts are under way by researchers (including one of us, J.L.G.) to examine the utility of TF-CBT with this underserved population.

Overcoming Potential Challenges

Some potential challenges in the implementation of the TF-CBT model include difficulty with youth or caregiver engagement, lack of appropriate caregiver, caregiver trauma history, avoidance in beginning the trauma narrative, and crises of the week.

Difficulty With Youth Engagement

When clinicians encounter resistant youth, this is often a failure of engagement. Clinicians are encouraged to explore that youth's interests as well as whether there are potential trauma reminders inherent in the therapy setting and/or therapy relationship that may need to be explored. Often, if you simply provide youth with psychoeducation about trauma, trauma reactions, and information about ways in which TF-CBT can help them feel better, they are surprised to learn that they are not alone, that treatment works, and that healing is possible. As with any treatment approach, TF-CBT greatly values the critical importance of the therapeutic relationship.

Caregiver Engagement or Lack of Caregiver

The critical role of parents is emphasized early in treatment by clinicians expressing the view the parents are the copilot for the TF-CBT process, assisting children in learning of coping skills and encouraging children in the trauma-focused components of treatment. Interventions targeted at specialized training for clinical staff, such as engaging youth and families training for clinicians, have been used successfully with some TF-CBT implementation efforts (McKay et al. 2004) and have increased retention rates for TF-CBT services. There are some instances in which a caregiver is unavailable to participate in treatment (e.g., residential setting, parent's own mental health). In these situations, TF-CBT can still be done by focusing on the youth-only components. Research has shown that even when a caregiver is not included in treatment, TF-CBT is still effective in improving a child's symptoms (Cohen and Mannarino 2015). Similarly, TF-CBT can be used with youth in foster care or in residential treatment; clinicians are encouraged to think creatively about the caregiver role because there may be instances in which others (e.g., direct care staff, other family members) serve in the caregiver role in treatment. For youth in foster care, clinicians are encouraged to incorporate foster parents to the extent that it is feasible to do so (Dorsey et al. 2014).

Caregiver Trauma History

Intergenerational transmission of trauma occurs frequently, and caregiver trauma history is a common barrier to treatment. If clinicians find themselves getting off track when working with a child because a parent's trauma history is interfering with treatment (e.g., the parent is so triggered by his or her own experiences that it is difficult to focus on the child's experience), this is a good indication that the parent may need his or her own referral for individual trauma-focused therapy. Occasionally, clinicians may find that it is the caregiver's trauma history that has directly or indirectly led to the traumatization or maltreatment of the child (e.g., failure to protect), as discussed in the following vignette.

Clinical Vignette

Seven-year-old Carmen was in treatment for exposure to domestic violence: physical abuse by her father and suspected emotional abuse from both her mother and her father. Carmen initially was highly symptomatic, with behavioral difficulties (e.g., aggressive outbursts), nightmares, and mood disturbance, as well as disrupted attachment and relationships (e.g., with her mother and peers and at school). Although Carmen was progressing in treatment, her mother, Rosa, continued to struggle with engagement in treatment and greatly minimized the role of trauma in Carmen's behavior and emotional functioning. Rosa's prevailing thought was "Carmen is doing this negative behavior to spite me." Additionally, Rosa continued to expose Carmen to numerous unhealthy caregivers (e.g., various boyfriends). After the clinician spent additional time with Rosa discussing the family history, it was revealed that Rosa continued to be symptomatic from both her role as a victim in the domestic violence by Carmen's father and a lengthy history herself of severe child abuse, including sexual abuse, physical abuse, and exposure to domestic violence. Her prevailing thought was, "It happened to me…what Carmen went through isn't nearly as bad as what I went through…I turned out just fine." Unfortunately, in addition to Rosa's minimization of the impact of trauma on (and her failure to protect) her daughter, her unresolved trauma continued to interfere with her ability to effectively parent and keep Carmen safe.

If it is determined that the parent or caregiver is not meeting the child's basic physical or emotional needs outside of the therapy sessions, clinicians should follow the guidelines in the state where they live regarding child protective or child welfare concerns and should file reports when necessary to ensure the child's safety. In addition, clinicians should provide proper referral for caregivers who require treatment for their own trauma(s).

Avoidance in Starting the Trauma Narration Process

Should youth have difficulty beginning the trauma narration, clinicians are encouraged first to consider whether enough gradual exposure has been conducted prior to beginning the trauma narrative. The beginning of the trauma narration should not be the first time that the child has, for example, used the words "sexual abuse" or talked about "when your uncle shot your daddy." Second, clinicians are also advised to consider their own avoidance in engaging in the trauma narrative process. Third, the trauma narration component should include materials and media that youth are comfortable with (e.g., using music or art materials or allowing the clinician to be the child's "secretary"). The clinician should provide the youth an age-appropriate rationale for beginning the trauma narration, and the narration should be completed at a pace that the child is comfortable with, beginning with nontraumatic information and material that is less traumatic to discuss and leading up to talking about more difficult material.

Crises of the Week

Clinicians are encouraged to view crises of the week, or COWs, as opportunities to practice the TF-CBT PRAC skills. For example, a patient whose COW involved breaking up with her boyfriend and who subsequently had difficulty focusing in class because of the recurring thought "nobody will ever love me the way he did" was able to practice relaxation skills or cognitive coping skills that challenged the inaccurate and unhelpful thought. COWs can also be used as opportunities to draw a connection to the youth's trauma experience, as outlined in the following vignette.

> When 14-year-old Johnny, who had a history of severe physical abuse and exposure to domestic violence in his home, swore and punched a locker after someone accidentally bumped into him in the hallway, he received a detention and experienced disruption in his relationships with his peers. In addressing this COW, Johnny's clinician worked with him to provide additional psychoeducation to help him understand that the unanticipated touch in the hallway served as a trauma reminder, engaging his body's alarm system or fight/flight/freeze response. Johnny and his clinician practiced coping skills that he could use in the event that this were to happen in the future, including problem-solving strategies, relaxation skills, and other affective regulation skills.

Sociocultural and Policy Implications

The research base on TF-CBT has grown exponentially in the last 10 years, adding to the evidence for the effectiveness of TF-CBT in treating mental health and behavior-related trauma symptoms across geographic, ethnic, religious, and socioeconomic groups and across treatment settings (Cohen and Mannarino 2015; Cohen et al. 2017). TF-CBT has been implemented successfully with male and female youth in urban, suburban, and rural environments and has demonstrated success with white, African American, and Hispanic children from all socioeconomic environments. TF-CBT has been adapted to address the unique needs of the Hispanic and Latino population and with individuals who are hearing impaired or deaf. There have been multiple TF-CBT dissemination efforts in a variety of languages worldwide, including in several African countries, the Netherlands, Norway, Australia, Japan, and Germany. (For a review of these studies, see Cohen and Mannarino 2015; Cohen et al. 2017; Griffin et al., in press.)

Additionally, TF-CBT is able to be disseminated at a fraction of the cost in comparison with other treatment models, with data supporting its use in reducing costs for the larger managed care system (Greer et al. 2014). As such, it is more cost-effective to train providers in various adaptations to TF-CBT for special populations rather than train them in newer treatments (with less evidence) designed specifically for those groups. In addition, integrating TF-CBT training into existing training programs or academic settings is less costly when attempting to train clinicians in practice at agencies with productivity requirements.

Conclusion

Although a number of treatments address childhood trauma, no treatment has a larger evidence base than TF-CBT, with RCTs in both clinic- and community-based settings. TF-CBT is a phase-based, components-based, time-limited, cost-effective treatment that is designed to be provided in a flexible manner to address the unique needs of each youth and family—all elements that are valuable when working with trauma-exposed children in a complex mental health and managed care system. TF-CBT, like any treatment, has its limitations and is not a panacea for all of the emotional, behavioral, or psychological needs of youth and their families who have experienced trauma. However, when conducted with fidelity, it is highly effective in reducing a variety of trauma-related symptoms in both youth and caregivers, improving youth and caregiver competencies, and promoting healing and resiliency.

KEY CONCEPTS

- Trauma-focused cognitive-behavioral therapy is a trauma treatment for children ages 3–18 who have experienced single or multiple traumas, including youth with complex trauma experiences and their nonoffending caregiver.

- TF-CBT is a components- and phase-based treatment that emphasizes proportionality and incorporates gradual exposure into each component.

- TF-CBT consists of several core treatment components that can be represented by the acronym PRACTICE, including psychoeducation and parenting skills, relaxation training, affective expression and modulation/regulation, cognitive coping, trauma narrative and cognitive processing of the trauma narrative, in vivo exposure, conjoint (parent-child) sessions, and enhancing safety and future development.

- TF-CBT is considered the most efficacious and well-supported intervention for childhood trauma.

Discussion Questions

1. Which patients are appropriate for TF-CBT?

2. What outcomes are to be expected when TF-CBT is completed with a patient?

3. How important is caregiver involvement in TF-CBT?

4. What are potential barriers in TF-CBT and what are some suggested strategies to address these barriers?

Suggested Readings

Cohen JA, Mannarino AP: Trauma-focused cognitive behavior therapy for traumatized children and families. Child Adolesc Psychiatr Clin N Am 24(3):557–570, 2015 26092739

Cohen JA, Mannarino AP, Deblinger E: Trauma-Focused CBT for Children and Adolescents: Treatment Applications. New York, Guilford, 2012

Cohen JA, Mannarino AP, Deblinger E: Treating Trauma and Traumatic Grief in Children and Adolescents, 2nd Edition. New York, Guilford, 2017

de Arellano MA, Lyman DR, Jobe-Shields L, et al: Trauma-focused cognitive-behavioral therapy for children and adolescents: assessing the evidence. Psychiatr Serv 65(5):591–602, 2014 24638076

References

Bartlett JD, Griffin JL, Spinazzola J, et al: The impact of a statewide trauma informed care initiative in child welfare on the well-being of children and youth with complex trauma. Child Youth Serv Rev 84:110–117, 2018

Berger V, Gehart-Brooks DR: Feelings Jenga. J Family Psychother 11(1):81–85, 2000

Cohen JA, Mannarino AP: Trauma-focused cognitive behavior therapy for traumatized children and families. Child Adolesc Psychiatr Clin N Am 24(3):557–570, 2015 26092739

Cohen JA, Deblinger E, Mannarino AP, et al: A multisite, randomized controlled trial for children with sexual abuse-related PTSD symptoms. J Am Acad Child Adolesc Psychiatry 43(4):393–402, 2004 15187799

Cohen JA, Mannarino AP, Murray LK: Trauma-focused CBT for youth who experience ongoing traumas. Child Abuse Negl 35(8):637–646, 2011 21855140

Cohen JA, Mannarino AP, Deblinger E: Trauma-Focused CBT for Children and Adolescents: Treatment Applications. New York, Guilford, 2012a

Cohen JA, Mannarino AP, Kliethermes M, et al: Trauma-focused CBT for youth with complex trauma. Child Abuse Negl 36(6):528–541, 2012b 22749612

Cohen JA, Mannarino AP, Jankowski K, et al: A randomized implementation study of trauma-focused cognitive behavioral therapy for adjudicated teens in residential treatment facilities. Child Maltreat 21(2):156–167, 2016 26747845

Cohen JA, Mannarino AP, Deblinger E: Treating Trauma and Traumatic Grief in Children and Adolescents, 2nd Edition. New York, Guilford, 2017

de Arellano MA, Lyman DR, Jobe-Shields L, et al: Trauma-focused cognitive-behavioral therapy for children and adolescents: assessing the evidence. Psychiatr Serv 65(5):591–602, 2014 24638076

Dorsey S, Pullmann MD, Berliner L, et al: Engaging foster parents in treatment: a randomized trial of supplementing trauma-focused cognitive behavioral therapy with evidence-based engagement strategies. Child Abuse Negl 38(9):1508–1520, 2014 24791605

Drewes A, Cavett A: Play applications and skills components, in Trauma-Focused CBT for Children and Adolescents: Treatment Applications. Edited by Cohen JA, Mannarino AP, Deblinger E. New York, Guilford, 2012, pp 105–123

Fraser JG, Lloyd SW, Murphy RA, et al: Child exposure to trauma: A comparative effectiveness review of parenting and trauma-focused interventions for child maltreatment. J Dev Behav Pediatr 34:353–368, 2013 23588113

Greer D, Grasso DJ, Cohen A, et al: Trauma-focused treatment in a state system of care: is it worth the cost? Adm Policy Ment Health 41(3):317–323, 2014 23334468

Griffin JL, Murray LM, Cohen JA, et al: Therapy for the Child Sexual Abuse Victim: Medical Response to Child Sexual Abuse, 2nd Edition. Florissant, MO, STM Learning (in press)

King NJ, Tonge BJ, Mullen P, et al: Treating sexually abused children with post-traumatic stress symptoms: a randomized clinical trial. J Am Acad Child Adolesc Psychiatry 39(11):1347–1355, 2000 11068889

Konanur S, Muller RT, Cinamon JS, et al: Effectiveness of trauma-focused cognitive behavioral therapy in a community-based program. Child Abuse Negl 50:159–170, 2015 26318778

McKay M, Hibbert R, Hoagwood K, et al: Integrating evidence-based engagement interventions into 'real world' child mental health settings. Journal of Brief Treatment and Crisis Intervention 4:177–186, 2004

Murray LK, Skavenski S, Kane JC, et al: Effectiveness of trauma-focused cognitive behavioral therapy among trauma-affected children in Lusaka, Zambia: a randomized clinical trial. JAMA Pediatr 169(8):761–769, 2015 26111066

O'Connor K: The Color-Your-Life technique, in Handbook of Play Therapy. Edited by Schaefer CE, O'Connor KJ. New York, Wiley, 1983, pp 251–258

Scheeringa MS, Weems CF, Cohen JA, et al: Trauma-focused cognitive-behavioral therapy for posttraumatic stress disorder in three- through six-year-old children: a randomized clinical trial. J Child Psychol Psychiatry 52(8):853–860, 2011 21155776

10

Cue-Centered Therapy

Hilit Kletter, Ph.D.

CUE-CENTERED THERAPY (CCT) is a manual-based treatment protocol intended for youth ages 8–18 years who have experienced repeated exposure to traumatic events (Carrion 2016). CCT consists of 15 weekly individual sessions (3 or 4 of the 15 sessions are joint sessions with the caregiver) designed to last approximately 50 minutes each. The aim of this intervention is to address vulnerability to emotional problems for which the accumulation of stressors throughout life (allostatic load; see McEwen 2000) was a precursor. In addition, CCT focuses on such domains as social support, strengthening the caregiver-child relationship (attachment), and improving emotional and behavioral regulation. It is an integrative approach combining elements from cognitive, behavioral, psychodynamic, expressive, and family therapies.

The main goal of CCT is to build strength and resilience by empowering the child through knowledge regarding the relationship between history of trauma exposure and current maladaptive behaviors. Children and caregivers learn about the significance of traumatic stress, how adaptive responses become maladaptive, how to cope with rather than avoid ongoing stress, and the importance of verbalizing their life experiences.

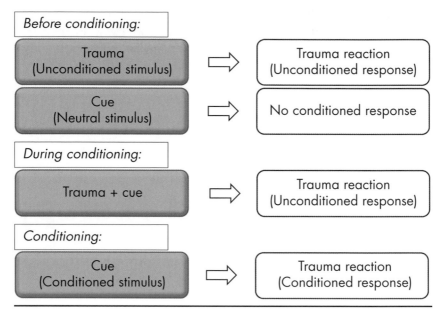

FIGURE 10–1.   Trauma conditioning process.

The treatment process involves overall competence building, reduction of physical symptoms of anxiety, modification of cognitive distortions, and facilitation of emotional expression. In CCT, youth and caregivers learn to recognize and effectively manage maladaptive responses that occur in response to traumatic reminders (cues).

CCT incorporates several unique components. First, through use of a life timeline, CCT aims to address the impact of allostatic load, the "wear and tear" on the body as a result of the accumulation of circumscribed traumatic events as well as other daily or life stressors. Youth are at risk for developing trauma symptoms when the allostatic load exceeds physiological and psychological resources. Second, several CCT sessions focus on teaching both youth and caregivers about the conditioning process that occurs through learning (classical conditioning) when an individual is exposed to repeated trauma, which results in increased sensitivity of fear and anxiety networks (Figure 10–1). Third, CCT combines an insight-oriented approach and use of visual icons to link trauma history, emotions, cognitions, physiological reactions, and behaviors to help the child overcome compartmentalization of these constructs. Although the main focus in CCT is on the child, caretakers are involved in certain sessions, including psychoeducation on stress and trauma, midtherapy update from the child, identification of cues, and facilitation of exposure.

There are four phases of treatment within CCT. Phase 1 includes a thorough assessment of both trauma-specific and comorbid symptoms along with an assessment of social support and the child and family's functioning before, during, and after the traumatic event(s). Psychoeducation on trauma reactions, the development of traumatic cues through classical conditioning, research showing the effectiveness of trauma interventions, and treatment components is then provided to the child and caregiver. The final part of this phase is development of a coping toolbox, with some of the tools taught by the therapist and some developed by the child. After the tools are taught and practiced, the child chooses which to include in his or her toolbox. This maximizes the likelihood that the child will use the tools.

Phase 2 involves creation of a traumatic stress history narrative, with the goal of having the child verbalize circumstances, emotions, body sensations, and behavioral responses. As the child recalls the traumatic experiences, the therapist assists in identification of emotions, thoughts, physiological reactions, and cues related to those experiences. In addition, the therapist completes a life timeline to map out all the events that the child can recall and asks the child to rate these events as positive, neutral, or negative. This shared exercise helps place the traumatic events in the greater context of the child's life. Following completion of the facilitated narrative, the therapist assists the child in restructuring cognitive distortions using the information and strategies taught in phase 1.

Phase 3 begins with a joint session with caregiver and child to update the caregiver on the child's progress, share skills learned, and prepare for upcoming exposure to traumatic cues. The therapist then meets with the child alone to finalize the list of cues to work on and prepare for exposure by identifying how cues currently have an impact on emotions, cognitions, physiological reactions, and behaviors. The therapist also helps the child identify alternative responses from the coping toolbox that he or she would like to try out during the exposure. The final three sessions of this phase involve gradual exposure to traumatic cues: imaginary, in-session simulation, and in vivo.

The final phase of CCT begins with revisiting the traumatic stress history narrative. The child is asked to retell the story while incorporating the skills learned in CCT to note any changes in quality and content of the narrative as well as shifts in emotions and cognitive distortions. The final sessions in this phase are dedicated to termination. The first termination session is done with caregiver and child together to discuss the child's strengths, summarize treatment progress, and provide recommendations as needed. The final termination session is done with the child

TABLE 10–1.   CCT components

Phase 1

Session 1: Psychoeducation

Sessions 2 and 3: Mindfulness, relaxation, and cognitive tools

Phase 2

Sessions 4 and 5: Chronic traumatic stress history

Sessions 6 and 7: Cognitive reformulation and emotional processing

Phase 3

Session 8: Midtherapy update

Session 9: Approaching cues

Session 10: Imaginary exposure to cues

Session 11: In-session exposure to cues

Session 12: Evaluation of in vivo exposure assignment

Phase 4

Session 13: Revisiting the chronic traumatic stress history

Session 14: Termination session with child and caregiver

Session 15: Termination session with child only

alone to review skills learned, discuss how coping tools may be used in the future, and answer any remaining questions. A complete list of sessions covered in CCT is provided in Table 10–1. Each session has specific goals to be met; however, there is flexibility for the therapist to draw on his or her own strengths in determining how to reach those goals.

CCT Research

To date, there has been one randomized controlled trial (RCT) of CCT (Carrion et al. 2013). Sixty-five youth from 13 high-risk schools in San Francisco and East Palo Alto were randomly assigned to CCT or a wait-list control group. Assessments were conducted pretreatment, midtreatment, and posttreatment as well as at 3-month follow-up. Results showed reduced posttraumatic stress (both by child and caregiver report), anxiety, and depression and an overall improvement in functioning as rated by the therapists. In addition, caregivers had differential reductions in anxiety and depression. These gains were maintained at 3-month follow-up. An example of improvement after CCT is given in the following vignette.

Clinical Vignette

Luisa is a 15-year-old Latina female referred for treatment following a fire that destroyed her family's home. She presented with extreme anxiety, frequent crying, lack of eye contact and turning away while talking, sucking her thumb, and low frustration tolerance. She was twice placed in juvenile hall for instigating fights with her peers. At the start of CCT, Luisa developed a coping toolbox to help her manage her anxiety and anger. She discovered that her love of art was a great way to help her relax. Her life timeline revealed that Luisa had been exposed to numerous traumatic events aside from the fire, including her father's alcoholism, domestic violence, her mother's hospitalization and diagnosis of a psychotic disorder, Luisa's gang involvement, and the death of her close friend by a revenge killing of fellow gang members.

Luisa was at first highly guarded and kept her narrative focused on the fire. As CCT helped her link her experiences with her current behaviors, she allowed herself to talk for the first time about the impact of her friend's death. Through cognitive reframing, she changed from believing that it was not acceptable to demonstrate fear or sadness to allowing herself to experience these emotions and knowing that she had control over them. She was also able to shift her thinking of feeling responsible for what happened to her friend. Luisa learned how cues may elicit responses similar to trauma reactions and that some of these responses are maladaptive. She identified her friend's brother and the neighborhood where the shooting occurred as cues. Gradual exposures enabled her to confront these cues. At the end of treatment, Luisa was far more confident, her school attendance and grades improved, she cared more about her appearance, and her father reported that she was managing her anger better even when he tried to push her buttons to see how she would react.

Developmental Approaches to CCT

Preschool-Age Children

Given the cognitive concepts covered in the treatment, CCT was standardized for use with youth ages 8 years and older. However, I have used it in a clinical setting with a child as young as 4 years. To make CCT adaptable for preschoolers, greater involvement of caregivers is necessary to support the skills learned. Because young children may have difficulty sustaining attention for a full 50 minutes, shorter sessions may need to be considered, or sessions may need to include breaks between teaching moments. Because CCT is a talk therapy, greater incorporation of play and art is recommended for teaching concepts.

Stories may also be helpful; for example, with one patient who was particularly fond of trains, I used the *Thomas the Train* books (e.g., Awdry

2007) to initiate discussion on emotion identification and expression. The visual aids included in the CCT manual can be used to convey concepts without need for much language. Session content may further need to be simplified or made more concrete. For example, the verbal descriptions of emotion intensity on the feelings thermometer, introduced as one of the coping strategies, may be substituted with drawings of faces or colors (e.g., green for "good/happy," yellow for "so-so," red for "bad/scared/angry/worried") to depict the emotion.

Finally, because abstract thinking is only just emerging in this age group (Scheeringa et al. 2001), the cognitive reformulation sessions may be particularly difficult. In place of the cognitive reformulation techniques, puppets may be used to demonstrate talking back to anxious thoughts, drawings may be used to illustrate destruction of negative thoughts, or the child can be helped to identify "good" experiences to focus on in place of anxious thoughts (Minde et al. 2010).

School-Age Children

CCT was developed with the school-age group in mind; thus, not many modifications are needed. Suggestions include providing teachers with a copy of the coping toolbox and instructing them on how these tools can be implemented in the classroom. Because behavioral issues are a common symptom in this age group, caregivers may need additional assistance with setting of consistent limits and management of acting-out behaviors. Play and art are still relevant to this age group in helping to promote cooperation and sustaining focus. Although school-age youth are better able to grasp the concept of cognitive reframing, thought bubbles or cartoons may assist in further solidifying this skill. Finally, relevant to all developmental levels but found to be particularly helpful for this group, therapists can create a booklet of the CCT session worksheets to give to the child at end of treatment to reinforce his or her progress and continued practice of skills.

Adolescents

It is natural for adolescents to begin to pull away from their parents as they establish their own identity and self-reliance. Thus, it is important to make a special effort to involve caregivers of this age group in CCT treatment. It is important to note that the limit on sessions involving caregivers in CCT does not stem from a lack of recognition of how crucial their involvement is but rather from the understanding that if caregivers have limitations on their ability to be involved, the youth may still be treated.

Although CCT targets many of the sequelae resulting from trauma exposure, it does not directly address substance use, self-injurious behaviors, and suicidality, behaviors that can be more prominent among traumatized adolescents. If any of these behaviors are present, a risk assessment is warranted to determine whether other treatment interventions that specifically address these behaviors may be needed prior to engagement in CCT. In this day and age, technology makes a wealth of information readily available, and savvy adolescents are susceptible to researching their own symptoms to self-diagnose. However, much of what they discover may be misinformation. CCT includes suggestions for handouts to provide trauma education to caregivers, and this can be expanded to provide adolescents with their own relevant recommended readings. Finally, the emphasis of CCT on empowerment of youth as their own agents of change is especially salient to this age group in restoring self-efficacy and finding meaning from their traumatic experiences.

Transitional-Age Youth

Transitional-age youth (TAY; ages 16–24 years) who experience chronic traumatic experiences often lack reliable and dependable connections that can help them transition into adulthood and learn the skills necessary for independent living. In the initial phase of CCT, the social support assessment can help TAY in identifying sources of support. The coping strategies taught in CCT will likely need to be supplemented with teaching of life skills such as résumé writing, financial management, and interview skills. Because traumatized TAY generally have not had the opportunity to learn these skills, the skills may appear insurmountably daunting, and thus it may be beneficial to incorporate them into exposures along with traumatic cues. Finally, in addition to learning the components of CCT, TAY may need assistance with connection to resources such as stable housing, vocational training, education, and employment.

Overcoming Challenges to CCT Implementation

Trauma treatment with youth presents many unique challenges. Among them is that it is generally an adult who decides the child needs treatment rather than the child seeking it himself or herself. Thus, youth do not always enter treatment as willing participants. In addition, traumatized youth have a wide range of reactions. Other challenges might include how

TABLE 10–2.   CCT treatment challenges and possible solutions *(continued)*

Challenge	Solutions
4. Child has difficulty starting the narrative	• Use what you know from assessment to provide a prompt such as "Tell me about the time that ____." If the child gets stuck, you can ask, "Then what?" "How are you feeling?" or "What do you think about that?" • Begin with more benign events from the life timeline. Proceed chronologically so that there is a natural progression to traumatic and other events. • When possible, have the child describe life prior to any traumatic history. • The child can write the narrative or draw it out to get started. Eventually move toward verbalization.
5. Child has trouble identifying feelings or thoughts	• Ask, "What do you think other kids would think or feel?" • Use thought or feelings bubbles, cartoons, or stories.
6. Child does not complete take-home assignments	• Provide a written reminder to both child and caregiver. Some youth prefer the use of smartphones for reminders. • Complete homework together in session while avoiding judgment. • Identify obstacles to completion and problem-solve the obstacles. Help child determine when to practice and for how long.
7. Child has difficulty changing cognitive distortions	• Compare evidence for and against the thought. • Create a list of the child's positive traits. • Emphasize how the child got through the traumatic events. • Use the life timeline to challenge the thought that only bad things happen.

TABLE 10–2.   CCT treatment challenges and possible solutions *(continued)*

Challenge	Solutions
8. Child refuses to do exposures	• Give youth the control in identifying a small step he or she is willing to take to work toward confronting the cue.
	• It may be necessary to have caregivers sit in on exposures so the child feels more supported.
	• Do not force the child if he or she is absolutely resistant. Reinforce the child's efforts in coming to treatment and attempting change and approach from an angle of curiosity on how exposures could be facilitated.
9. Child has difficulty thinking of how coping strategies may be applied in the future	• Role-play possible scenarios and have child practice how to apply the developed tools.
	• Create a plan for what to do if a tool does not work and how to develop new ones.
10. Child has difficulty finding solutions to possible obstacles to use of tools	• Help the child think of how to modify the tool (e.g., practicing breathing less conspicuously).
	• If a certain tool cannot be used in a specific situation, have the child think of what other tools could be used instead.
	• If the child has a hard time remembering a tool, you can create a physical reminder of the toolbox, create a mnemonic to help the child remember the tool(s), or have the child write the tool(s) on a small notecard he and she can carry.
11. You are experiencing vicarious traumatization	• Engage in self-care: healthy eating, exercise, sleep.
	• Debrief with a colleague after hearing something particularly troublesome, preferably the same day.
	• Consider weekly consultation and case conferences and your own therapy.
	• Engage in relaxing activities and recognize your own limits.

cause the setting is familiar, and because large numbers of individuals can be reached (Jaycox et al. 2009). One cultural consideration for trauma treatment is variation in how symptoms may manifest. Thus, the addition of a physiological component within CCT may be especially salient to certain cultures in which trauma symptoms are experienced as more physical rather than psychological.

Policy Implications

Although there are a growing number of trauma interventions for youth and the components that ought to be included in these interventions are known, more funding is needed to encourage research on the development of algorithms to determine which interventions are most appropriate for which youth. To this end, I and my colleagues are currently conducting another RCT that will examine CCT along with trauma-focused cognitive-behavioral therapy and treatment as usual, which comprises flexible, integrated services offered at a community mental health agency. The aims of the study are to identify which treatment phases are most effective and which child characteristics predict treatment outcomes and to identify neuromarkers that may be predictive of treatment outcome. There is also a need for establishing more formal training standards for clinicians interested in practicing trauma interventions. Often, clinicians are not trained in evidence-based practices or do not receive adequate supervision to obtain proficiency in delivering these interventions.

Finally, because CCT is a more insight-oriented approach, placing more emphasis on educating youth and their families on how traumatic reactions come to develop, this education can also be adapted to help policy makers understand the causes and outcomes of trauma. Sharing this information with policy makers is critical in increasing awareness of why childhood trauma impacts development academically, socially, emotionally, and medically and the prevention and treatment services available to mitigate this impact.

Conclusion

CCT is a multimodal intervention proven effective in the reduction of trauma exposure symptoms and associated anxiety and depression in chronically traumatized youth. Although there are specific goals for each of the CCT components, the flexibility in how to attain those goals makes it feasible to adapt the treatment to various age groups and to use it in a variety of settings with any trauma type. There are many challenges to treating traumatized youth that increase when the trauma is chronic or ongoing. I have frequently been asked, "Are 15 sessions of CCT really enough to see improvement in these kids?" The simple answer is "yes." It is very easy to become sidetracked or to have trouble deciding where to even begin when doing trauma work, and that is exactly why treatments such as CCT are necessary to provide guidelines to clinicians on what they should focus on. CCT contributes to the growing number of trauma interventions available for youth; however, there is still a need to determine which components of these interventions are most essential as well as which interventions work best for which youth. In addition, greater accessibility of such interventions is needed both to clinicians and the populations they serve.

For clinicians, cost and time may be factors in determining whether or not to pursue training on such interventions. Furthermore, the availability of certain interventions may be limited by geographical location, and thus there is a need to determine how to best disseminate these treatments. Trauma-exposed youth may face similar obstacles in accessing available interventions. In addition, they may not know of the interventions available to them; more efforts are needed to increase public awareness. Finally, many clinicians do not receive proper training on these interventions; therefore, improved training standards are needed to ensure quality of care. These may include defining clear steps for how one learns an intervention as well as hours of practice required to demonstrate ability to deliver the intervention.

KEY CONCEPTS

- CCT offers a structured approach with specific goals for each session while also allowing clinicians flexibility in how to meet those goals.

- For youth experiencing chronic trauma, traumatic experiences should not be processed in isolation. CCT therefore shifts the focus to the allostatic load. The load is the "wear and tear" that the body experiences during accumulation of traumas and other stressors throughout life. If the load exceeds psychological and physiological resources, there is risk for development of trauma symptoms.

- CCT takes a more insight-oriented approach to educate youth and their families on how cues (traumatic reminders) develop through classical conditioning and impact current domains of functioning (emotions, cognitions, physiological reactions, and behaviors).

• Trauma is not one size fits all, and the population affected by trauma is equally heterogeneous. Therefore, clinicians need a variety of interventions to address the varying needs of traumatized youth.

Discussion Questions

1. How might you incorporate CCT into your practice and adapt it to the populations with whom you work?

2. Consider how the challenges encountered within CCT are similar to or different from the ones you have encountered. What solutions have worked for you?

3. In the case vignette, what cultural factors might need to be considered for Luisa and her family, and how would these factors affect how you would engage with them in treatment?

Suggested Readings

Carrion VG: Cue-Centered Therapy for Youth Experiencing Posttraumatic Symptoms: A Structured Multimodal Intervention, Therapist Guide. New York, Oxford University Press, 2016

Carrion VG, Hull K: Treatment manual for trauma-exposed youth: case studies. Clin Child Psychol Psychiatry 15(1):27–38, 2010 19914939

Carrion VG, Kletter H, Weems CF, et al: Cue-centered treatment for youth exposed to interpersonal violence: a randomized controlled trial. J Trauma Stress 26:654–662, 2013 24490236

References

Awdry RW: Go, Thomas Go! New York, Random House, 2007

Carrion VG: Cue-Centered Therapy for Youth Experiencing Posttraumatic Symptoms: A Structured Multimodal Intervention, Therapist Guide. New York, Oxford University Press, 2016

Carrion VG, Kletter H, Weems CF, et al: Cue-centered treatment for youth exposed to interpersonal violence: a randomized controlled trial. J Trauma Stress 26:654–662, 2013 24490236

Cook A, Spinazzola J, Ford J, et al: Complex trauma in children and adolescents. Psychiatr Ann 35(5):390–398, 2005

Jaycox LH, Stein BD, Amaya-Jackson L: School-based treatment for children and adolescents, in Effective Treatments for PTSD: Practice Guidelines From the International Society for Traumatic Stress Studies, 2nd Edition. New York, Guilford, 2009, pp 327–345

McEwen BS: Allostasis and allostatic load: implications for neuropsychopharmacology. Neuropsychopharmacology 22(2):108–124, 2000 10649824

Minde K, Roy J, Bezonsky R, et al: The effectiveness of CBT in 3–7 year old anxious children: preliminary data. J Can Acad Child Adolesc Psychiatry 19(2):109–115, 2010 20467547

Scheeringa MS, Peebles CD, Cook CA, et al: Toward establishing procedural, criterion, and discriminant validity for PTSD in early childhood. J Am Acad Child Adolesc Psychiatry 40(1):52–60, 2001 11195563

11

Child-Parent Psychotherapy

Alicia F. Lieberman, Ph.D.
Chandra Ghosh Ippen, Ph.D.
Miriam Hernandez Dimmler, Ph.D.

CHILD-PARENT PSYCHOTHERAPY (CPP) is a relational treatment for children in the birth to 5 years age range who are showing mental health or behavioral disturbances or are at risk for these difficulties as the result of exposure to traumatic events, environmental adversities, parental mental illness, and/or harmful parenting practices. The treatment goal is to help parents create physical and emotional safety for the child and the family by promoting an age-appropriate partnership between parent and child. Treatment is deemed successful when parents become the child's reliable protectors and consistently guide the child toward the three key components of early mental health: developmentally expectable affect regulation, safe and satisfying relationships, and pleasurable engagement in exploration and learning. When the family situation involves risk or actual harm to physical and/or emotional safety, the primary treatment focus involves helping the child and the parent learn realistic appraisals of threat and effective responses to danger in order to increase the parent's competence and the child's trust in the parent as a protector (Lieberman et al. 2015). CPP is informed by a commitment to incorporate the cultural values of the family into every aspect of the treatment.

Internalizing Reality: How the Environment Affects the Child-Parent Relationship

John Bowlby made an extraordinary contribution to the understanding of developmental psychopathology when he stated that reality matters and that the parents' physical and emotional availability and competence as protectors from danger are key ingredients in fostering young children's secure attachments and mental health (Bowlby 1969). By placing the function of attachment in the evolutionary context of protection from predators, attachment theory highlights the pathogenic potential of environmental threats in the absence of reliable access to a safe caregiver. Over and above the dangers posed by natural predators, however, there is extensive research documenting high levels of exposure to traumatic events in infancy and early childhood, including mortality and morbidity as the result of accidental injury, physical abuse, domestic violence, and community violence (for a review, see Lieberman et al. 2011).

In light of these realities, a core CPP component involves screening for exposure to frightening and dangerous events and assessing their impact on the child's physical well-being and emotional life (Lieberman et al. 2015). CPP helps parent and child identify and address sources of danger and fear, practice safe and rewarding patterns of relating, and cultivate perceptions of themselves and each other as capable and worthy of love and protection. Using joint child-parent sessions as the format of treatment, the CPP therapist relies on spontaneously emerging behaviors, interactions, and free play as ports of entry to the creation of a goal-corrected partnership (Bowlby 1969) by translating the meaning of the child's behavior for the parent and facilitating the child's age-appropriate understanding of the parent's motives.

The Foundational Phase: Assessment and Engagement

Infants, toddlers, and preschoolers are affected deeply by what happens to them, to their parents, and to people close to them, particularly when these events involve unresolved fear. Bowlby (1988) highlighted the pathogenic effects on the child of "knowing what you are not supposed to know and feeling what you are not supposed to feel," with the risk of dissociation, depersonalization, and splitting defense mechanisms when the child is not allowed to disclose frightening experiences. CPP has adopted the guiding value of "speaking the unspeakable," modeling an attitude of supportive interest in exploring the impact of trauma exposure on the child and on the parent. This approach is characteristic of most trauma-informed treatment approaches, which share the therapeutic goals of helping traumatized individuals put their trauma experience in the context of other aspects of their lives, normalize their experience, differentiate between remembering and reliving the traumatic event, and restore healthy engagement with developmental goals (Marmar et al. 1993). What is unique to CPP is the extension to the treatment of infants, toddlers, and preschoolers of this explicit therapeutic focus on addressing the emotional impact of trauma.

The prevailing notion among adults and even treatment providers is that very young children are too cognitively immature to notice or to be affected psychologically by traumatic events. On the contrary, clinical and research experience documents that trauma exposure has profound physiological, emotional, social, and cognitive effects on children in the birth to 5 years age range (for a review, see Lieberman et al. 2011).

The foundational phase of CPP consists of an assessment and engagement period (4–6 sessions) designed to gather information and cultivate parental engagement in treatment on behalf of the child. It includes individual sessions with the parent with the goal of co-creating a treatment plan based on a shared understanding of the child's needs and on the family's cultural values. Information gathering includes the presenting problem, background of the referral to treatment, demographic information, the child's developmental timetable and individual differences, risk and protective factors in the family constellation, and child-rearing cultural values and practices. The parent is asked about specific traumatic and stressful events, both in the child's life and in the life of each of the child's primary caregivers. The foundational phase also includes observation of the parent and child during structured and/or free play situations, observation of the child in interaction with the therapist or another assessor during a structured and/or free play situation, assessment of the child's developmental functioning using structured tools or clinical observation, and assessment of the child's functioning in alternative settings or with other caregivers.

Clinicians who are first learning CPP often raise the concern that addressing traumatic events early in treatment may frighten the parent and/

or the child and interfere with the formation of a therapeutic alliance. On the contrary, CPP outcome research indicates that therapeutic engagement and progress are facilitated when treatment incorporates frank and supportive acknowledgment of the adversities that affect the family members' emotional states. As a result, a core CPP competency is the therapist's skill and comfort in addressing traumatic events.

The foundational phase culminates in an individual session with the parent(s) to cocreate a treatment formulation and treatment plan. The feedback session includes the *formulation triangle*, in which the therapist helps the parent understand the possible connections between the stresses and trauma in the child's life and the child's symptoms and explains how treatment will address these key causal connections (Figure 11–1). If the parent's own trauma history and mental health disturbances emerge during the foundational phase as an important etiological factor in the child's functioning, the therapist proposes a parent's formulation triangle by describing how the parent's difficult life experiences may influence his or her current individual functioning, perception of the child, and parenting practices. These conversations serve as the basis for a treatment plan that is created jointly by the therapist and the parent and includes an agreement about how to describe treatment to the child.

Core CPP Treatment: Introducing the Child to CPP

The first joint session with parent and child recapitulates the treatment plan agreed on during the feedback session. The therapist and the parent jointly introduce the formulation triangle to the child, using words and actions that are geared to the child's developmental stage (see Figure 11–1).

Treatment Considerations: Children's Developmental Stage

The clinical case formulation takes into account the young child's developmental stage. Babies are clearly not in a position to understand a verbal explanation of the formulation triangle, and their treatment involves helping the parent learn to read and respond to the child's affective signals and exploring the emotional obstacles the parent may encounter in this process. Beyond infancy, even barely verbal toddlers can be remarkably responsive to a

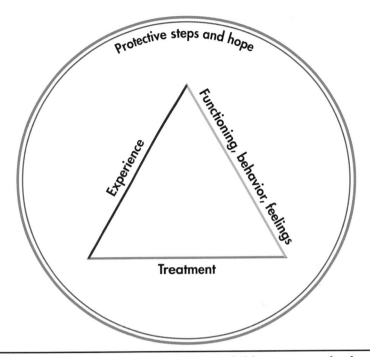

FIGURE 11–1.   Introducing the child to child-parent psychotherapy: the formulation triangle.

Source.   Lieberman AF, Ghosh Ippen C: "Introducing Child-Parent Psychotherapy to Children and Their Caregivers." Unpublished manuscript, Department of Psychiatry, University of California, San Francisco, San Francisco, CA, 2014.

brief explanation of what happened to them and are able to use simple words to describe how sad or mad they are and can show how they feel about what happened. When the toddler or preschooler is able to use language and symbolic play to describe experiences and articulate feelings, the treatment focus shifts to make the child an active participant in the treatment.

The CPP developmental framework incorporates the normative developmental anxieties originally identified by Freud (1959) and elaborated more recently by Marans (2005) and Pynoos et al. (1999)—namely, fear of separation and loss, fear of losing the parents' love, fear of body damage, and fear of moral condemnation or not living up to the expectations of one's social group. Once established, these fears last throughout the life course and may reemerge when the adult is feeling vulnerable because of internal or external circumstances. In situations of trauma and adversity, reality serves as a confirmation of the child's normative fears: many children *are* abandoned, insufficiently loved, physically harmed, and told that they are "bad." Whether their fears are based on fantasy or on real life events, children manifest their overwhelming emotions through behaviors that often trigger rejecting or punitive parental responses (e.g., the child cries inconsolably; has unmanageable tantrums; becomes aggressive, reckless, or defiant; withdraws; shows a constriction of emotional expression; loses developmental milestones; or engages in self-endangering behaviors). Parents, in turn, may feel ineffectual, unloved, and disrespected by their child, reexperiencing in adulthood the developmentally appropriate fears now experienced by their child. CPP therapists strive toward a simultaneous understanding of the child's and the parent's emotional experiences as efforts to cope with these universal fears.

Parents' Developmental Stage

Development lasts a lifetime, and the parents' developmental stage is also incorporated into how treatment is formulated and conducted. The ability to function adequately in adult roles is an important component of a parent's ability to care adequately for the child. Treatment sometimes needs to focus on helping with urgent material needs, family crisis, or parental mental health problems that interfere with effective parenting. CPP therapists use a variety of interventions to maintain a dual focus on the child's and the parent's experience, including collateral individual sessions with the parent or referring the parent to other resources as clinically indicated.

Role of Play

Play reflects young children's efforts to make meaning from their experiences. Children use play to express their understanding of what is happening, enact their wishes and their fears, and experiment with a range of outcomes as they strive to cope with their reality (Erickson 1964). CPP is similar to other child psychotherapies in encouraging play, but it differs from other approaches in seeing play as an opportunity for the child and the parent to *play together* in order to foster emotional closeness and as a vehicle to cocreate trauma narratives and protective narratives that address the relevant emotional issues confronting them.

Theoretical Influences

The origins of CPP go back to psychoanalytic infant-parent psychotherapy and the eloquent metaphor of "ghosts in the nursery" (Fraiberg et al. 1975) to describe the intergenerational transmission of psychopathology. This paradigm has been expanded to include "angels in the nursery" (Lieberman et al. 2005) as a metaphor to explore experiences of love and acceptance as a necessary counterbalance to the focus on unresolved conflict of the ghosts in the nursery approach. Hope is a key ingredient in all treatment but is the most crucial ingredient to counter the despair of trauma. In CPP, the parent and the child are helped to retrieve benevolent memories from the past or to create together new supportive moments that in time become memories that nurture trust, pleasure, and joy. In this way, CPP incorporates the attachment theory emphasis on the importance of secure attachments in creating a healthy personality structure (Bowlby 1969).

Theory and clinical strategies from the field of adult and child trauma are an important influence when the child and/or the parent have experienced traumatic events (Pynoos et al. 1999), and cognitive-behavioral strategies are often used to guide cognitive change and effect behavioral change. The philosophical outlook encompassing these different perspectives is the conviction that hope and a positive engagement with the activities of living are the primary components of any successful therapeutic endeavor.

Intervention Modalities

As a cross-disciplinary approach, CPP uses a range of modalities informed by developmental psychology, psychoanalytic/attachment theory, trauma, cognitive-behavioral psychotherapy, and social learning theory.

Translating Behavioral Meanings Using Play, Body Sensations, Physical Contact, and Language

Adverse and traumatic experiences shape perception, and many problems in the child-parent relationship originate in distortions or misunderstandings in the meaning that parent and child give to each other's behavior. Young children hold the developmentally appropriate conviction that the parents are all-powerful and that the child is responsible for the parent's moods and behaviors. In response to trauma, the child might correctly or incorrectly think that the parent made the traumatic event happen or failed to protect on purpose or that the child is responsible for the traumatic event because of his or her behavior or thoughts. CPP uses words, play, physical affection, and other means of communication to acknowledge and provide support for accurate perceptions and to correct misperceptions by describing the motives and function of child and parent behaviors, as well as to build trust and expand empathic understanding.

The therapeutic setting includes toys chosen according to the child's developmental stage and the goals of treatment. These toys allude to relationship themes (e.g., a family of dolls that match the child and family's ethnicity, farm animals, wild animals), nurturing and self care (e.g., toy food, kitchen and eating utensils), the specific stressors endured by the child (e.g., police cars, ambulance), and healing (e.g., medical kit). Toy selection may change in the course of treatment in response to evolving therapeutic needs. The focus is on encouraging play that involves the child with the parent. The clinician participates as requested by the child and serves as narrator and translator of the play themes, with the goal of clarifying meanings and scaffolding emotional growth.

Language is used to put feelings into words that help the child and the parent understand, channel, and manage intense emotions. The body is the primary locus of intense emotion and the driver of unmanageable action. The CPP therapist helps child and parent focus on body sensations to move their attention from impulsive action to reflection and affect regulation by naming sensations and feelings and helping to trace their origins and meanings.

Affectionate physical contact builds trust and conveys love between parent and child. When the child is frightened or upset, a hug can speak louder than words. For example, Tyler, a 4-year-old boy, asked his mother, "Will you leave me if I am bad?" She was able to hold him tightly and reassure him of her love. Tyler had assumed that his mother made his father leave and was afraid she would do the same to him. Her hug and reassurance came with a clear explanation, helped along by the therapist's guidance: "Your daddy is a grown-up, and he left because he was not safe. You are a little boy, and you are still learning what is OK and what is not. I will teach you, and I will never leave you."

Using Unstructured Reflective Developmental Guidance

CPP uses unstructured developmental guidance in response to the needs of the moment. It does not follow a prescribed curriculum, and it is reflective in the sense that it encourages the parent to integrate thinking and feeling into a new a more empathic understanding of development. The example above, involving Tyler's somatic response to his mother's trauma narrative and the resolution that followed, incorporated developmental guidance that included reframing, empathy, and a clear explanation of the different expectations from fathers and from little boys. In addressing the emotional impact of stressful or traumatic events, psychoeducation about normative responses can normalize child and parent responses and make both the child and the parent feel accepted and understood.

Modeling Appropriate Protective Behavior

When modeling protective action, the therapist takes an active role in countering punitiveness and deflecting or stopping potentially dangerous behavior. Modeling protective behavior is particularly important when parents and children have distorted perceptions of danger and safety as the result of chronic experiences of violence or other trauma. When the parent has been the perpetrator of trauma, young children's ability to recognize and protect themselves from danger is severely derailed. In this situation, the therapist's protective action in the moment not only serves to provide safety but also shows a commitment to help the parent learn how to protect the child.

Take, for example, the case of Stella, a 2-year-old girl. During therapy one day, Stella quickly opened the playroom door and started to run down the hall while her mother, Kim, stayed in her seat. The therapist ran down the hall in hot pursuit, retrieved Stella, held her close, and said, "I can't let you run away. You have to stay with your mom and me." Back in the office, the theme turned to what had just happened and became an opportunity to link the therapist's protective action to developmental guidance to Kim about the importance of retrieving young children when they run away in order to keep them safe.

Applying Insight-Oriented Interpretation

Exploring the unconscious or symbolic meaning of behavior can increase self-understanding and can be effective with parents as well as with young children who have acquired receptive language. Supportive, well-timed interpretations can increase parental awareness of motives, negative attributions, and behaviors that interfere with the parents' ability to nurture and protect their children. Interpretations can also help young children who blame themselves for the traumatic event(s) or for their parents' problems by promoting a more accurate understanding of causality and of their own role in the family.

In the example of Stella described in the previous subsection, Kim responded to the therapist's offer of developmental guidance with the dismissive comment, "She always does that; I am sick and tired of her running away." The therapist understood this statement as an expression of Kim's emotional rejection of her child and commented, "Is it easier sometimes when she is not there because it gives you a breather?" This sympathetic, supportive acknowledgment of maternal ambivalence enabled Kim to start disclosing her doubts about her capacity to love her child and deepened the scope of the therapeutic work.

Addressing Traumatic Reminders

Treatment must address traumatic play and other manifestations of traumatic stress whenever trauma exposure emerges as a possible source of the child's mental health problems. This therapeutic modality enables the child to narrate the traumatic event through play, drawings, or verbal description and provides relaxation exercises to address somatic reexperiencing and behavioral reenactments. In many situations, the child and the parent are traumatized by the same events, such as in the case of car accidents, community violence, and domestic violence. In other situations, the parent may experience vicarious trauma from witnessing or learning about what happened to the child, such as when the child was abused by the other parent or was attacked by a dog. Treatment in these cases needs to address the impact of the trauma on the parents as well, including appropriate referrals when necessary.

In the case of Stella, an incident emerged in the course of treatment in which Stella had run out of the house and into the street when frightened by her parents' fighting. A neighbor retrieved Stella, brought her to her own house, and did not return her until hours later, after the parents had calmed down. Learning about this situation enabled the therapist to help Stella's mother, Kim, understand her daughter's running away as a way of remembering this frightening event and a request for help in feeling safe. Addressing Stella's running away as a traumatic reminder helped Kim respond with greater empathy to behavior she had originally perceived as misbehavior.

Retrieving and Creating Benevolent Memories

Bringing to conscious awareness what William Harris (personal communication, May 2004) called *beneficial cues* serves a therapeutic function by expanding the perception of goodness in the self and others. Beneficial cues can be defined as moments of well-being that serve as reminders for experiences of being supported and cherished and that promote self-worth. Remembering moments of receiving loving care can give parents the motivation to provide such experiences to the child. Therapy also provides a setting for the creation of new memories that offer a sense of trust, pleasure, and self-worth when such memories from the past are not readily available.

In the case of Stella, Kim's anger at the neighbor who retrieved Stella from the street and kept her in her house for several hours was assuaged when the therapist asked about her usual relationship with this neighbor. Kim's face softened as she said, "She is my auntie. She used to keep me in her house when my parents fought." This memory of protection gave new meaning to the neighbor's action in protecting the child.

Providing Emotional Support

Therapist emotional support is a shared component of all psychotherapies. Emotional support is expressed through words and actions that convey positive regard, realistic hope that the treatment goals can be achieved, permission for self-expression, encouragement of reality testing, and genuine therapist satisfaction in response to the child and parent's achievements of developmental milestones and personal goals. Emotional support is particularly important in the treatment of parents and children facing poverty and discrimination because it affirms the parents' and the child's right to dignity and respect as integral members of society.

Using Crisis Intervention, Case Management, and Concrete Assistance

Therapist involvement in trying to alleviate oppressive or dangerous life circumstances and problems of living can help parents become more receptive to mental health treatment. Crisis intervention is often the immediate therapeutic action when the child is referred soon after a traumatic event such as maltreatment, community violence, or an accident. Ensuring safety is the first order of business in these circumstances, and concrete interventions can give the beleaguered parents a sense that change for the better may be possible as the result of treatment. Therapist engagement may include advocacy with different agencies, consultation with the child care provider to prevent expulsion of the child for inappropriate behavior, mediation between the parent and child protective services if questions of abuse or neglect arise, or referral to other needed services.

Empirical Evidence

CPP is accredited as an evidence-based treatment by the Substance Abuse and Mental Health Services Administration (SAMHSA) National Registry of Evidence-Based and Promising Practices. CPP efficacy is empirically documented in five randomized trials that included samples of anxiously attached toddlers of impoverished, unacculturated Latina mothers with trauma histories; toddlers of depressed mothers (Cicchetti et al. 2000); maltreated infants and maltreated preschoolers in the child protection system; toddlers of mothers with clinical depression; and preschoolers exposed to domestic violence (see Lieberman et al. 2015). These five randomized trials included more than 500 racially and ethnically diverse children in households ranging from poverty to middle-class backgrounds and populations of maltreated infants, toddlers, and preschoolers in the child welfare system and preschoolers exposed to an average of five traumatic events.

Findings showed improvements in a variety of domains, including reduced child and maternal symptoms, more positive child attributions (of parents, themselves, and relationships), improvements in the mother-child relationship and the child's attachment security (Lieberman et al. 1991), and improvements in child cognitive functioning (see Lieberman et al. 2015). In one follow-up study with children who had open cases in the child welfare system, preschoolers in the CPP group had a 2% placement in foster care 1-year posttreatment, compared with 21% in the comparison group. In an effectiveness study with preschoolers in foster care who received CPP and matched controls who received treatment as usual at the Illinois Department of Child and Family Services, the CPP group had 50% fewer placement changes than the comparison group (see Lieberman et al. 2015 for a review).

Training and Community Dissemination

The CPP treatment manual is now in its second edition, with updated fidelity forms (Lieberman et al. 2015). CPP is disseminated nationally through the Early Trauma Treatment Network, a center of the SAMHSA National Child Traumatic Stress Network (NCTSN) that involves the collaboration of four university-based programs: the Child Trauma Research Program at the University of California, San Francisco (lead program); Child Witness to Violence at Boston Medical Center; the Child Violence Exposure Program at Louisiana State University Health Sciences Center; and the Infant Team at Tulane University School of Medicine. The training of clinicians in CPP is conducted within the NCTSN learning collaborative model, which combines didactic teaching with competence training through case-focused consultation for 18 months. In addition to learning collaboratives, CPP is taught through internships and fellowships for master's level, doctoral, and postdoctoral students. CPP currently has 55 CPP trainers in 30 states who maintain peer consultation through listserv exchanges and twice-monthly conference calls for fidelity and cultural and system adaptations. Since 2011, 96 implementation-level CPP trainings were conducted in more than 30 states. International outreach includes implementation-level trainings in Australia, Colombia, Israel, and the Scandinavian countries.

Conclusion

In summary, CPP is an attachment- and trauma-informed treatment for children in the birth to 5-year age range and their families, with particular focus on underserved and impoverished populations. CPP practitioners are committed as a group to enhancing the mental health of children and families with histories of marginalization and historical trauma as a vehicle for enhancing individual well-being and increasing public investment to redress the impact of adversity on children, families, and communities.

KEY CONCEPTS

- Trauma exposure has been identified as a significant pathogenic factor in early childhood.
- Parents are vehicles for the intergenerational transmission of trauma and healing.
- Early identification of trauma is an essential component of effective assessment and treatment for young children with developmental, behavioral, and mental health problems.
- The formulation triangle in child-parent psychotherapy (CPP) has the function of helping the child and the parents understand the possible causal connections between trauma exposure and presenting symptoms and explains the role of treatment in alleviating the impact of trauma.
- CPP focuses on addressing traumatic reminders in the parent-child relationship, everyday functioning, and the child's play.

Discussion Questions

1. Why does CPP use joint child-parent sessions as the format for psychotherapy?

2. What is the formulation triangle?

3. What is the rationale for identifying and addressing trauma exposure in the initial phase of treatment?

4. What is the function of the CPP foundation phase?

5. What are the basic modalities of CPP?

Suggested Readings

Lieberman AF, Ghosh Ippen C, Van Horn P: Don't Hit My Mommy! A Manual for Child-Parent Psychotherapy With Young Children Exposed to Violence and Other Trauma. Washington, DC, Zero to Three Press, 2015
Pynoos RS, Steinberg AM, Piacentini JC: Developmental psychopathology of childhood traumatic stress and implications for associated anxiety disorders. Biol Psychiatry 46:1542–1554, 1999
Scheeringa M, Zeanah CH: A relational perspective on PTSD in early childhood. J Trauma Stress 14(4):77–815, 2011 11776426

References

Bowlby J: Attachment and Loss, Vol I: Attachment. New York, Basic Books, 1969
Bowlby J: The Secure Base: Parent-Child Attachments and Healthy Human Development. New York, Basic Books, 1988
Cicchetti D, Rogosch FA, Toth SL: The efficacy of toddler-parent psychotherapy for fostering cognitive development in offspring of depressed mothers. J Abnorm Child Psychol 28(2):135–148, 2000 10834766
Erikson E: Childhood and Society, 2nd Edition. Oxford, UK, Norton, 1964
Fraiberg S, Adelson E, Shapiro V: Ghosts in the nursery: a psychoanalytic approach to the problems of impaired infant-mother relationships. J Am Acad Child Psychiatry 14(3):387–421, 1975 1141566
Freud S: Inhibitions, symptoms and anxiety (1926), in The Standard Edition of the Complete Psychological Works of Sigmund Freud, Vol 20. Translated and edited by Strachey J. London, Hogarth Press, 1959, pp 87–156
Lieberman AF, Weston DR, Pawl JH: Preventive intervention and outcome with anxiously attached dyads. Child Dev 62(1):199–209, 1991 2022136

Lieberman AF, Padrón E, Van Horn P, et al: Angels in the nursery: the intergenerational transmission of benevolent parental influences. Infant Ment Health J 26(6):504–520, 2005 28682485

Lieberman AF, Chu A, Van Horn P, et al: Trauma in early childhood: empirical evidence and clinical implications. Dev Psychopathol 23(2):397–410, 2011 23786685

Lieberman AF, Ghosh Ippen C, Van Horn P: Don't Hit My Mommy: A Manual for Child-Parent Psychotherapy With Young Children Exposed to Violence and Other Trauma. Washington, DC, Zero to Three Press, 2015

Marans S: Listening for Fear: Helping Kids Cope, From Nightmares to the Nightly News. New York, Henry Holt, 2005

Marmar C, Foy D, Kagan B, et al: An integrated approach for treating posttraumatic stress, in American Psychiatric Press Review of Psychiatry, Vol 12. Edited by Oldham JM, Riva MB, Tasman A. Washington, DC, American Psychiatric Press, 1993, pp 238–272

Pynoos RS, Steinberg AM, Piacentini JC: A developmental psychopathology model of childhood traumatic stress and intersection with anxiety disorders. Biol Psychiatry 46:1542–1554, 1999 10599482

12

Eye Movement Desensitization and Reprocessing and Dialectical Behavior Therapy

Stephanie Clarke, Ph.D.
Sanno E. Zack, Ph.D.

EYE MOVEMENT desensitization and reprocessing (EMDR) and dialectical behavior therapy (DBT) represent two powerful integrative treatment approaches that consider posttraumatic sequelae from a broader perspective than posttraumatic stress disorder (PTSD) as defined by the *Diagnostic and Statistical Manual of Mental Disorders*, 5th Edition (DSM-5; American Psychiatric Association 2013). The approaches differ in their current phases of development and evaluation, areas of emphasis, and unique strengths in addressing youth trauma. In this chapter, we review the evidence base, theoretical underpinnings, developmental considerations, challenges and controversies, and proposed future directions for each approach.

Eye Movement Desensitization and Reprocessing

EMDR is a unique approach to youth trauma treatment for several reasons (Shapiro 1989). First, EMDR integrates elements of psychodynamic and cognitive-behavioral therapy (CBT), two traditions with long histories and differing strengths. Second, targets go beyond the strict DSM-5 (American Psychiatric Association 2013) definition of PTSD, with trauma defined broadly as anything that impacts the psyche negatively, derails healthy development, and continues to affect the individual's functioning (Adler-Tapia and Settle 2017). Thus, studies of the application of EMDR to patients with PTSD focus on traumatic memories and associated material but also target any experiences that contribute to traumatic symptomatology (e.g., negative cognitions). For example, if a patient who seeks treatment for PTSD feels unsafe as a result of a sexual assault and during the course of treatment, a childhood memory of feeling unsafe when learning to swim arises spontaneously, it is included in treatment and processed using standard EMDR techniques. Third, psychodynamic elements of the approach incorporate somatic processing theory and practice, something not explicitly found in most other trauma approaches. Finally, the simultaneous development of the approach for youth and adults is an advantage in that developmental considerations were present from the start rather than developed through downward extension.

Empirical Support

A robust body of evidence supporting EMDR for PTSD in adults has led to its endorsement as a treatment of choice for PTSD by the American Psychiatric Association (2004) and the U.S Department of Veterans Affairs and U.S. Department of Defense (2004). A comparatively small but growing body of literature examining EMDR with traumatized youth yields promising results. In fact, EMDR and trauma-focused cognitive-behavioral therapy (TF-CBT) are the only PTSD treatments currently recommended for traumatized children and adolescents by the World Health Organization 2013), and EMDR is considered a PTSD treatment of choice for children and adolescents by the Substance Abuse and Mental Health Services Administration and the California Evidence-Based Clearinghouse for

Child Welfare (CEBC). The International Society of Traumatic Stress Studies rates EMDR as an evidence level B treatment for children and adolescents with PTSD (Foa et al. 2009).

Compared with the 20 published randomized control trials (RCTs) of TF-CBT, there are currently 8 published RCTs investigating EMDR for youth (see Table 12–1). These studies demonstrate that EMDR is far superior to both treatment as usual (TAU) and waitlist control. Additionally, EMDR has been found to be comparable and in some areas superior to CBT and TF-CBT comparison groups, with EMDR resulting in treatment gains in fewer sessions (e.g., Jaberghaderi et al. 2004). Further, EMDR does not require homework, a potential advantage for youth who struggle with negative school histories, low motivation, or insufficient caregiver support to follow through on the between-session assignments required in other treatments. In addition to the 8 RCTs, more than 20 mixed-design studies support EMDR as a treatment for posttraumatic symptoms in youth (see meta-analysis by Rodenburg et al. 2009). Findings of these additional studies need to be interpreted cautiously given the lack of randomization and comparison groups. In concert with the RCTs, studies collectively point to the efficacy, effectiveness, and efficiency of EMDR for youth with posttraumatic sequelae.

History and Underlying Theory

The adaptive information processing (AIP) theory underlying EMDR holds that just as the body possesses natural, automatic processes for healing physical ailments, there is a similar automatic process for healing from difficult emotional experiences, which are believed to be held at multiple physiological levels in the body. The AIP theory posits that an automatic information processing system incorporates new experiences into extant memory networks, affective arousal is diminished as it is processed, and new information is used adaptively to guide future behavior. In EMDR, this process is referred to as *adaptive resolution*. When a trauma occurs, this natural process is disrupted. Trauma memories and associated cognitions, perceptions, and sensations are encoded into emotional networks without having been processed and brought to adaptive resolution because the body's automatic processes are overwhelmed in response to a traumatic experience. These dysfunctionally encoded elements give rise to posttraumatic symptomatology when they are activated or triggered. Thus, a dysfunctional cognition (e.g., I'm not worthy of being loved) is viewed as a symptom of unprocessed traumatic material rather than a cause of posttraumatic symptoms; in other words, symptoms are treated

TABLE 12–1. Study characteristics of randomized controlled trials examining use of EMDR with traumatized children and adolescents

Reference (country)	Group	Symptoms or diagnosis	Trauma type	N, age, gender	Number of sessions	Intervention effects
Ahmad et al. 2007 (Sweden)	Wait list	PTSD diagnosis (DSM-IV)	Various; history of other traumas allowed	N=33, 6–16 years (M=10), 58.8% female	8	Significant improvement in treatment group's PTSD symptoms, especially reexperiencing symptoms
Chemtob et al. 2002 (United States)	Wait list	PTSD diagnosis (DSM-IV)	Natural disaster (Hurricane Iniki); unknown if other traumas	N=32, 6–12 years (M=8.4), 22 females	3	56.3% of participants no longer met criteria for PTSD; gains maintained at 6-month follow-up
de Roos et al. 2011 (Netherlands)	CBT	PTSD diagnosis (DSM-IV) or partial PTSD (two of three symptoms)	Explosion; history of other traumas allowed	N=52, 4–18 years	Up to 4	CBT and EMDR group PTSD symptoms improved significantly; EMDR required fewer sessions; improvement maintained at 3 months
Diehle et al. 2015 (Netherlands)	TF-CBT	PTSD diagnosis (DSM-IV-TR) or partial PTSD (two of three symptoms)	Various; history of other traumas allowed	N=48, 8–18 years (M=13), 38% male	8	Comparable symptom reduction across EMDR and CBT groups

TABLE 12–1. Study characteristics of randomized controlled trials examining use of EMDR with traumatized children and adolescents *(continued)*

Reference (country)	Group	Symptoms or diagnosis	Trauma type	N, age, gender	Number of sessions	Intervention effects
Jaberghaderi et al. 2004 (Iran)	CBT	PTSD symptoms	Sexual abuse; history of other traumas allowed	N=19, 12–13 years, all females	Up to 12	Similar symptom reduction in PTSD and behavioral symptoms; results achieved in EMDR group took half the number of sessions than CBT group
Kemp et al. 2010 (Australia)	Wait list	PTSD diagnosis (DSM-IV-TR) or partial PTSD (two of three symptoms)	Motor vehicle accident; excluded if maltreatment history	N=27, 6–12 years (M=9), 15 males	4	Participants meeting 2 of 3 PTSD criteria dropped from 100% to 25% post-treatment; treatment gains maintained at 3- and 12-month follow-up
Soberman et al. 2002 (United States)	TAU	PTSD symptoms	NA	N=29, 10–16 years, all males	TAU plus 3 EMDR sessions	EMDR group showed significant reduction in memory-related distress and positive trend toward reduction of traumatic stress symptoms
Wanders et al. 2008 (Netherlands)	CBT	Behavioral problems, low self-esteem, distressing memories	NA	N=26, 8–13 years (M=10), all males	4	Comparable gains in behavior and self-esteem, with EMDR group exhibiting larger improvement in target behavior; gains maintained at 6-month follow-up

Abbreviations. CBT=cognitive-behavioral therapy; EMDR=eye movement desensitization and reprocessing; NA=not available; PTSD=posttraumatic stress disorder; TAU=treatment as usual; TF-CBT=trauma-focused cognitive-behavioral therapy.

as evidence of unprocessed material that needs to be brought to adaptive resolution.

The goal of EMDR is to access, stimulate, and reprocess dysfunctionally encoded information so it can be integrated into healthy emotional networks. This is achieved through exposure and reprocessing in the context of optimal physiological conditions brought about by bilateral stimulation (BLS). BLS refers to visual, auditory, or tactile external movement that provides alternating stimulation to each side of the body, thus eliciting alternating activation of each side of the brain. The most common form of BLS is eye movements (EMs): the therapist moves his or her fingers or hand from side to side and instructs the patient to follow with his or her eyes. The function of BLS is to stimulate brain areas associated with sensation, perception, emotion, cognition, and any other trauma-related symptoms for the purposes of innervating the body's natural mechanisms for processing that were thwarted as a result of being overwhelmed by traumatic experience.

Controversy and Debate: AIP Theory

Despite the evidence base supporting EMDR, there is debate as to the core active ingredients that account for symptom change, specifically, the role of AIP and BLS. Although EMDR as a package has strong empirical support, AIP remains a largely untested hypothesis. Some researchers (e.g., Schubert and Lee 2009) argue that BLS is unnecessary because it is the exposure component of EMDR that leads to trauma symptom reduction. Despite the controversy, 14 studies comparing EMDR with and without EMs have demonstrated efficacy of EMs in EMDR for enhanced processing of distressing memories, yielding moderate to large effect sizes (for a review of the potential explanations for these findings, see meta-analysis by Lee and Cuijpers 2013).

Developmental Approaches and Considerations

EMDR can be used across the lifespan beginning at age 2 years and is applied over eight phases using a standardized protocol (Table 12–2). Although therapists generally move through the eight EMDR phases in sequence, the process is often circular, so it is common to return to previous phases (e.g., to enhance the patient's resources if she or he is struggling to tolerate the later phases of treatment). Table 12–3 summarizes developmentally appropriate techniques and adaptations for use of EMDR with children (Adler-Tapia and Settle 2009b; Adler-Tapia and Settle 2017).

TABLE 12–2. Eight phases of EMDR

Treatment phase	Purpose and procedures
1. History taking, case conceptualization, and treatment planning	Identify the presenting problem (focus on self-perceptions, cognitions, emotions, and physical sensations relating to traumatic experience).
	Provide general EMDR psychoeducation
	Create *targeting sequence plan* (inventory of traumatic material) organized by *negative cognition* (NC) (e.g., I'm not good enough)
2. Preparation	Provide more specific psychoeducation about EMDR and BLS
	Inventory and/or install resources, mastery experiences, and self-capacities with the application of BLS
	Identify BLS that works best for patient
	Identify patient's stop signal and create safe/calm space
3. Assessment	Identify *target image* (i.e., scene or picture representing worst part of trauma) and its associated emotions, bodily sensations, and negative cognitions (e.g., I am in danger)
	Generate *positive cognition* (PC) (what the patient would like to believe, e.g., I am safe now) and rate the PC on the validity of cognition (VOC) scale (1=completely false to 7=completely true)
4. Desensitization	Patient attends to target image, NC, and trauma-related emotions and cognitions while therapist applies BLS
	Take SUDS rating of trauma-related emotion and continue BLS until SUDS rating is 0
	Can last one session to several months
5. Installation	Patient focuses on PC previously identified while therapist applies BLS
	Evaluate VOC after each set of saccades and continue BLS until VOC rating is 7
6. Body scan	Use BLS to target any bodily sensations present when patient thinks or talks about the trauma until resolved
7. Closure	A target is considered complete, or closed, when SUDS rating is 0, VOC rating is 7, and body scan is clear
8. Reevaluation	Review all targets and if all are in closure phase, commence discharge planning

Abbreviations. BLS=bilateral stimulation; EMDR= eye movement desensitization and reprocessing; SUDS=Subjective Units of Distress Scale.

TABLE 12–3. Techniques and adjustments for the use of EMDR with children

Phase	Procedure(s)	Infants, toddlers, and preschoolers	School-age children
1. History taking, case conceptualization, and treatment planning		Assess developmental achievements and deficits Enhance parental attunement Provide parent management (e.g., limit setting)	Assess developmental achievements and deficits Enhance parental attunement Provide parent management (e.g., model healthy expression and regulation of emotion, provide psychoeducation about normative adolescent behaviors)
2. Preparation	Emotion literacy	NA	Use emotional facial expression materials Use trace of child's body and ask child to color or place bandage on places where he or she might hurt (e.g., heart, stomach) Use body sensations and other clues for labeling emotions accurately

TABLE 12–3. Techniques and adjustments for the use of EMDR with children *(continued)*

Phase	Procedure(s)	Infants, toddlers, and preschoolers	School-age children
2. Preparation *(continued)*	Emotion regulation skills	Emphasize contact with parents (e.g., being held or rocked) Have the parent hold child while child mimics parent's breathing Teach paced breathing through counting, blowing up balloon and letting air out slowly, or blowing bubbles	Teach paced breathing Use guided imagery of favorite place using all senses Use butterfly hugs Create a physical imaginary container for difficult emotions, experiences, and/or coping skills Use an image or a drawing of a remote control to change the channel or reduce the volume (emotion) Teach ways to discharge emotion that do not get child into trouble (e.g., jumping jacks) Elicit story of time child felt strong emotion (e.g., anger) but did not get in trouble to enhance mastery feelings and explore coping skills child already possesses

TABLE 12–3.   Techniques and adjustments for the use of EMDR with children *(continued)*

Phase	Procedure(s)	Infants, toddlers, and preschoolers	School-age children
3. Assessment	Identifying target and target image	Parent tells preverbal child's story Preschoolers and some toddlers can relay story verbally (story with the "scary stuff," "bad thoughts," and "yucky feelings") or through art (drawing, coloring) or play (e.g., dollhouse and figures) Preschoolers and perhaps toddlers can use toys or coloring to reflect worst part of target	Children can identify the target verbally or through play, puppets, drawings, etc. Use terms "bad thought" and "good thought" rather than NC and PC Use Thoughts Kit for Kids to help identify NCs and PCs Address VOC by drawing a seven-step bridge and asking where the child stands between the good feeling and the bad feeling Take SUDS ratings by moving hands together and far apart until child describes the "size" of the emotion

TABLE 12–3. Techniques and adjustments for the use of EMDR with children *(continued)*

Phase	Procedure(s)	Infants, toddlers, and preschoolers	School-age children
4. Desensitization	Processing	For preverbal children, parent relays event If toddler or preschooler is stuck, use cognitive or motor interweave	Test limits after child reports SUDS rating of 0 If child is stuck, use cognitive or motor interweave
	BLS	Attempt eye movements through use of hand or object of interest to child (e.g., toy) Apply tactile BLS through parent tapping or gently squeezing child's arms, legs, or feet; use NeuroTek device (buzzies)	Use eye movements, tactile BLS (buzzies), or auditory BLS or therapist can tap on hands

TABLE 12–3. Techniques and adjustments for the use of EMDR with children *(continued)*

Phase	Procedure(s)	Infants, toddlers, and preschoolers	School-age children
5. Installation	PC plus BLS	Parent gives child positive feedback, focusing on "good feeling" (rather than PC) For verbal children who are capable, help child generate "good thought"	Reduce frequency of VOC rating
6. Body scan		Parent or therapist provides BLS head to toe to "tap out the owies" For children who are able, they can apply tactile BLS with their hands or using the buzzies "wherever it hurts or feels yucky"	Describe body scan as X-ray for distress or discomfort or as an imaginary magnifying glass

Abbreviations. BLS=bilateral stimulation; NA=not applicable ; NC=negative cognition; PC=positive cognition; SUDS=Subjective Units of Distress Scale; VOC=validity of cognition.

Infants, Toddlers, and Preschoolers

As in any treatment with young children, parents of preschoolers are heavily involved in the application of EMDR and functionally serve as co-therapists. In phase 1, the therapist enhances parental attunement to the child and addresses any other parenting concerns while assessing the ways in which trauma may have derailed developmental processes. Standard protocols such as the stop signal are also adapted to be developmentally appropriate (e.g., rather than saying "stop," the child may hold up his or her hand). The safe/calm space may also incorporate the parent or use child-friendly media (e.g., the child can draw the safe space, or the safe space can be an actual space created in the room or on the parent's lap). In phase 2, the therapist may teach age-appropriate relaxation skills to titrate affect such as simplified breathing instructions or soothing through contact with the parent.

In phases 3 and 4, the parent tells the preverbal child's story using the child's communication style. Toddlers and preschoolers can tell their stories through a variety of methods (e.g., drawing or coloring, re-creation with toys), with or without parental help. Eye movements and/or tactile BLS can also be applied in a number of developmentally sensitive ways. The NeuroTek device (also known as *buzzies*) has two buzzing paddles the child holds as he or she applies alternating tactile BLS. In phase 5, a "good feeling" or "good thought" rather than a positive cognition that is appropriate for the child's developmental level is installed through use of BLS. In phase 6, the parent, therapist, or child provides BLS head to toe rather than the therapist applying BLS only if the patient indicates bodily distress or discomfort, thus relieving identification and communication burdens for young children.

School-Age Children

Parents' involvement in sessions with school-age children is more variable and dependent on the child's desires. The therapist, however, still assesses and enhances the parents' attunement to the child, addresses any other parenting concerns, and assesses the ways in which trauma may have derailed development. In phase 2, a primary goal is to teach the school-age child skills for managing strong emotions. Relaxation and calming techniques, such as breathing strategies, are typically part of the teaching. Guided imagery while applying BLS can also be used. Another relaxation skill, called the *butterfly hug*, is a type of BLS in which the child crosses his or her arms and alternates tapping on his or her arms while visualizing what he or she is observing as passing by like clouds as he or she takes deep breaths.

There are also developmentally adapted skills for titrating and distancing from intense or overwhelming emotions, such as physical or imaginary containers and metaphors for turning down intensity of emotions or leaving an emotional experience (e.g., remote control for TV). Children are taught how to express intense emotions without getting into trouble by learning new words to describe how they feel, and they are taught safe and appropriate ways to discharge intense energy underlying such emotions as anger and frustration. Emotional literacy and body awareness are also important skills to teach and strengthen given that children are asked to identify emotions and bodily sensations during the later phases of EMDR. Mindfulness of body sensations can first be taught by explaining in developmentally appropriate language that hurts on the outside of the body can sometimes be seen as bruises or scrapes, but hurts can happen inside, too. Therapists can provide psychoeducation about somatic symptoms, for example, noting that stomachaches can arise from eating something or from feeling afraid or worried.

In phase 3, school-age children can generally describe the target and target image verbally but can also be given the option to express them in other ways (e.g., art). As with younger children, the therapist uses alternative terms ("good thought" and "bad thought") instead of positive cognition (PC) and negative cognition (NC), which may not make sense to the child. The validity of cognition (VOC) rating of the good thought and Subjective Units of Distress Scale (SUDS) rating of emotion can also be adjusted for different developmental levels with truncated and less complex or more visually based scales. Ana Gomez's Thoughts Kit for Kids consists of pictures and games that can be used to facilitate elicitation of the NC, PC, and associated VOC (Gomez 2009).

During phase 4, an additional challenge with children can occur when processing stops as a result of the child reporting that nothing is coming up or nothing is changing. In this circumstance, a cognitive interweave (i.e., question or statement offered by the therapist) can be used. It is recommended that the therapist first try less intrusive interventions, such as changing the direction or speed of BLS. The concept of a *motor interweave* was also developed by child therapists to jump-start processing when a child is stuck. This is based on the idea that young children often store memories in sensory-motor format, and processing may continue when the child is given permission to take any adaptive actions he or she was unable to perform during the trauma (e.g., yelling for help or running across the room). Note that children often process targets much faster than a therapist anticipates, in part because the traumatic experience has far fewer associations than it might with an adult, who has a much longer life history. Finally, a common challenge is children inadvertently learning that by stating they are no longer noticing distress, they can move on from BLS and reprocessing. It is therefore important to test the limits with children, perhaps going for a bit longer after a child fails to endorse discomfort or distress.

Preadolescents and Adolescents

Although procedures for each phase are fundamentally the same for adolescents and adults, there are some important considerations for this age group. First, adolescents need to be given the opportunity to be interviewed separately from their parents during phase 1 because it is imperative to ask all adolescents about topics that may be difficult to discuss in the presence of parents (e.g., substance use, sexual activity). It is also important to get a sense of what the adolescent would like to improve in his or her life and to discuss how EMDR might be able to address the adolescent's concerns. Because parent-child conflict is often at its peak in adolescence, it is important to assess and to help the family make any repairs or adjustments.

The first and second phases may require more sessions than is typical for younger children in order to build a strong alliance. In phase 2, it is important to do a thorough assessment of emotion recognition and regulation skills because adolescents may seem similar to adults, but within the population there is a wide range of emotional literacy and coping skills for identifying and managing strong emotion. Teenagers may need greater intervention in these areas. For phase 3, Gomez's previously mentioned Thoughts Kit for Kids can be used with younger adolescents to help identify the NC and PC and to provide easier ways of rating the PC's VOC.

Comparative Summary of Developmental Considerations

Practice guidelines from the World Health Organization (2013) differentiate EMDR from TF-CBT and other CBT approaches to trauma in the following ways, which reflect attunement to the young child's development: First, EMDR does not require a coherent and detailed trauma narrative or description of the event, which may be impossible for very young children owing to undeveloped expressive language abilities. Second, without the need for a detailed narrative, the number of treatment sessions is potentially reduced. EMDR also does not directly challenge negative or dysfunctional beliefs, which can be a particularly difficult undertaking for preadolescent children. It also does not require extended exposure, which can make it more palatable to children and families. Finally, EMDR does not include homework assignments, thus reducing burden on the family and child. In sum, EMDR has the potential to be a shorter and easier treatment for children to complete.

Sociocultural and Policy Implications

EMDR is proposed as a potentially effective treatment for historically un-derserved and hard to treat populations as determined by the CEBC, such as children in foster care and welfare programs, despite notable challenges such as the potential lack of a consistent caregiver and the need to treat each session as it may be the last owing to unexpected moves or alterna-tive placements (Adler-Tapia and Settle 2012). For children who remain with parents who have been abusive toward them, there is an integrative EMDR and family therapy approach to help parents strengthen the at-tachment relationship with their child, understand the child's behavior through the AIP model, and learn effective parent management skills (Wesselmann et al. 2014). The ability to provide treatment in the absence of a consistent caregiver and uncertainty of future sessions and to help families repair relationships damaged by abusive behavior constitute ma-jor contributions to underserved child and family health and well-being and could reduce mental health care costs in the long term.

Dialectical Behavior Therapy

DBT was developed as a treatment for adults with chronic suicidal ide-ation and self-injurious behavior (Linehan 1993) and is currently the gold standard for treating individuals diagnosed with borderline personality disorder (BPD). Although DBT was not developed as a trauma treatment per se, it is well documented that BPD and PTSD are highly comorbid. This finding is in keeping with the biosocial model underlying DBT, which posits that chronic environmental invalidation, the most extreme of which is trauma (e.g., childhood maltreatment), underlies the dysregula-tion observed in this population.

The treatment of trauma was historically addressed directly in DBT through a phase-based approach, with PTSD being the identified primary target of phase II treatment once life-threatening symptoms of self-harm and suicidal behavior have been eliminated or reduced and stabilized. More recently, however, PTSD has become a formal target earlier in treatment (Harned et al. 2012). DBT has been adapted for adolescents with multiproblem behaviors (Miller et al. 2007), and the conceptualization and handling of PTSD and trauma sequelae within the adolescent population raises meaningful questions and areas for further research and clinical protocol development.

Trauma and Suicidal Behavior in Adolescents

Recent meta-analysis examining findings from 28 studies demonstrated a significant link between PTSD and suicidal behavior (i.e., thoughts, plans, and acts relating to suicide) in adolescents (Panagioti et al. 2015). Suicide is the third leading cause of death among adolescents, pointing to an urgent need to develop treatment approaches that address suicidal behavior and related trauma symptomatology. PTSD treatment guidelines unequivocally recommend treating suicidal behavior before engaging in trauma work for both adults and children because there is concern that the affective intensity often associated with exposure work in trauma treatment may exacerbate nonsuicidal self-injury (NSSI) behavior (deliberate, self-inflicted damage of bodily tissue) and suicidal behavior (Ford and Cloitre 2009). As a result, evidence is limited for the efficacy of gold standard youth trauma treatments, such as TF-CBT, for children and adolescents with suicidal behavior because these individuals are typically excluded from treatment studies. This is problematic, however, because it means that the treatment fails to address a large subset of the highest-risk youth. Trauma symptomatology and suicidal behavior are often inextricably linked in that flashbacks, nightmares, or trauma cues and reminders may act as the catalyst that precipitates suicidal behavior for some youth. A more successful approach to treatment might involve simultaneous treatment of both PTSD and suicidal behavior.

History and Underlying Theory

DBT can be conceptualized as a behavioral therapy that incorporates third-wave mindfulness approaches and a dialectical philosophy and asks patients to hold that seemingly opposite ideas can be true at the same time. In DBT, this includes accepting where one is with one's current struggles while also working toward change. The biosocial theory underlying DBT suggests that symptoms of extreme emotion dysregulation and impulsivity associated with NSSI result from a combination of (hardwired, biological) emotion sensitivity coupled with an invalidating environment where one's emotions are ignored, deemed bad or incorrect, or belittled, leading to transactional interactions in which emotional response is further escalated.

Developmental Approaches and Considerations

DBT for Adolescents

Standard DBT was adapted by Rathus and Miller (2002) to treat suicidal behavior and NSSI behavior in adolescents, decrease maladaptive behavior, and increase behavioral coping skills. DBT for adolescents (DBT-A) comprises the same components of standard DBT (Linehan 1993) (see Table 12–4 for standard DBT components), with a few recommended adaptations (Miller et al. 2007). First, duration of treatment is reduced from 1 year to 16 weeks. This varies across studies, with RCTs in Norway and the United States using a 6-month protocol. Second, weekly skills groups are multifamily, such that one or both parents must attend each week with the adolescent, and additional family therapy is provided as necessary. Finally, a "Walking the Middle Path" skills module was added, which aims to minimize parent-adolescent conflict and power struggles and to improve communication.

A growing number of studies have examined the effect of Rathus and Miller's (2002) DBT-A protocol on adolescents engaging in NSSI behavior (Fleischhaker et al. 2011; James et al. 2015; Mehlum et al. 2014; Rathus and Miller 2002; Tørmoen et al. 2014; Woodbury and Popenoe 2008). To date, however, there is only one published RCT of DBT-A. Mehlum and colleagues' (2014) RCT demonstrated that Norwegian adolescents receiving DBT versus TAU exhibited a reduction in self-harm frequency, suicidal ideation, and depressive symptoms, with reduced self-harm continuing at 1-year follow-up (Mehlum et al. 2016). The first United States–based RCT of DBT-A, the Collaborative Adolescent Research on Emotions and Suicide (CARES) study, found DBT-A to lead to significantly greater reductions in suicide attempts and NSSI at the end of treatment than individual and group supportive therapy (McCauley et al. 2018). Thus, with two RCTs supporting the efficacy of DBT-A in reducing NSSI and suicide attempts, DBT-A is the first empirically supported treatment for decreasing NSSI and repeated suicide attempts in youth based on criteria for well-established treatments commonly used in the field (Chambless and Ollendick 2001).

TABLE 12–4. Components of stage 1 standard DBT

Component	Function	Structure
Individual psychotherapy (at least one session per week)	Enhance capacities related to skills modules 1. Apply skills to patient's unique circumstances 2. Improve motivation and reduce dysfunctional behavior 3. Structure the environment to reinforce effective behavior and positive change	Treatment hierarchy: 1. Life-interfering behavior 2. Therapy-interfering behavior 3. Quality-of-life-interfering behavior
Group skills training (one session per week)	Teach the following skills: 1. Mindfulness 2. Distress tolerance 3. Emotion regulation 4. Interpersonal effectiveness	1. Mindfulness exercise 2. Homework review 3. Teaching of new skill
Telephone coaching (available 24/7)	1. Help with skills application in context (e.g., in a crisis) 2. Should be made unavailable for 24 hours after patient engages in self-injurious behavior	Brief, focused calls for 1. Skill use in a crisis 2. Addressing therapist-patient rupture 3. Reporting good news
Therapist consultation team (one session per week)	Support therapist's motivation, adherence, and effectiveness	1. Mindfulness exercise 2. Clinical concerns, including therapist's therapy-interfering behavior

DBT and Trauma Treatment for Adults

Researchers and clinicians focusing on traumatized adults who engage in NSSI and suicidal behavior have been grappling with the reality that postponing exposure treatment for trauma in order to address suicidal behavior first is complicated by the fact that PTSD symptoms are often underlying, prompting, or exacerbating suicidal behavior. The DBT prolonged exposure (DBT PE; see Table 12–5) protocol was developed to address the strong association between PTSD and suicidal behavior. Although PTSD and other comorbid disorders are typically not targeted directly in stage 1 DBT, given the challenges to waiting a full year before addressing trauma sequelae, the DBT PE protocol was developed to manualize the implementation of PE therapy for PTSD in the context of standard stage 1 DBT.

The DBT PE protocol (Harned and Linehan 2008) was first published in two case studies, which documented that patients' PTSD symptoms were significantly reduced and that patients did not engage in self-injurious behavior during the exposure portion of treatment. Importantly, these findings provided preliminary evidence that PTSD treatment could be safely and effectively implemented with individuals struggling with suicidal and self-harming behaviors. In a preliminary evaluation with a larger sample size, Harned and colleagues (2012) examined the impact of the DBT PE protocol on women with BPD, PTSD, and current or recent serious NSSI behavior. At the end of treatment, the majority of participants no longer met criteria for PTSD, and, additionally, there were significant reductions in suicidal ideation. Importantly, again, there was no systematic evidence to suggest that engaging in prolonged exposure during stage 1 DBT exacerbated self-injurious behavior or use of crisis services. In a pilot RCT comparing the DBT PE protocol with standard DBT (Harned et al. 2014), DBT PE led to significant improvements in PTSD symptoms and reductions in suicidal and NSSI behavior as compared with participants in the DBT treatment–only group. This finding provides evidence to support the notion that PTSD symptoms may underlie self-injurious behavior for many patients and points to the need for further studies examining concurrent treatment of both PTSD and self-injurious behavior, particularly for youth.

DBT and Trauma Treatment for Adolescents

Given promising early support for DBT PE for adults, as well as the considerable evidence linking suicidality and PTSD for a subset of youth, developing and testing a protocol to formally incorporate trauma treatment into DBT for adolescents with PTSD and suicidal behavior is warranted.

TABLE 12–5.   Inclusion criteria and treatment approaches for DBT PE protocol

---

To be eligible for DBT PE studies, patients must meet the following criteria:

1. Cannot be at imminent risk for suicide
2. Must have 2 or more months of no suicide attempts or NSSI
3. Must exhibit ability to refrain from NSSI in face of past triggers for those behaviors
4. Cannot be engaging in any major therapy-interfering behaviors
5. Must have identified PTSD as their highest-priority target
6. Must be able to experience the intense affect associated with exposure work without attempts to escape it

The following DBT strategies are incorporated into PE:

1. Monitoring of negative reactions to exposure (e.g., urges to engage in self-injurious behavior)
2. Assessment and treatment of problems arising as a result of exposure (e.g., dissociation)
3. Infusion of therapist strategies, such as dialectics, validation, and irreverence, in sessions

---

Abbreviations.   DBT=dialectical behavior therapy; NSSI=nonsuicidal self-injury; PE=prolonged exposure; PTSD=posttraumatic stress disorder.

Source.   Harned et al. 2012.

Just as PE is the gold standard treatment for PTSD in adulthood, TF-CBT is currently the gold standard trauma treatment for children and adolescents (Cohen et al. 2017). Research examining the incorporation of TF-CBT into standard DBT would be a major contribution to clinical practice and the empirical evidence base.

The development of DBT PE began with a case study series to assess safety and feasibility of trauma treatment with an actively or recently self-harming, suicidal patient population. To date, there is one published parallel case example with an adolescent known to these authors. Berk and colleagues (2014) incorporated TF-CBT into standard DBT treatment with a 16-year-old adolescent girl who was sexually abused at age 12 by an extended family member and whose PTSD symptoms served as a trigger for self-harm and suicidal ideation. Treatment involved the completion of 6 months of stage 1 DBT-A followed by the application of TF-CBT, modified to incorporate relevant DBT concepts and to not duplicate overlapping skills. Treatment was effective in both eliminating self-harm and suicidal behavior and resolving clinical symptoms of PTSD. This case example can serve as a strong starting point for laying out a proposed treatment protocol. In this case, however, TF-CBT elements followed completion of stage 1 DBT, which may or may not be necessary or optimal as the standard for all cases. The ideal timing for formal trauma treatment integration is an open empirical question, given the need to establish adequate safety and sufficient coping skills for the teenager to manage the intensity of trauma-focused treatment while also taking into account that the PTSD may be serving as the primary trigger or precipitant to self-harm and suicidal behavior.

Proposed Protocol for Adolescents: DBT TF-CBT

In this subsection, we propose a parallel protocol to that created by Harned and colleagues (2012) for adults with PTSD and suicidal behavior or BPD, incorporating TF-CBT into standard DBT for adolescents (Figure 12–1).

Assessment and Precommitment

When PTSD or significant trauma symptoms are evident in the clinical picture for an adolescent with suicidal and/or self-harming behavior, providing psychoeducation regarding trauma, PTSD, and their relation to emotion dysregulation and suicidal and other behavioral problems is an opportunity to enhance treatment motivation, particularly for young people, during the precommitment phase of DBT. Psychoeducation in itself serves as low-grade exposure by explicitly defining types of trauma, speaking aloud about trauma as a concept, explaining PTSD symptoms, and helping the adolescent to identify and rate the intensity of his or her trauma symptoms using such measures as the UCLA PTSD Index (Elhai et al. 2013) or the Clinician-Administered PTSD Scale for DSM-5—Child/Adolescent Version (CAPS-CA-5; Pynoos et al. 2015). Having the patient rate his or her symptoms gives the clinician the opportunity to see in real time how the adolescent is coping with trauma-related affect and can reveal important behaviors (e.g., avoidance, dissociation) to target at a later time in treatment. Psychoeducation about trauma should also be incorporated into the explanation of the DBT biosocial model that is typically provided to adolescents and their caregivers during this phase, with the goal of providing validation and a framework within which teenagers and their families can begin to understand the teenager's difficulties from a nonpathologizing, behavioral standpoint.

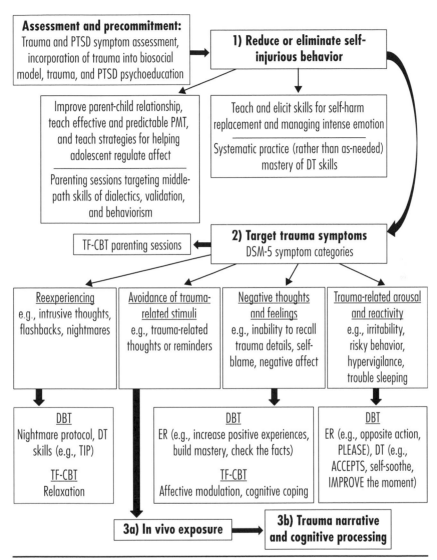

FIGURE 12–1. Proposed dialectical behavior therapy (DBT) trauma-focused cognitive-behavioral therapy (TF-CBT) protocol.

Abbreviations. ACCEPTS=activities, contributing, comparisons, emotions, pushing away, thoughts, sensations; DT=distress tolerance; ER=emotion regulation; IMPROVE=imagery, meaning, prayer, relaxation, one thing in the moment, vacation, encouragement; PLEASE=[treat] physical illness, [balance] eating, [avoid mood] altering drugs, [balance] sleep, exercise, [build] mastery; PMT=parent management training; PTSD=posttraumatic stress disorder; TIP=temperature, intense exercise, progressive relaxation.

posures given the adolescent's recent history of self-injurious behavior. Once the patient is able to tolerate these exposures in the presence of the therapist and demonstrate effective use of coping strategies for affective dysregulation, exposure challenges can be assigned as homework with an explicit reminder to the adolescent that the therapist is available for phone coaching prior to, during, and after the exposure challenge. In fact, it might be beneficial to plan the day and time of the exposure so the therapist can ensure he or she is available, especially during initial exposure challenges assigned as homework.

Construction of the trauma narrative and cognitive reprocessing occur in step 3, either in tandem with exposure challenges or sequentially, depending on the adolescent's level of anxiety about the narrative. Of note, TF-CBT allows for in vivo exposure to occur prior to the construction of the trauma narrative, although typically, in vivo exposure is conceptualized as optional and follows the narrative. Given the observation by Harned and colleagues (2012) that DBT patients often rate talking about the trauma the highest on their in vivo target list, beginning in vivo exposure before the narrative in DBT TF-CBT is recommended.

Retaining Core DBT Elements Throughout

Throughout the proposed second and third steps of DBT TF-CBT, the overarching framework of DBT is maintained, including the dialectical stance, use of motivational enhancement and engagement strategies such as irreverence, the weekly use of diary cards to track any increase in NSSI urges or suicidal ideation, and the chaining of any such behaviors that occur. Coaching calls should also be continued, with the option of support for trauma exposures. If affective arousal from the exposure and reprocessing phases precipitates reemergence of self-injurious behavior, this immediately becomes the focus of session, in keeping with the DBT hierarchy. Harned and colleagues (2012, 2014) found that self-injurious behavior decreased as a result of completing the DBT PE protocol; however, when a patient did engage in self-injurious behavior in the exposure and reprocessing phases, they suspended this phase briefly until the patient was able to again refrain from these behaviors.

Sociocultural and Policy Implications

Paradoxically, under-resourced adolescents and families may be most in need of DBT given that environmental stressors play a role in the biosocial model, yet they are often the patients who are least able to access DBT services. The multicomponent structure of DBT makes it a high-resource approach, which may limit its use in community settings owing to limited state funding and intensive therapist training requirements in the context of high clinician turn-over typical of these settings (Carmel et al. 2014). However, studies show that adults receiving DBT in community settings exhibit significantly reduced psychiatric- and crisis-related emergency department visits, psychiatric inpatient visits, and use of several other crisis services (e.g., Comtois et al. 2007). Thus, the model is, in fact, highly cost-effective if invested in by agencies. Carmel and colleagues (2014) evaluated barriers and proffered solutions to implementing standard DBT, and extension of this type of research to adolescent DBT programs will be useful because funding comprehensive DBT up front is likely to reduce mental health costs in the long run.

KEY CONCEPTS

- Adaptive information processing, the primary theory underlying eye movement desensitization and reprocessing (EMDR), posits that the body possesses natural, automatic processes for healing from difficult emotional experiences. Typically, new experiences are automatically processed into memory networks, diminishing affective arousal and adaptively guiding future behavior. In the case of trauma, this process is disrupted, and memories, sensations, and cognitions from the event are stored in the body in an unprocessed manner, showing up as trauma symptoms.

- Bilateral stimulation (BLS) refers to visual, auditory, or tactile external movement that activates each side of the brain by alternating stimulation to each side of the body. The most common form of BLS is eye movements. BLS is used in EMDR to activate the body's natural mechanism for processing difficult emotion that was disrupted as a result of being overwhelmed by traumatic experience.

- Dialectical behavior therapy prolonged exposure (DBT PE) is an approach to treating co-occurring posttraumatic stress disorder (PTSD) and suicidal or self-injurious behavior in adults by adapting gold standard prolonged exposure trauma treatment into dialectical behavior therapy.

- DBT trauma-focused cognitive-behavioral therapy (DBT TF-CBT) refers to a proposed approach outlined by the authors to treat co-occurring PTSD and suicidal or self-injurious behavior in youth. The model parallels that of DBT PE for adults and incorporates trauma-focused cognitive-behavioral therapy into dialectical behavior therapy for teenagers.

Discussion Questions

1. Given the strong evidence base for multiple approaches to youth trauma treatment, including EMDR and TF-CBT, how might clinicians most effectively decide which approach to use for which youth?

2. Is the controversy surrounding the mechanistic role of BLS in EMDR a meaningful one? Should we commit to further research regarding the role of BLS in EMDR for traumatized youth, or is the finding of effective treatment outcomes sufficient?

3. Given that DBT-A is a 16-week to 6-month treatment, should the incorporation of TF-CBT for comorbid PTSD be held until stage 1 DBT is completed, or are the advantages sufficient to start TF-CBT once suicidal behavior and NSSI are stable?

4. How can stakeholders such as insurance companies and government payers be best incentivized to invest in DBT for under-served populations given its capacity to address the highest-risk behaviors in traumatized adolescents? Or should adaptations be made to reduce the resource load?

Suggested Readings

Adler-Tapia R, Settle C: Evidence of the efficacy of EMDR with children and adolescents in individual psychotherapy: a review of the research published in peer-reviewed journals. J EMDR Res Prac 3(4):232–247, 2009

Adler-Tapia R, Settle C: EMDR and the Art of Psychotherapy with Children: Infants to Adolescents, 2nd Edition. New York, Springer, 2017

Berk M, Shelby J, Avina C, Tangeman K: Dialectical behavior therapy for suicidal and self-harming adolescents with trauma symptoms, in Evidence-Based Approaches for the Treatment of Maltreated Children, Vol 3. Edited by Timmer S, Urquiza A. New York, Springer, 2014, pp 215–236

Linehan MM: Cognitive-Behavioral Treatment of Borderline Personality Disorder. New York, Guilford, 1993

References

Adler-Tapia R, Settle C: Evidence of the efficacy of EMDR with children and adolescents in individual psychotherapy: a review of the research published in peer-reviewed journals. J EMDR Res Prac 3(4):232–247, 2009a

Adler-Tapia R, Settle C: Healing the origins of trauma: an introduction to EMDR in psychotherapy with children and adolescents, in Treatment of Traumatized Adults and Children. Edited by Rubin A, Springer DW. Hoboken, NJ, Wiley, 2009b, pp 349–417

Adler-Tapia R, Settle C: EMDR for the treatment of children in the child welfare system who have been traumatized by abuse and neglect, in Programs and Interventions for Maltreated Children and Families at Risk. Edited by Rubin A. Hoboken, NJ, Wiley, 2012, pp 141–160

Adler-Tapia R, Settle C: EMDR and the Art of Psychotherapy with Children: Infants to Adolescents, 2nd Edition. New York, Springer, 2017

Ahmad A, Larsson B, Sundelin-Wahlsten V: EMDR treatment for children with PTSD: results of a randomized controlled trial. Nord J Psychiatry 61(5):349–354, 2007 17990196

American Psychiatric Association: Practice Guideline for the Treatment of Patients With Acute Stress Disorder and Posttraumatic Stress Disorder. Washington, DC, American Psychiatric Association, 2004

American Psychiatric Association: Diagnostic and Statistical Manual of Mental Disorders, 5th Edition. Arlington, VA, American Psychiatric Association, 2013

Berk M, Shelby J, Avina C, et al: Dialectical behavior therapy for suicidal and self-harming adolescents with trauma symptoms, in Evidence-Based Approaches for the Treatment of Maltreated Children, Vol 3. Edited by Timmer S, Urquiza A. New York, Springer, 2014, pp 215–236

Carmel A, Rose ML, Fruzzetti AE: Barriers and solutions to implementing dialectical behavior therapy in a public behavioral health system. Adm Policy Ment Health 41(5):608–614, 2014 23754686

Chambless DL, Ollendick TH: Empirically supported psychological interventions: controversies and evidence. Ann Rev Psychol 52:685–716, 2001 11148322

Chemtob CM, Nakashima J, Carlson JG: Brief treatment for elementary school children with disaster-related posttraumatic stress disorder: a field study. J Clin Psychol 58(1):99–112, 2002 11748599

Cohen JA, Mannarino AP, Deblinger E: Treating Trauma and Traumatic Grief in Children and Adolescents, 2nd Edition. New York, Guilford, 2017

Comtois KA, Elwood L, Holdcraft LC, et al: Effectiveness of dialectical behavior therapy in a community mental health center. Cognit Behav Pract 14:406–414, 2007

de Roos C, Greenwald R, den Hollander-Gijsman M, et al: A randomised comparison of cognitive behavioural therapy (CBT) and eye movement desensitisation and reprocessing (EMDR) in disaster-exposed children. Eur J Psychotraumatol 2(1):5694–6705, 2011 22893815

Diehle J, Opmeer BC, Boer F, et al: Trauma-focused cognitive behavioral therapy or eye movement desensitization and reprocessing: what works in children with posttraumatic stress symptoms? A randomized controlled trial. Eur Child Adolesc Psychiatry 24(2):227–236, 2015 24965797

Elhai JD, Layne CM, Steinberg AS, et al: Psychometric properties of the UCLA PTSD Reaction Index part II: investigating factor structure findings in a national clinic-referred youth sample. J Trauma Stress, 26(1):10–18, 2013 23417874

Fleischhaker C, Böhme R, Sixt B, et al: Dialectical behavior therapy for adolescents (DBT-A): a clinical trial for patients with suicidal and self-injurious behavior and borderline symptoms with a one-year follow-up. Child Adolesc Psychiatry Ment Health 5(1):3, 2011 21276211

Foa EB, Keane TM, Friedman MJ, et al: Effective Treatments for PTSD: Practice Guidelines of the International Society for Traumatic Stress Studies. New York, Guilford, 2009

Ford JD, Cloitre M: Best practices in psychotherapy for children and adolescents, in Treating Complex Stress Disorders: An Evidence-Based Guide. Edited by Courtois CA, Ford JD. New York, Guilford, 2009, pp 59–81

Gomez AM: Thought Kits for Kids, 2009. Available at https://anagomez.org/node/156. Accessed July 20, 2018.

Harned MS, Linehan MM: Integrating dialectical behavior therapy and prolonged exposure to treat co-occurring borderline personality disorder and PTSD: two case studies. Cognit Behav Pract 15:263–276, 2008

Harned MS, Korslund KE, Foa EB, et al: Treating PTSD in suicidal and self-injuring women with borderline personality disorder: development and preliminary evaluation of a dialectical behavior therapy prolonged exposure protocol. Behav Res Ther 50(6):381–386, 2012 22503959

Harned MS, Korslund KE, Linehan MM: A pilot randomized controlled trial of dialectical behavior therapy with and without the dialectical behavior therapy prolonged exposure protocol for suicidal and self-injuring women with borderline personality disorder and PTSD. Behav Res Ther 55:7–17, 2014 24562087

Jaberghaderi N, Greenwald R, Rubin A, et al: A comparison of CBT and EMDR for sexually abused Iranian girls. Clin Psychol Psychother 11(5):358–368, 2004

James S, Freeman KR, Mayo D, et al: Does insurance matter? Implementing dialectical behavior therapy with two groups of youth engaged in deliberate self-harm. Adm Policy Ment Health 42(4):449–461, 2015 25199812

Kemp M, Drummond P, McDermott B: A wait-list controlled pilot study of eye movement desensitization and reprocessing (EMDR) for children with post-traumatic stress disorder (PTSD) symptoms from motor vehicle accidents. Clin Child Psychol Psychiatry 15(1):5–25, 2010 19923161

Lee CW, Cuijpers P: A meta-analysis of the contribution of eye movements in processing emotional memories. J Behav Ther Exp Psychiatry 44(2):231–239, 2013 23266601

Linehan MM: Cognitive-Behavioral Treatment of Borderline Personality Disorder. New York, Guilford, 1993

McCauley E, Berk MS, Asarnow JR, et al: Efficacy of dialectical behavior therapy for adolescents at high risk for suicide: a randomized clinical trial. JAMA Psychiatry 75(8):777–785, 2018 29926087

Mehlum L, Tørmoen AJ, Ramberg M, et al: Dialectical behavior therapy for adolescents with repeated suicidal and self-harming behavior: a randomized trial. J Am Acad Child Adolesc Psychiatry 53(10):1082–1091, 2014 25245352

Mehlum L, Ramberg M, Tørmoen AJ, et al: Dialectical behavior therapy compared with enhanced usual care for adolescents with repeated suicidal and self-harming behavior: outcomes over a one-year follow-up. J Am Acad Child Adolesc Psychiatry 55(4):295–300, 2016 27015720

Miller AL, Rathus JH, Linehan MM: Dialectical Behavior Therapy With Suicidal Adolescents. New York, Guilford, 2007

Panagioti M, Gooding PA, Triantafyllou K, et al: Suicidality and posttraumatic stress disorder (PTSD) in adolescents: a systematic review and meta-analysis. Soc Psychiatry Psychiatr Epidemiol 50(4):525–537, 2015 25398198

Pynoos RS, Weathers FW, Steinberg AM, et al: Clinician-Administered PTSD Scale for DSM-5-Child/Adolescent Version. Washington, DC, National Center for PTSD, 2015

Rathus JH, Miller AL: Dialectical behavior therapy adapted for suicidal adolescents. Suicide Life Threat Behav 32(2):146–157, 2002 12079031

Rodenburg R, Benjamin A, de Roos C, et al: Efficacy of EMDR in children: a meta-analysis. Clin Psychol Rev 29(7):599–606, 2009 19616353

Schubert S, Lee CW: Adult PTSD and its treatment with EMDR: a review of controversies, evidence, and theoretical knowledge. J EMDR Pract Res 3(3):117–132, 2009

Shapiro F: Efficacy of the eye movement desensitization procedure in the treatment of traumatic memories. J Trauma Stress 2(2):199–223, 1989

Soberman J, Greenwald R, Rule DL: A controlled study of eye movement desensitization and reprocessing (EMDR) for boys with conduct problems. Aggress Maltreat Trauma 6:217–236, 2002

Tørmoen AJ, Grøholt B, Haga E, et al: Feasibility of dialectical behavior therapy with suicidal and self-harming adolescents with multi-problems: training, adherence, and retention. Arch Suicide Res 18(4):432–444, 2014 24842553

U.S. Department of Veterans Affairs; U.S. Department of Defense: VA/DoD Clinical Practice Guideline for Management of Post-traumatic Stress. Publ 10Q-CPG/PTSD-04. Washington, DC, Veterans Health Administration, 2004

Wanders F, Serra M, de Jongh A: EMDR versus CBT for children with self-esteem and behavioral problems: a randomized controlled trial. J EMDR Prac Res 2(3):180–189, 2008

Wesselmann D, Schweitzer C, Armstrong S: Integrative Team Treatment for Attachment Trauma in Children: Family Therapy and EMDR. New York, Norton, 2014

Woodbury KA, Popenoe EJ: Implementing dialectical behavior therapy with adolescents and their families in a community outpatient clinic. Cognit Behav Pract 15:277–286, 2008

World Health Organization: Guidelines for the Management of Conditions Specifically Related to Stress. Geneva, World Health Organization, 2013

CHAPTER

13

Mindfulness and Yoga

John P. Rettger, Ph.D.

IN THIS CHAPTER, I explain how mindfulness and yoga methods can be used to support development, address stress and trauma, and promote wellness among youth and their caretakers. The reader should bear in mind that this is a new field of study, and scientific studies are preliminary and empirical understanding remains in its infancy.

Defining Mindfulness

Mindfulness is "the awareness that arises by paying attention on purpose, in the present moment, and non-judgmentally" (Kabat-Zinn 2013, p. 394). Further, mindfulness reconnects the individual to his or her natural human capacity to live with curiosity, acceptance, trust, patience, compassion, generosity, and gratitude (Kabat-Zinn 2013). Therapists using mindfulness-based approaches may emphasize working holistically with youth through focusing on their mental, physical, emotional, and, if appropriate, spiritual experiences.

Mindfulness includes formal and informal practices. Formal mindfulness includes structured practices such as meditation and yoga. Informal practice is the performance of everyday activities mindfully. For example, you can wash the dishes as a chore, or you can perform the activity with a fuller sensory awareness of the scent of the soap, the temperature of the water, the sound of the clanking dishes, the sight of the bubbles, and the lingering taste in the mouth from having eaten. To cultivate this type of philosophical orientation in psychotherapy requires the therapist to practice mindfulness as well.

Mindfulness of the Therapist

Mindfulness therapists, scholars, and instructors are adamant that those wishing to instruct mindfulness must have an established and ongoing practice of mindfulness themselves (Saltzman and Goldin 2008; Segal et al. 2013). For example, the developers of mindfulness-based cognitive therapy (MBCT) recommend that aspiring teachers should first be a participant in an MBCT course and have a daily practice for at least 1 year before they begin to instruct the material. Practicing mindfulness provides a depth of experiential understanding of what it takes to commit to the practice (Segal et al. 2013) and work through roadblocks.

Developing a Mindfulness Practice

Given the centrality of a personal mindfulness practice for clinicians who wish to use mindfulness with patients, a few tips are offered on initiating one's own practice.

1. Enroll as a participant in a mindfulness-based stress reduction (MBSR) or MBCT class. These classes provide a structured and comprehensive approach to developing a practice. It is easier at first to practice in group settings.
2. If you are interested in yoga, it is helpful to locate a local center and start with classes designated for beginners. Consult with the staff if you are pregnant or have any medical conditions or injuries.
3. Choose a time of day when you can practice consistently.
4. If you are meditating and practicing yoga at home, create a special space where the only activity you perform there is meditation or yoga.
5. Put all electronics and phones on silent mode and kept out of view unless you are using them for a guided video practice (in which case all notifications should be turned off).

6. Similarly, inform all family members or roommates that you are entering into practice and are not to be disturbed. Work with your family on any child care needs so you are not interrupted during your practice time. Pets also may like to join in on yoga time; you can choose to include them or not.
7. Remember to bring mindfulness into your everyday activities and relationships.

For the reader interested in definitions of specific mindfulness practices and their application, Table 13–1 provides a brief overview.

Empirical Support

Mindfulness has been investigated for decades in adult populations, and researchers have recently shifted toward identifying mediating variables in MBSR and MBCT (Gu et al. 2015). In their recent review, Gu et al. (2015) identified cognitive and emotional reactivity, mindfulness, rumination, and worry as mechanisms in mindfulness-based interventions. For clinical outcomes, they identified mindfulness, rumination, and worry as significant mediators. These findings bear relevance for working with youth exposed to trauma, considering the role of reactivity, rumination, and worry in this population. Early results with youth suggest that mindfulness-based interventions are "feasible, beneficial, and well-accepted by youth" (Perry-Parrish et al. 2016, p. 174). In a recent review, Perry-Parrish and colleagues (2016) reported positive outcomes across broad domains, including reduction in elevated blood pressure; improved attention and executive function; and improvements across interpersonal functioning, self-awareness, anxiety, depression, coping, somatization, self-hostility, posttraumatic stress symptoms, and global psychiatric functioning.

Stress and Trauma

Exposure to stress and varying degrees of trauma is an inevitable part of human experience. For instance, at some point, all human beings experience loss, sickness, death, and challenging emotions such as despair, intense sadness, or anxiety. Human history and the contemporary world have no shortages of war, disease, hunger, natural disasters, and devastating forms of human abuses. Despite these significant adversities, there are always some individuals who survive without eventually developing posttraumatic stress disorder, whereas others do not (van der Kolk et al. 1996).

TABLE 13–1.   Mindfulness practices and applications

Practice	Description	Key applications, tips, and further reading
Awareness of breath (AOB)	AOB is a foundational mindfulness practice that holds the breath as the "anchor" or focus point of the meditation. Breathing always occurs in the present moment; therefore, it is the ideal anchor. AOB is performed seated, standing, or lying down for any duration of time: shorter period for novices, longer for more seasoned practitioners. Breathing through the nose is preferred over mouth breathing but is not necessary. The aim is to breathe completely through the lungs and the belly, utilizing the full capacity of the lungs to get oxygen moving through the body.	AOB is an essential practice to calm the nervous system. It helps to direct focus and attention and clear the mind. Long, slow, and deep breathing helps to create calm. For younger children, the use of "breathing buddies" (a stuffed animal) can be beneficial, as can other learning props as visuals. Attention can be directed using either hands on the sides of the ribs (feel the rib cage move with the breath) or one hand on belly and one hand on heart (breathe into these areas and move the hands with the breath to ensure appropriate depth of breathing). Further reading: "Anchor Breath: A Breathe Activity" in Cohen Harper 2015

TABLE 13–1. Mindfulness practices and applications *(continued)*

Practice	Description	Key applications, tips, and further reading
Body scan	Scanning the body directs the attention to move through the entire body.	Body scanning is helpful in overcoming a sense of disconnection and numbing from the physical body.
	Attention is paid to each system (e.g., digestive, respiratory) in the body and the five senses.	It can be useful for learning to sense where emotions, stress, and tension are held in the body.
	Body scanning can be performed in any physical position, but lying down is preferred.	It is beneficial to people struggling to accept their body as it is.
	It can be combined with AOB, and themes of gratitude for the body can be woven in.	Skillful application and preparatory work are advised for trauma survivors because of risk of traumatic memories emerging.
	It can also be performed during the final relaxation pose in yoga.	Use of developmentally appropriate language in describing anatomical parts is essential.
		Further reading: see Willard 2016
Mindful eating meditation	Mindful eating teaches the rediscovery of eating as a form of nourishment and sensual pleasure.	Mindful eating focuses on the five senses, using taste last in exploring the food object.
	It cultivates awareness of proper portion size.	Classically, it is taught with a raisin.
	It generates gratitude for ecology and sustainability and for food as a life force.	The clinician should consider culturally and developmentally appropriate food to use in introducing the practice.
	It teaches interconnectedness through realization of the logistics of food cultivation: from the sun, rain, oceans, farmers, ranchers, and those who produce the food that arrives on one's plate.	The clinician should encourage the patient to practice mindful eating at one meal daily.
	It increases awareness of nutrition, satiety, and how one feels after eating certain foods.	Mindful eating can also be practiced with beverages, such as decaffeinated herbal tea.
		Further reading: Saltzman and Goldin 2008; Willard 2016

TABLE 13–1.   Mindfulness practices and applications (continued)

Practice	Description	Key applications, tips, and further reading
Lovingkindness and compassion practices	Lovingkindness and compassion are highly effective and structured approaches for overcoming fear and cultivating healing emotions of love, forgiveness, kindness, and compassion. Skillful approaches begin with "objects" of meditation that are easiest to work with (when working on forgiveness, it is best to start with minor transgressions rather than major ones). These practices work to release toxic "energy," such as hatred, resentment, and envy, from the body. These practices can generate more positive emotions, relationships, and contentment, thus improving physical well-being and quality of life. They can be applied to oneself or others.	Caution in application is needed so as not to avoid deeper psychological healing work that is necessary. Skillful instruction needs to occur so as to avoid generating misunderstandings about forgiveness work (e.g., forgiveness is more about freeing oneself from unhelpful attachments to the perpetrator(s) or event rather than suggesting anything was OK about what happened). It is helpful to match the appropriate meditation to the appropriate situation and use adaptations for developmental stage and cultural relevancy, including religious and spiritual orientation. For younger children, the clinician may incorporate actual physical actions (e.g., acts of kindness to friends) or artwork to symbolize the individual persons included in the meditation for pre-abstract or concrete thinkers. Modify the language and instructional style to match the instructor's natural teaching style. Further reading: Saltzman and Goldin 2008

TABLE 13–1. Mindfulness practices and applications (*continued*)

Practice	Description	Key applications, tips, and further reading
Yoga movement	Yoga increases breath and body awareness, strength, concentration, and physical well-being.	Mindful yoga tends to be more intentional in movement, slower, and tailored to meet the needs of individual students.
	It teaches the connection between breathing and physiological states.	When developmentally adapted to use fun and relevant imagery, yoga is highly effective for engaging students.
	Different categories of yoga postures can be used to change the physical energy level.	Adaptations should be made for trauma survivors.
	Yoga can be used to overcome some mental, emotional, and physical challenges and limitations.	When working with youth, sequencing should be intentional to consider the role of sex, gender, and interpersonal dynamics in group settings.
	It can be used to build and strengthen a sense of community in groups.	The instructor should be trained and knowledgeable regarding safety and posture modifications and physical assists; physical assists should be used extremely cautiously with youth because of concerns regarding touch in therapy and school settings.

Note. For further reading, see Cohen Harper 2015.

Trauma is an experience that occurs when an individual or group is exposed to or directly experiences an extremely stressful event that threatens their life or safety. Trauma impacts people through symptoms that alter the physiological, psychological, existential, and spiritual domains of human beings. For example, the flight/fight/freeze response may be continuously ramped up unnecessarily, thus contributing to physiological dysregulation. Intrusiveness may impair focus, avoidance can impact normal activities, negative emotions can zap happiness, and hyperarousal can disturb relaxation. Life meaning and purpose can diminish, and a sense of connectedness to self, others, nature, and spirit or a higher power can diminish. Children and youth are particularly vulnerable because of the sensitivity of the developing brain and because of their physical vulnerability. At each developmental phase, there are central features and critical functions being developed that mindfulness and yoga practitioners should consider in tailoring interventions.

Mindfulness and Trauma Therapy

There are several strategies suggested by Tara Brach, a Buddhist psychologist and prominent mindfulness teacher, that therapists can use in a mindfulness-oriented therapy approach to trauma (Brach 2015). These strategies can be integrated into other treatment modalities, as described in the clinical vignette at the end of this section. The initiation of mindfulness-oriented therapy involves steps to provide the patient with resources. An important first step is for the therapist to establish a safe and caring relationship with the patient (Brach 2015). This relationship forms the foundation for the therapy journey. Brach suggests that this relationship serves as an important *outer refuge* for the patient. This means that therapists, through both their actual physical presence in the room and their more subtle, energetic therapeutic presence, can serve as a source of comfort and safety for patients as they progress through treatment.

An essential next step is to work with the patient on his or her ability to safely reconnect to and accept himself or herself (Brach 2015). Brach writes that it is through the therapist's authentic validation of the youth that the patient can learn to cultivate self-acceptance, which serves as a foundation of establishing an *inner refuge*, or the patient's own internal sense of safety, self-soothing, and connection to his or her innate goodness. Another essential ingredient is to "de-shame" the trauma. This involves working to heal the self-blame and self-hatred that may be connected to the trauma experience and that is further reinforced through negative self-talk over time. This is an essential aspect of trauma processing work. Youth may feel that they are responsible for having had something bad happen. For example, a youth exposed to domestic violence may feel that he or she could have done something more to protect the victimized parent. It is important to let the youth know that he or she did what he or she should have done in order to manage and survive the traumatic experience. Through this process, the youth can eventually learn to internalize the positive voice and presence of the therapist and build an inner refuge.

From a mindfulness perspective, the establishment of inner refuge essentially involves the youth having the experience of a reawakening of the natural loving state of his or her own heart (Brach 2015). This awakening can be developed through mindfulness practices such as *lovingkindness*, which is a meditative strategy to deliberately train self-compassion and overcome fear and worry. Other strategies for developing the ability to self-soothe and self-regulate include guided visualizations focused on the cultivation of lovingkindness, self-compassion, and acceptance. For example, when fear is present, the youth can visualize loved ones who represent safety and strength. Visualizing these loved ones is a process of calling forward one's "helpers." These helpers can be evoked during difficult moments. For example, working through challenging affect and trauma processing, the youth can invoke the helpers to help him or her stay connected to the affect and trauma processing. Youth may think of loving family members or friends or familiar characters such as superheroes as helpers.

Similarly, "safe places" can be imagined and evoked. In my work with youth, some safe places that patients have thought of include favorite neighborhood parks, lakes, and summer vacation spots. It is helpful to work directly with youth on learning how to evoke these images (Brach 2015). The therapist can guide youth to visit this place in their mind and report on what they see, hear, touch, smell, and taste (if applicable). The youth could even produce an art piece visualizing this location. A last example would be the use of memories of times when the youth was successful and strong in a specific situation. Working with these memories helps to cultivate the mindfulness foundation of self-trust and self-reliance. The youth can see how he or she has had positive experiences of mastery and effectiveness. The therapist can point out the moments in therapy in which the patient is demonstrating progress and mastering these resourcing practices and working through scary and difficult emotions and content with bravery.

The following vignette illustrates how these types of techniques can be integrated into trauma therapy with a teenager who tended to "check out" or dissociate during trauma processing work.

Clinical Vignette

Mary is a 14-year-old female referred by a parent for trauma therapy after the tragic death of her younger sibling. Mary was not convinced that therapy was useful for her but agreed to give it a try, mostly to please her parents. Considerable work had been undertaken to prepare Mary for processing the trauma narrative. The primary treatment approach being used was trauma-focused cognitive-behavioral therapy. Mary had completed psychoeducation related to traumatic grief, exercises in stress reduction, and relaxation training, as well as affect identification, expression, and modulation. Mary was able to complete a written trauma narrative. However, when it came time in the therapy to read the narrative to the therapist and work with it in more detail, Mary would shut down. She looked away, covered her face with her hair, moved slowly side to side in her swivel chair, and was unresponsive to the therapist's attempts to engage with her. The therapist, relying on his own mindfulness practice and training, thought to ask Mary if she would be willing to try an exercise that might help her. Mary agreed.

The therapist asked Mary to look around the office and tell him five different things she saw, then four things, then three, all the way to one. Then he asked if she could tell him different things she heard, then four, again all the way to one. Mary was able to successfully complete this exercise. She enjoyed the challenge of having to identify unique objects of focus throughout the practice. It was through the process of connecting to her sensory experience, in the present moment, in the immediate physical environment, that she was able to pull herself back from her state of disconnection and was able to recenter herself and come back to a state of self-regulation. She even smiled and laughed during the exercise because she found it difficult to name novel things and not repeat herself.

Several of the foundations discussed earlier are present in this vignette. The exercise required Mary to shift her awareness to the external, present moment context and to be a curious observer of her surrounding environment in very specific ways in order to identify novel sights, sounds, and objects. This essentially was a variation of a seeing and hearing sensory meditation. A major difference was that Mary was asked to communicate her observations in the moment to the therapist, which also helped to reestablish the therapy relationship in the moment. The therapist embodied several characteristics of a mindful practitioner in this therapy moment, remaining centered, patient, compassionate, nonjudgmental, and nonanalytical toward Mary and her experience. The therapist was also able to not get caught in striving toward meeting therapy objectives and pushing the patient forward. Rather, he was able to let go, come back to his own breathing, and join Mary where she was in the moment.

Mindfulness for Youth

In the book *Growing Up Mindful*, Christopher Willard, a leading scholar in the field, suggests several recommendations on teaching mindfulness to youth (Willard 2016). Consistent with the discussion of trauma work in the previous section, Willard discusses the importance of establishing a strong relationship between teacher and student or between therapist and child. The relationship should be developed before the therapist even begins to introduce mindfulness practices. Care and attention must be used in constructing an authentic, positive, and trusting relationship. Therapists, particularly those working in time-limited settings, may feel rushed to start mindfulness. However, Willard suggests that moving too quickly may lead to resistance. Even more care to build a trusting relationship must be taken in trauma therapy. When resistance arises, Willard notes, it may be symptomatic of moving too quickly and not establishing a trusting relationship. In more challenging cases, the foundation of the therapist's own mindfulness practice is critical in remembering to pause, self-reflect, take a step back, and reexamine the relationship to determine how to move forward.

After establishment of a strong therapeutic relationship, Willard (2016) suggests that the practitioner engage in critical self-reflection to clarify what the real teaching or intervention agenda is. Often, he points out, this agenda has something to do with changing the child. The risk here is the unintentional communication to the child that there is something undesirable about him or her. This is a pitfall that can quickly arise in the context of school-based settings, where there is a lot of pressure to achieve outcomes and the teacher or clinician may be asked to justify diverting valuable instruction time toward mindfulness in place of academics. Propounding this issue is the likelihood that children are also simultaneously getting this type of treatment at home or elsewhere. Mindfulness practice is a safe space and should be set up in such a way that the child perceives it as a safe harbor from negativity and judgment. Again, having a strong foundation in mindfulness practice can alleviate the practitioner's worries about satisfying the demands of the system because of the trust developed in the practice itself.

Willard's (2016) third teaching is to use the wisdom gleaned from the relationship with the child to customize mindfulness toward the child's specific interests and strengths. If the child enjoys sports, incorporate athletic movements in yoga practice. If the child is engaged with the expressive arts, use colorful mandalas or clay to connect to the five senses. If the child is music oriented, he or she can play the drum to generate a rhythmic beat and focus his or her attention. Different learning styles can be accommodated, and the therapist should consider adaptations that may be appropriate for trauma-related cues that could be activated by any of the above activities and techniques. Of course, when using such cues in trauma treatment, the therapist should do so only after proper preparation.

Last, if the child is harder to engage, then use relevant positive role models with whom the youth can engage (Willard 2016). It is helpful to find culturally relevant examples of aspirational figures who participate in mindfulness, yoga, or other contemplative practices whom the youth will be excited about. For younger children, this involves using characters from television shows, books, or games. For older children, adolescents, and transitional-age youth (TAY), search the Internet to discover professional athletes and celebrities who practice yoga and meditation. A simple Internet search demonstrates that there is no shortage of celebrity examples. Table 13–2 summarizes key points regarding developmental applications of mindfulness.

Preschoolers

Preschoolers, or children between ages 3 and 6 years, are in the midst of an exciting time of psychological, emotional, and physical development (Davies 2011). The central features of development include play and a more logical and realistic view of reality, as opposed to the egocentricity and magical thinking that typified earlier development. These children's increased prosocial interactions and observations of adults will help them begin to develop empathy and perspective taking. The children are learning to communicate more of their attachment needs verbally. They are continuing to develop essential skills in the areas of social functioning and self-regulation, as well as a movement toward the development of a more complex sense of self and morality. Much can be written about all of these areas, and mindfulness interventions must be tailored to match each child's abilities.

One example of effective mindfulness intervention for preschoolers is a recent study of a mindfulness intervention for economically disadvantaged preschoolers. In a mixed-methods pilot randomized controlled trial, researchers evaluated a 12-week mindfulness intervention based on the Kindness Curriculum pioneered by the Center for Investigating Healthy Minds (Poehlmann-Tynan et al. 2016). The central features of this curriculum were breath and movement exercises; music; reading developmentally appropriate materials about kindness and caring; and activities centered on

TABLE 13–2. Developmental adaptations of mindfulness and yoga practice

Developmental age	Suggested adaptations
Preschoolers	Create a vibrant and fun classroom environment with short mindfulness and yoga practices.
	Assess the abilities of the child or group to determine appropriate length of practices.
	Animate the practices by using fun imagery, music, stories, and animal yoga poses with noises.
	Include instructional materials that use the five senses.
	Emphasize movement and kinesthetic practices over seated, stationary, meditation-type exercises.
	Try to include caregivers.
Middle childhood/ school age	Engage youth through movement.
	Increase practice time appropriately.
	Begin to initiate discussions on emotions to promote self-regulation capacities (Davies 2011).
	Initiate learning about empathy and create positive peer interactions to promote self-efficacy and self-esteem (Davies 2011).
	Use a meditation bell to teach present-moment sensory awareness.
Mature school-age youth, adolescents, and transitional-age youth	Invite students to practice and give them a choice in how they will participate.
	Consider the gender makeup and identities of the students, their continuing development of sexuality and romantic partnerships (Sanders 2013), and ways to adapt the physical classroom and exercises for physical and emotional safety.
	Match the practices to suit the needs of the youth.
	Consider peer groups and their impact on engagement.
	Promote learning of perspective-taking skills (Sanders 2013).
	Include positive decision making and positive peer interactions.

Note. For further reading on these adaptations in preschoolers, see Cohen Harper (2013); for adaptations for middle childhood and older, see Willard and Saltzman (2015); and for suggestions on engaging youth, see Willard (2016).

teaching emotional awareness, sharing, and kindness. The researchers suggested that mindfulness participation was linked to significant increases in attentional focus. Mindfulness students also outperformed control subjects on self-regulation skill enhancements at postintervention and maintained this performance at a 3-month follow-up. Interestingly, no changes in empathy or compassion were found in either group. However, it was noted that mentorship received by the control subjects might have boosted their empathy and compassion enough to wash out intervention group gains. The researchers also thought that the mindfulness dosage was too low.

Instructor interviews and classroom observations suggested that movement-based activities were the most engaging for the preschoolers (Poehlmann-Tynan et al. 2016) and that verbal instruction led to disengagement. The instruction was enhanced by use of breathing props, and the most engaging practice was "animal yoga." It was also suggested that mindfulness delivered after outdoor time enhances positive participation and that developmental adaptations are necessary to ensure that the curriculum matches the capabilities of the students.

School-Age Youth

School-age youth (middle childhood, age 6–12 years) experience a sensitive period of development in which they are refining motor skills and are gradually developing physically; in the brain, development of the frontal lobe of the cerebral cortex is accelerated (Davies 2011). For example, myelination is under way within the corpus callosum and subcortical regions, thus enhancing bilateral brain hemisphere communication (Mah and Ford-Jones 2012). Simultaneously, adaptive changes are also occurring in the cortical gray matter. As age increases, motor coordination and movement become more precise and brain function more efficient. Children are moving toward the concrete operational stage of cognitive development; are becoming less egocentric; and are beginning to develop morality, a social sense of self, and self-worth (Davies 2011). In healthy development, there is a budding sense of competence, which is associated with several positive learning outcomes. Disruptions in healthy development at this stage can stifle engagement and achievement. Researchers have also demonstrated the importance of the environment and nurturance to foster optimal brain development.

For example, in a longitudinal cohort investigation of child and adolescent brain development, researchers discovered a link between poverty and structural differences in brain regions tied to school readiness skills, with results being worse for the poorest children (Hair et al. 2015). Findings such as these point to a need for interventions that promote healthy brain development. Early research of a mindfulness intervention in adult brains demonstrated a connection between mindfulness practice and enhanced brain development in critical learning areas (Hölzel et al. 2011). Researchers need to use experimentation to determine if mindfulness can stave off the adverse effects of poverty and promote school readiness. Hair and colleagues' (2015) study also suggested the importance of extending interventions beyond the child to families and systems approaches. Poverty is a complicated factor to address in treatment, but one can wonder about the possibilities of creating a more compassionate society characterized by increased generosity to those in need of resources.

Following from these developmental considerations, mindfulness- and yoga-based approaches can be tailored to this age group by using activities that target the functions specified above. Three key points to consider in working with school-age youth are their level of affective and cognitive development, their existing capacity for attention, and interdependence within the family (Knowles et al. 2015).

Researchers have targeted this age group effectively. For example, in a study of 100 Canadian fourth and fifth graders who were taught 12 weekly (40–50 minute) lessons from the MindUp social and emotional learning (SEL) program (Schonert-Reichl et al. 2015), mindfulness students reported fewer symptoms of depression and peer-rated aggression. They also were scored higher by their peers on prosocial metrics and garnered more peer acceptance than control subjects in a social responsibility program. Further, mindfulness students outperformed the comparison group in cognitive control and stress physiology, empathy, perspective taking, emotional control, optimism, school self-concept, and mindfulness. Schonert-Reichl and colleagues' finding on skills related to empathy and perspective is interesting because Poehlmann-Tynan et al. (2016) noted a lack of significant findings in this area for preschoolers. Certainly, we cannot be sure whether it is factors related to mindfulness dosage or curriculum or whether it is age and maturity that are linked to this finding.

Essential mindfulness adaptations and practices that were taught in the MindUp program included everyday instruction at 3-minute time intervals three times per day. These interventions included breathing and sound and sensory awareness practices that targeted executive function and self-regulation. Appropriate literature was used to instruct the children in SEL themes such as empathy and positive emotions. To make these lessons more accessible, researchers had the children engage in experiential activities of acts of kindness and community service. The researchers addressed environmental factors by transforming classroom ecology into value qualities such as "belonging, caring, collaboration, and understanding others" (Schonert-Reichl et al. 2015, p. 55). A strength of this approach is that teachers work to transfer the SEL and mindfulness skills to the entire school day and to promote internalization and behavioral externalization of learning. The results of this study, despite limitations in the study design and analysis that may have favored intervention group results, demonstrate the potential of mindfulness practices, when implemented strategically with SEL, in promoting positive development in middle childhood.

Adolescence and Transitional-Age Youth

The time between adolescence and transitional age—which occurs approximately in the second decade and the earlier part of the third decade of life—is an exciting and potentially tumultuous period of development (Meeus 2016). This period is marked by the youth's emerging personality and identity development (Meeus 2016) and critical brain changes (Siegel 2015). It can be a very challenging period of development for youth and their caregiver(s) because of the complex interaction of biological, social, and brain development factors. A central domain of development at this stage is sexuality. For example, the sexual organs begin to develop toward adult maturity in both females and males. Often, self-consciousness and emotional vulnerability come with changing bodies and challenging social networks.

Occurring in unison with the above physical changes, less obvious alterations are happening in the brain. For instance, powerful neurobiological changes are occurring in the dopamine-related circuitry of the brain (Siegel 2015). This dopamine increase may drive adolescents toward euphoric and dangerous activities. Because of the intensity with which the teenage brain seeks reward, there is a risk for an increase in impulsivity, addiction, and hyperrationality, which is essentially another term for concrete thinking. This potentially dangerous form of tunnel vision comes at the expense of the teenager being able to think "big picture" and results from the minimizing of risk and glorification of potential rewards. Development is even more complicated considering the central role that friendships and social status play in the teenager's life.

Mindfulness- and yoga-based strategies can be used to potentially balance out the intensity of these developmental changes and to be a path toward greater self-esteem, self-reliance, acceptance, and stress management. Further, mindfulness and yoga can promote healthy decision making and successful navigation of academic and social pressures and challenges.

Like younger-age youth, teenagers can be successfully engaged in mindfulness and yoga by tailoring the instruction more specifically to the needs and interests of the individual teenager or by creating safe and engaging groups in which teenagers with similar needs are brought together. Given the sensitivity and self-consciousness teenagers may be feeling concerning their bodies, adaptations to mindfulness and yoga practices need to be made. One such adaptation may be consideration of the gender makeup and gender identities of the students. Because of physical and emotional safety reasons, females may feel safer in classes that do not include their male peers. For instance, females may not want males behind them in yoga practice because some postures have physically vulnerable shapes that youth may sexualize (e.g., downward-facing dog, a posture in which the hands and feet are on the floor and the hips are elevated, like an upside-down V shape). Males may not like other males or females behind them either. Therefore, it may be advantageous in group settings to set up the room in such a way so that no youth is located behind another youth. This kind of adaptation to the physical practice space is also a strategy for working in a way that is sensitive to traumatized youth.

Another adaptation is to permit and encourage those youths who wish to leave their eyes open in practices to do so. A hallmark feature of trauma is hypervigilance. Even though hypervigilance is being described as a symptom here, it should be conceptualized as a critical survival mechanism to be not ameliorated but controlled. Traumatized youth may wish to position themselves so that they can scan the environment for threats and ensure their safety. With targeted clinical treatment, hypervigilance can be regulated and used skillfully by the youth. If the instructor does a sufficient job in creating a safe environment, it may be that hypervigilance resolves on its own through mindfulness practice.

Another subgroup of teens that may need to be engaged is athletes. For this group, a more vigorous, cardiovascular- and movement-based yoga practice may be more engaging. In addition, although it seems contrary to the philosophy of mindfulness and yoga, I have observed youth being more successfully engaged through yoga groups that have been designated as "competitive."

Numerous research studies suggest potential benefits of yoga with high school students. In a randomized controlled trial in a New York City high school, students in yoga classes who were reported to have greater participation demonstrated a significantly higher GPA (Hagins and Rundle 2016). Earlier studies found statistically significant differences between yoga participants and control subjects on anger control, fatigue, and inertia (Khalsa et al. 2012); other studies have found similar results with regard to mood (Noggle et al. 2012) and memory (Sarokte and Rao 2013; Verma et al. 2014). It is worth reiterating that there are not enough studies in this area. In addition, several studies were conducted in India, which may not generalize very well to youth in other countries or cultures.

Conclusion

Mindfulness and yoga are two emerging holistic approaches to promoting healthy development and addressing developmental trauma and distress in youth. A vital factor in the authentic and successful delivery of contemplative interventions for youth is the personal mindfulness practice of the therapist. By drawing from developmental psychology and mindfulness and yoga protocols, tailored approaches have been developed to address specific needs of youth across developmental stages. There is an abundance of well-deserved enthusiasm among mindfulness practitioners as implementation efforts continue to grow rapidly. This growth must be matched by efforts to advance rigorous evaluation of youth mindfulness and yoga programs.

KEY CONCEPTS

- An essential factor in mindfulness interventions, if not the most important factor, is the self-practice of the teacher or therapist.
- Mindfulness and yoga interventions can be tailored to meet developmental and cultural needs of the individual child.
- Trauma-informed approaches include making physical adaptations to the environment as well as ensuring personal physical and emotional safety.

Discussion Questions

1. How might mindfulness interventions differ across treatment settings?

2. What are specific and unique factors of mindfulness that may vary across cultures?

3. What are a few examples of different treatment contexts in which mindfulness interventions might not be effective?

Suggested Readings

Greco LA, Hayes SC (eds): Acceptance and Mindfulness Treatments for Children and Adolescents: A Practitioner's Guide. Oakland, CA, New Harbinger, 2008

Willard C: Growing Up Mindful: Essential Practices to Help Children, Teens, and Families Find Balance, Calm, and Resilience. Boulder, CO, Sounds True, 2016

Willard C, Saltzman A (eds): Teaching Mindfulness Skills to Kids and Teens. New York, Guilford, 2015

References

Brach T: Healing traumatic fear: the wings of mindfulness and love, in Mindfulness-Oriented Interventions for Trauma: Integrating Contemplative Practices. Edited by Follette V, Briere J, Rozelle D, et al. New York, Guilford, 2015, pp 31–42

Cohen Harper J: Little Flower Yoga for Kids: A Yoga and Mindfulness Program to Help Your Child Improve Attention and Emotional Balance. Oakland, CA, New Harbinger, 2013

Cohen Harper J: Yoga: reaching heart and mind through the body, in Teaching Mindfulness Skills to Kids and Teens. Edited by Willard C, Saltzman A. New York, Guilford, 2015, pp 179–194

Davies D: Child Development: A Practitioner's Guide, 3rd Edition. New York, Guilford, 2011

Gu J, Strauss C, Bond R, Cavanagh K: How do mindfulness-based cognitive therapy and mindfulness-based stress reduction improve mental health and well-being? A systematic review and meta-analysis of mediation studies. Clin Psychol Rev 37:1–12, 2015 25689576

Hagins M, Rundle A: Yoga improves academic performance in urban high school students compared to physical education: a randomized controlled trial. Mind Brain Educ 10(2):105–116, 2016

Hair NL, Hanson JL, Wolfe BL, et al: Association of child poverty, brain development, and academic achievement. JAMA Pediatr 169(9):822–829, 2015 26192216

Hölzel BK, Carmody J, Vangel M, et al: Mindfulness practice leads to increases in regional brain gray matter density. Psychiatry Res 191(1):36–43, 2011 21071182

Kabat-Zinn J: Full Catastrophe Living: Using the Wisdom of Your Body and Mind to Face Stress, Pain, and Illness. New York, Bantam, 2013

Khalsa SBS, Hickey-Schultz L, Cohen D, et al: Evaluation of the mental health benefits of yoga in a secondary school: a preliminary randomized controlled trial. J Behav Health Serv Res 39(1):80–90, 2012 21647811

Knowles L, Goodman M, Semple R: Mindfulness with elementary-school-age children, in Teaching Mindfulness Skills to Kids and Teens. Edited by Willard C, Saltzman A. New York, Guilford, 2015 pp 19–41

Mah VK, Ford-Jones EL: Spotlight on middle childhood: rejuvenating the 'forgotten years'. Paediatr Child Health 17(2):81–83, 2012 23372398

Meeus W: Adolescent psychosocial development: a review of longitudinal models and research. Dev Psychol 52(12):1969–1993, 2016 27893243

Noggle JJ, Steiner NJ, Minami T, et al: Benefits of yoga for psychosocial well-being in a US high school curriculum: a preliminary randomized controlled trial. J Dev Behav Pediatr 33(3):193–201, 2012 22343481

Perry-Parrish C, Copeland-Linder N, Webb L, et al: Mindfulness-based approaches for children and youth. Curr Probl Pediatr Adolesc Health Care 46(6):172–178, 2016 26968457

Poehlmann-Tynan J, Vigna AB, Weymouth LA, et al: A pilot study of contemplative practices with economically disadvantaged preschoolers: children's empathic and self-regulatory behaviors. Mindfulness 7(1):46–58, 2016

Saltzman A, Goldin P: Mindfulness-based stress reduction for school-age children, in Acceptance and Mindfulness Treatments for Children and Adolescents: A Practitioner's Guide. Edited by Greco L, Hayes S. Oakland, CA, New Harbinger, 2008, pp 139–161

Sanders RA: Adolescent psychosocial, social, and cognitive development. Pediatr Rev 34(8):354–358, quiz 358–359, 2013 23908362

Sarokte AS, Rao MV: Effects of Medhya Rasayana and Yogic practices in improvement of short-term memory among school-going children. Ayu 34(4):383–389, 2013 24695779

Schonert-Reichl KA, Oberle E, Lawlor MS, et al: Enhancing cognitive and social-emotional development through a simple-to-administer mindfulness-based school program for elementary school children: a randomized controlled trial. Dev Psychol 51(1):52–66, 2015 25546595

Segal Z, Williams JM, Teasdale J: Mindfulness-Based Cognitive Therapy for Depression, 2nd Edition. New York, Guilford, 2013

Siegel DJ: Brainstorm: The Power and Purpose of the Teenage Brain. New York, Penguin, 2015

van der Kolk BA, McFarlane AC, Weisaeth L: Traumatic Stress: The Effects of Overwhelming Experience on Mind, Body, and Society. New York, Guilford, 1996

Verma A, Shete SU, Thakur GS, et al: The effect of yoga practices on cognitive development in rural residential school children in India. National Journal of Laboratory Medicine 3(3):15–19, 2014

Willard C: Growing Up Mindful: Essential Practices to Help Children, Teens, and Families Find Balance, Calm, and Resilience. Oakland, CA, Sounds True, 2016

Willard C, Saltzman A: Teaching Mindfulness Skills to Kids and Teens. New York, Guilford, 2015

14

Psychopharmacology

Craig L. Donnelly, M.D.
Roy Lubit, M.D., Ph.D.
Antra Bami, M.D.

POSTTRAUMATIC STRESS DISORDER (PTSD) is a complicated condition to both diagnose and treat and involves multiple neurobiological systems influencing cognitive, affective, and behavioral domains of functioning. PTSD was not originally recognized as a disorder in childhood but was subsequently found to be common among youth by applying adult diagnostic criteria in child and adolescent populations. Epidemiological studies show a high prevalence of PTSD in children: about 13.4% of youth exposed to trauma will develop some posttraumatic symptoms (Copeland et al. 2007). One of the major revisions made in the *Diagnostic and Statistical Manual of Mental Disorders*, 5th Edition (DSM-5; American Psychiatric Association 2013) is the inclusion of a developmentally sensitive set of criteria for diagnosis that has been shown to yield approximately three to eight times more children qualifying for PTSD compared with DSM-IV (Scheeringa et al. 2012) as well as more precise target symptoms.

The clinical presentation of PTSD in childhood is extraordinarily heterogeneous, often with a bewildering array of symptoms. This is especially true for traumatic experiences that occur prior to or around the establishment of language in children, where trauma may be "encoded" in motor or emotional memories and may thus "prime" stress-related brain hypothalamic-pituitary-adrenal axis responsivity and other physiological responses that are elicited in the absence of language-based memory recall (Mylle and Maes 2004; Pfefferbaum 2005).

Although there has been a significant growth in the understanding and categorization of PTSD symptoms in children over the different iterations of DSM, there continues to be a dearth of empirical support in the pediatric treatment literature for any psychopharmacological treatment strategy. Therefore, many current medication treatments are extrapolated from adult psychopharmacological evidence or are based on regional standard of care and/or expert consensus.

Once an accurate diagnosis of PTSD has been made, target symptom clusters must be identified and stratified on the basis of severity and whether the individual is likely to be responsive to pharmacological interventions versus those needing psychotherapeutic interventions. Treatment choices are dependent on such factors as severity of symptoms (e.g., hallucinations, severe flashbacks or dissociation, nightmares), degree of functional impairment, acuity of symptom onset, degree of psychological distress associated with symptoms, and patient and family preference. Pharmacotherapy at times is warranted even in the absence of psychotherapy when symptoms are severe enough to impair functioning of the child or the child's capacity to engage in psychotherapy or when competent psychotherapy is unavailable. It should be noted that, just as in medication treatment, when psychotherapy is inexpertly applied or misapplied, it may be harmful to patients.

The approach to pharmacological treatment for PTSD is guided by the understanding of the neurobiology of trauma (Bremner et al. 1993; Charney et al. 1993; Langeland and Olff 2008). There is a delicate interplay of physiological systems, including the immune system, the neuroendocrine system, and the central nervous system (CNS), in regulating cognition, memory, and behavior, that is thought to be disrupted in PTSD (Asnis et al. 2004; De Bellis and Putnam 1994; Foa et al. 1999; Friedman and Southwick 1995; Stein et al. 2006; Yehuda 1998). Within the CNS, the primary mediators of stress response implicated in PTSD include the adrenergic, dopaminergic, serotonergic, γ-aminobutyric acid/benzodiazepine, opioid, and N-methyl D-aspartate (NMDA) neurotransmitters (Friedman and Southwick 1995). Understanding the effect of medications on these systems can help guide the appropriate pharmacological interventions. Furthermore, as demonstrated by Copeland and colleagues

(2007) in a study of 1,420 children ages 9–13 years, children exposed to trauma had almost double the rates of a comorbid psychiatric disorder than children who were not exposed to trauma. Therefore, it is common-place in treatment of PTSD to use several agents to target separate clusters of symptoms of PTSD and/or the accompanying comorbidities.

Serotonergic Agents

The neurotransmitter serotonin (5-hydroxytryptamine) is widely distrib-uted in the CNS and is an important neurotransmitter in psychiatric symptoms commonly associated with PTSD. These include aggression, obsessive or intrusive thoughts, alcohol and substance abuse, anxiety, de-pression, and suicidal behavior (Friedman 1990). Panic attacks, dissocia-tive episodes, and flashbacks appear to be related to serotonin function as well (Southwick et al. 1994), therefore making serotonin a key target for intervention.

The selective serotonin reuptake inhibitors (SSRI) sertraline and par-oxetine have U.S. Food and Drug Administration (FDA) indications for PTSD in adults (Brady et al. 2000; Marshall et al. 2001). In children, the SSRIs fluoxetine, sertraline, and fluvoxamine are approved for obsessive-compulsive disorder, and fluoxetine is also approved for depression. However, no SSRIs have FDA approval for use in children with PTSD be-cause evidence to strongly support their safety and efficacy in childhood is still lacking.

In a 24-week double-blind randomized placebo-controlled trial, Stod-dard et al. (2011) examined the ability of sertraline to prevent the onset of PTSD symptoms in 26 burn victims ages 6–20 years. Sertraline 25–150 mg/day was found to be somewhat more effective than placebo according to the parent reports, but the opposite was found in the child self-reports. Although the reason for the aberrant findings of the child report data re-mains unclear, it is important to keep in mind that a high placebo response rate appears to be more common in child and adolescent medication trials of CNS disorders such as depression and non-PTSD anxiety compared with adult trials (Bridge et al. 2009).

In a large multicenter double-blind randomized controlled trial by Robb et al. (2010), children ages 6–17 years who met DSM-IV criteria for PTSD from a variety of trauma exposures were administered sertraline 50–200 mg/day over a 10-week study period. The authors concluded that the treatment efficacy of sertraline was not superior to placebo in the treatment of PTSD in children and adolescents. Significantly, the positive results from adult trials may not be generalizable to childhood PTSD. A similar conclusion was drawn by Cohen et al. (2007), who examined sertraline 50–200 mg/day in a randomized clinical trial with 24 participants with PTSD ages 10–17 years old. They found comparable results for trauma-focused cognitive behavioral therapy (TF-CBT) plus sertraline versus TF-CBT plus placebo, with a statistically significant reduction in PTSD symptoms but no difference between the two groups.

Seedat et al. (2001) looked at use of citalopram 20 mg/day over a 12-week open-label trial in 8 patients ages 12–18 years with moderate to severe PTSD. The patients showed a 38% reduction in PTSD symptoms on the Clinician Administered PTSD Scale (CAPS); however, self-reported depressive symptoms did not improve. In another study, Seedat et al. (2002) used citalopram 20–40 mg/day in an 8-week open-label trial with 24 children and adolescents and 14 adults to compare outcomes in the two groups. The CAPS and Clinical Global Impressions–Severity (CGI-S) scores at endpoint showed a significant reduction in mean scores in both groups, indicating improvement in core symptoms of PTSD, but no difference was found in outcomes between groups.

Despite these data, in clinical practice, SSRIs appear to be generally safe, broad-spectrum agents and are therefore widely used off label in children with PTSD because many of these children exhibit symptoms associated with serotonergic dysregulation such as anxiety, depression, obsessional thinking, compulsive behaviors, aggression, and alcohol or substance abuse (Friedman 1990).

Common side effects seen in these studies were gastrointestinal symptoms, behavioral activation, epistaxis, headache, and akathisia, but in general these medications are well tolerated and safe. However, it should be noted that there is a black box warning regarding increased suicidal ideation and behavior in children treated with SSRIs based on studies of these agents with depression. Treatment should proceed with adequate safety monitoring in place, especially in the early months of treatment.

Other serotonergic agents are used more rarely for treating PTSD in children, including tricyclic antidepressants (imipramine, nortriptyline) and the serotonin-norepinephrine reuptake inhibitor venlafaxine. Robert et al. (1999) reported on the use of low-dose imipramine (1 mg/kg) to treat symptoms of acute stress disorder in children with burn injuries, particularly flashback-related sleep maintenance and insomnia. However, Robert and colleagues (2008) demonstrated that placebo was just as effective as fluoxetine or imipramine in children and adolescents when used for acute stress disorder. Venlafaxine was found to have good efficacy and safety in short-term treatment of PTSD when compared with placebo (Davidson et al. 2006).

Nefazodone, a 5HT type 2 receptor antagonist that was studied by Domon and Andersen (2000) in an open-label trial with adolescents with PTSD, was found to be particularly effective in reducing symptoms of hyperarousal, anger, aggression, insomnia, and concentration. However, nefazadone is rarely used in children and adolescents because of an FDA black box warning about the potential for developing hepatic failure.

Alpha Agonists

The catecholamines norepinephrine, epinephrine, and dopamine are involved in sympathetic arousal, anxiety, frontal lobe activation, mood regulation, reward dependence, working memory, and affect thinking and perceiving as well as behavioral arousal. Adrenergic agents such as the α_2 agonists clonidine and guanfacine, the α_1 antagonist prazosin, and the β antagonist propranolol have been shown to reduce sympathetic arousal, which is associated with the fight/flight/freeze reaction in mammals, a common reaction to trauma or threat. These medications may be effective in the treatment of hyperarousal, impulsivity, behavioral activation, sleep problems, and nightmares associated with PTSD (Akinsanya et al. 2017; De Bellis and Putnam 1994; Langeland and Olff 2008).

In an open-label trial of 17 children with severe chronic PTSD (13 male, 4 female; mean age 10.4, range 6.0–14.2) relatively low doses of clonidine (0.05–0.10 mg two times daily) were found to provide significant improvement in anxiety, arousal, concentration, mood, and behavioral impulsivity (Perry 1994). Harmon and Riggs (1996) reported that the use of a clonidine transdermal patch effectively reduced PTSD symptoms in all 7 patients (preschoolers, ages 3–6 years, who had severe physical and/or sexual abuse and neglect) in their open-label trial. In a single case study, Horrigan and Barnhill (1996) reported the effectiveness of guanfacine, an α-adrenergic agent, in reducing PTSD-associated nightmares in a 7-year-old child who had been exposed to extreme levels of domestic violence and physical abuse at the hand of her father. Both clonidine and guanfacine are commonly used, relatively safe agents and may be a first consideration for treatment of youth with PTSD.

In an uncontrolled A-B-A design study, Famularo et al. (1988) found that propranolol 2.5 mg/kg/day significantly reduced PTSD symptoms over the 5 weeks of treatment in 8 of 11 children with physical, sexual, or both types of abuse. Intrusion and arousal symptoms appeared to be the most responsive. In a single case study, Brkanac et al. (2003) noted that prazosin 4 mg nightly caused a cessation of nightmares and global clinical improvement in a 15-year-old adolescent with PTSD. In a systematic review of prazosin 1–4 mg nightly in children and adolescents, Akinsanya et al. (2017) identified 6 case reports of children 7–16 years who showed marked improvement in nightmares, hyperarousal, and intrusive symptoms of PTSD. In three of the cases, discontinuation of prazosin resulted in increased intensity and frequency of PTSD-associated nightmares in children and adolescents who had reported remission of these nightmares while taking prazosin.

In adults, both clonidine and propranolol also have demonstrated success in treating PTSD symptoms such as nightmares, insomnia, and hyper-startle as well as intrusive memories and general hyperarousal. Reduction of CNS adrenergic tone through use of these agents to target reexperiencing and hyperarousal symptoms is a rational treatment strategy. Additionally, the α_2-adrenergic agents may be more effective than the psychostimulants for symptoms of attention-deficit/hyperactivity disorder (ADHD) in maltreated or sexually abused children with PTSD because they exert a "dampening down" effect on noradrenergic-mediated arousal symptoms (De Bellis and Putnam 1994). This presynaptic autoreceptor decrease in noradrenergic tone is in addition to the ADHD-beneficial effect by enhancing noradrenergic tone through stimulating postsynaptic α_2 receptors. De Bellis' group hypothesized that α_2 presynaptic receptor blockade, such as provided by clonidine or guanfacine, may modulate or reduce noradrenergic tone in the locus coeruleus—an activation center for arousal—and thus reduce PTSD symptoms of hyperarousal, in addition to treating ADHD symptoms. Stimulants, unlike the α agonists approved for ADHD treatment, lack this property.

Dopaminergic Agents

There have been several reports in the literature regarding use of dopamine-blocking agents for symptoms of PTSD in youth. Horrigan and Barnhill (1999) conducted an open-label trial using risperidone in 18 boys (mean age 9.28 years) in residential treatment for PTSD and significant comorbid psychiatric disorders (83% of the children were diagnosed with ADHD and 35% with bipolar disorder). They found that 13 of the boys experienced a remission of PTSD symptoms with risperidone. Meighen and colleagues (2007) reported a case series of three very young children (ages 2–3) diagnosed with acute stress disorder who were treated with risperidone. They found a significant reduction in hyperarousal, reexperiencing, and dissociative symptoms as well as an improvement in emotional responsiveness. In a case report of a 13-year-old boy with chronic PTSD related to sexual abuse and neglect, Keeshin and Strawn (2009) reported significant improvement of PTSD symptoms (decreased intrusive and hyperarousal symptoms) with adjunctive use of risperidone, although his treatment was complicated by transient hyperprolactinemia.

Stathis et al. (2005) reported the effectiveness of quetiapine 50–200 mg/ day in a 6-week case series of six adolescents 15–17 years old who met criteria for PTSD in a youth detention center. They found significant reduction in overall PTSD symptoms and a reduction in dissociation, anxiety, depression, and anger using the Trauma Symptom Checklist for Children. Clozapine (mean daily dose 102 mg/day) was reported to reduce polypharmacy with mood stabilizers and antidepressants in a residential population of adolescents with diagnosis of bipolar affective disorder, intermittent explosive disorder, and PTSD (Kant et al. 2004). In a case series of six adolescent males with treatment-resistant chronic PTSD and psychotic symptoms, clozapine 400–800 mg/day led to an overall improvement in psychiatric symptoms by clinician rating and self-report and behavioral presentation in four of the six adolescents treated (Wheatley et al. 2004).

Given the significant side-effect profile of atypical dopaminergic-blocking neuroleptics and scant evidence as to their utility in PTSD, these agents should be reserved for only the most debilitating cases when other agents have failed or when symptoms of paranoid behavior, parahallucinatory phenomena, intense flashbacks, self-destructive behavior, explosive or overwhelming anger, psychotic symptoms, severe self-mutilation, or aggressiveness are limiting recovery.

Miscellaneous Medications in the Treatment of Pediatric PTSD

Trauma exposure may induce sensitization or initiate kindling phenomena in limbic nuclei in the human CNS. A number of successful open-label trials have been conducted with anti-kindling/anticonvulsive agents with adult PTSD patients. As used in psychiatry to target affective disorders, lithium, carbamazepine, and divalproex sodium may also reduce extreme mood lability and anger dyscontrol found in PTSD.

Looff et al. (1995) reported on the use of carbamazepine 300–1,200 mg/ day (serum levels 10–11.5 µg/mL) in 28 children and adolescents with sexual abuse histories, half of whom had comorbid ADHD, depression, oppositional defiant disorder (ODD), or polysubstance abuse and were treated with concomitant medications such as methylphenidate, clonidine, sertraline, fluoxetine, or imipramine. By treatment end, 22 of 28 patients were free of PTSD symptoms. The remaining 6 improved significantly in all PTSD symptoms except abuse-related nightmares.

Anticonvulsants are commonly used in children and adolescents with seizure disorders or severe mood instability such as seen in bipolar disorder. These medications may be a useful intervention for debilitating avoidance or numbing, hyperarousal, and sleep dysregulation in children with PTSD or when overwhelming anger and aggressive explosiveness predominate. Steiner et al. (2007) conducted a randomized controlled trial comparing high-dose divalproex sodium (500–1,500 mg/day) with low-dose divalproex sodium (250 mg/day) in 12 juvenile offenders (ages unclear) with conduct disorder and PTSD. The high-dose divalproex sodium group had significantly greater reduction in intrusion and avoidance symptoms compared with the low-dose group.

There are several double-blind, placebo-controlled trials evaluating use of topiramate as monotherapy as well as adjunctive treatment for PTSD in adults, with some positive data (Tucker et al. 2007; Yeh et al. 2011). However, there are no clinical trials to date examining the efficacy of topiramate in the pediatric population.

The brain areas that are involved in the stress response also mediate motor behavior, affect regulation, arousal, sleep, startle response, attention, and cardiovascular function. Hence, it is not unusual for traumatized children, particularly those exposed to chronic trauma such as maltreatment, to exhibit a constellation of anxiety affective symptoms plus ADHD and other disruptive behavior symptoms. Some clinicians will consider the use of α agonists in these situations, hoping to avoid stimulant-induced potential exacerbation of anxiety and PTSD. Anecdotal experience suggests that many traumatized children have favorable responses to α agonists as well as to psychostimulants such as methylphenidate or dextroamphetamine. The symptoms best targeted are hyperactivity, impulse dyscontrol, and attention impairment. Bupropion is often considered a second-line agent for ADHD symptoms and may be a useful agent when affect dysregulation or depressed mood co-occurs with ADHD symptoms in children with PTSD (Daviss 1999).

It is important to remember that there is not necessarily a one-to-one correspondence between pharmacological effect and neurotransmitter system. For example, SSRIs may effectively reduce PTSD-related symptoms that are not essentially serotonergic in nature, owing to the complex interrelations between neurobiological systems. Much work remains to be done to identify which medications in which patients for which PTSD symptom constellations are indicated as first-line treatments.

In adults, benzodiazepines such as alprazolam have been shown to increase the risk of consolidating or worsening PTSD, perhaps by interfering with extinction of the fear memories or by impairing new learning (Rothbaum et al. 2014). However, benzodiazepines also carry risks of abuse and can cause paradoxical reactions in children and generally should be avoided in the treatment of PTSD in youth.

Using medications affecting memory to enhance TF-CBT is a rational strategy for treating PTSD in youth. Medications have been used to augment psychotherapy in three ways: by decreasing distressing symptoms and making it easier for the victim to speak about the trauma, by enhancing extinction learning during exposure therapy, and by blocking (negative) memory reconsolidation after reactivation of traumatic memories during therapy.

Extinguishing the exaggerated fear response via narrative creation during TF-CBT involves new learning. D-cycloserine, a partial NMDA agonist that may enhance learning, has been found to facilitate TF-CBT when given 90 minutes prior to virtual reality exposure in short-term therapy but not when used chronically (Rothbaum et al. 2014).

Antihistaminergic agents such as diphenhydramine or hydroxyzine and the complex antihistaminergic/antiserotonergic agent cyproheptadine have been reported anecdotally to exert anxiolytic and sleep-promoting effects in children with PTSD-related anxiety and sleep onset problems. Whether they have a role to play in primary treatment of PTSD symptoms or enhancing the effect of TF-CBT remains an open question.

Conclusion

Skills-based psychotherapy has more robust efficacy data than medication in the treatment of PTSD in children and adolescents (Keeshin and Strawn 2014). There are many gaps in the current state of knowledge about the psychopharmacology of pediatric PTSD. Empirical evidence is not systematic and is scant. Clinicians should take a rational approach when choosing pharmacological treatment of pediatric PTSD based on a convergence of evidence from the adult and child/adolescent literature as well as an understanding of the basic neurobiological mechanisms of the pharmacological agents and their impact on target symptoms.

When selecting pharmacological agents for pediatric PTSD, it is helpful to work stepwise, beginning with an accurate diagnosis of PTSD or subsyndromal PTSD symptoms that are significantly debilitating. Second, comorbid conditions such as depression, ADHD, ODD, anxiety, or attachment disorder must be identified. Third, clinicians must identify the target symptoms for treatment and specify reasonable treatment goals (e.g., reduction in sleep latency, frequency of nightmares, or avoidance behavior). Fourth, selection of therapeutics entails segregation of targets for psychosocial (e.g., TF-CBT) versus biological (e.g., pharmacological) intervention. These will often overlap. Both psychoeducation and TF-CBT should usually be in place before consideration is given to pharmacotherapy. Ideally, TF-CBT, including narrative exposure, skills, and trauma processing, is used in individual or group treatment, often in combination with family-oriented support or psychodynamically based interventions. Parents may need their own individual treatment as well.

Medications are unlikely to be effective in settings where trauma exposure or abuse is ongoing in the life of a child or when there is no framework in place for dealing with the aftermath of traumatic experiences. Unfocused, loosely conceived psychotherapy is to be avoided because it can inadvertently act to retraumatize and can be harmful. Pharmacological intervention can be used to facilitate psychotherapy by decreasing hyperarousal and avoidance. Medication intervention should be considered early in the treatment process when severe and debilitating symptoms are present that are limiting function or interfering with therapy.

When selecting pharmacological interventions in pediatric PTSD, the most debilitating symptoms should be treated first, balanced with a weighing of the symptoms most likely to be responsive to pharmacotherapy. Reduction in even one symptom (e.g., insomnia) may provide significant relief and improvement in overall functioning. Targeted multipharmacotherapy should be used when necessary.

As a general approach, treatment should begin with a broad-spectrum agent such as an SSRI, which covers symptoms of affect dysregulation, panic, comorbid depression, and anxiety. SSRIs are the only agents that appear to be consistently effective for avoidance, numbing, and dissociation symptoms. If ADHD symptoms are also present, the adjunctive use of a stimulant, an α agonist, or the antidepressant bupropion should be considered. The α agonists clonidine and guanfacine and the β antagonist propranolol, as well as the tricyclic antidepressant imipramine and the antihistamine cyproheptadine, should be considered if insomnia, hyperstartle, or hyperarousal symptoms are problematic.

In cases of SSRI nonresponse, consideration should be given to using venlafaxine or duloxetine because these serotonin-norepinephrine reuptake inhibitors have some consensus support for their use and appear to be relatively safe (but note the black box warning for suicidality). Dopaminergic agents such as risperidone, aripiprazole, or quetiapine should be reserved for severe cases of PTSD in which aggression, hallucinations, or severe mood instability are present. Inevitably, more effective pharmacological interventions will be identified as systematic clinical trials are undertaken in children and adolescents with PTSD.

KEY CONCEPTS

- DSM-5 has expanded PTSD criteria to better fit younger children.
- PTSD presentations in youth are exceedingly variable and often have complex comorbidities.
- PTSD symptoms should be clearly delineated; separation of target symptoms appropriate for psychotherapy versus psychopharmacology is essential for successful treatment.
- The best evidence for PTSD treatment in youth is for trauma-focused cognitive-behavioral therapy, and medication should not be viewed as a replacement for skills-based therapy.
- Selective serotonin reuptake inhibitors and serotonin-norepinephrine reuptake inhibitors are broad-spectrum agents but have at best low efficacy. These medications should be used with care to reduce symptoms, to facilitate therapy and social engagement, and to reduce avoidance.
- Clonidine and guanfacine are often considered first in treating hyperarousal symptoms in youth with PTSD.
- D-cycloserine, which improves memory, may enhance extinction learning from TF-CBT.

Discussion Questions

1. What are the first and second medication considerations for PTSD in youth and what risks do they carry?

2. What place do antipsychotics, mood stabilizers, and benzodiazepines have in the treatment of PTSD in youth?

3. How can medications be helpful in children as augmenting agents for therapy or to help abort the development of PTSD?

Suggested Readings

Beckers T, Kindt M: Memory reconsolidation interference as an emerging treatment for emotional disorders: strengths, limitations, challenges, and opportunities. Annu Rev Clin Psychol 13:99–121, 2017 28375725

Birur B, Math SB, Fargason RE: A review of psychopharmacological interventions post-disaster to prevent psychiatric sequelae. Psychopharmacol Bull 47(1):8–26, 2017 28138200

Donnelly C: Psychopharmacology for children and adolescents, in Effective Treatments for PTSD, 2nd Edition. Edited by Foa EB, Deane TM, Friedman MJ, Cohen JA. New York, Guilford, 2008, pp 687–704

Hruska B, Cullen PK, Delahanty DL: Pharmacological modulation of acute trauma memories to prevent PTSD: considerations from a developmental perspective. Neurobiol Learn Mem 112:122–129, 2014 24513176

Wilkinson JM, Carrion VG: Pharmacotherapy in pediatric PTSD: a developmentally focused review of the evidence. Curr Psychopharmacol 1(3): 252–270, 2012

References

Akinsanya A, Marwaha R, Tampi RR: Prazosin in children and adolescents with posttraumatic stress disorder who have nightmares: a systematic review. J Clin Psychopharmacol 37(1):84–88, 2017 27930498

American Psychiatric Association: Diagnostic and Statistical Manual of Mental Disorders, 5th Edition. Arlington, VA, American Psychiatric Association, 2013

Asnis GM, Kohn SR, Henderson M, et al: SSRIs versus non-SSRIs in post-traumatic stress disorder: an update with recommendations. Drugs 64(4):383–404, 2004 14969574

Brady K, Pearlstein T, Asnis GM, et al: Efficacy and safety of sertraline treatment of posttraumatic stress disorder: a randomized controlled trial. JAMA 283(14):1837–1844, 2000 10770145

Bremner JD, Davis M, Southwick SM, et al: Neurobiology of posttraumatic stress disorder, in American Psychiatric Press Review of Psychiatry, Vol 12. Edited by Oldham JM, Riba Tasman A. Washington, DC, American Psychiatric Press, 1993, pp 183–204

Brkanac Z, Pastor JF, Storck M: Prazosin in PTSD. J Am Acad Child Adolesc Psychiatry 42(4):384–385, 2003 12649625

Bridge JA, Birmaher B, Iyengar S, et al: Placebo response in randomized controlled trials of antidepressants for pediatric major depressive disorder. Am J Psychiatry 166(1):42–49, 2009 19047322

Charney DS, Deutch AY, Krystal JH, et al: Psychobiologic mechanisms of posttraumatic stress disorder. Arch Gen Psychiatry 50(4):295–305, 1993 8466391

Cohen JA, Mannarino AP, Perel JM, et al: A pilot randomized controlled trial of combined trauma-focused CBT and sertraline for childhood PTSD symptoms. J Am Acad Child Adolesc Psychiatry 46(7):811–819, 2007 17581445

Copeland WE, Keeler G, Angold A, et al: Traumatic events and posttraumatic stress in childhood. Arch Gen Psychiatry 64(5):577–584, 2007 17485609

Davidson J, Rothbaum BO, Tucker P, et al: Venlafaxine extended release in posttraumatic stress disorder: a sertraline- and placebo-controlled study. J Clin Psychopharmacol 26(3):259–267, 2006 16702890

Daviss WB: Efficacy and tolerability of bupropion in boys with ADHD and major depression or dysthymic disorder. Child Adolesc Psychopharmacol Update 1(5):1–6, 1999

De Bellis MD, Putnam FW: The psychobiology of childhood maltreatment. Child Adolesc Psychiatr Clin N Am 3:663–678, 1994

Domon SE, Andersen MS: Nefazodone for PTSD. J Am Acad Child Adolesc Psychiatry 39(8):942–943, 2000 10939221

Famularo R, Kinscherff R, Fenton T: Propranolol treatment for childhood posttraumatic stress disorder, acute type: a pilot study. Am J Dis Child 142(11):1244–1247, 1988 3177336

Foa EB, Davidson JR, Frances A: Treatment of posttraumatic stress disorder. J Clin Psychiatry 66(suppl 16):1–76, 1999

Friedman MJ: Interrelationships between biological mechanisms and pharmacotherapy of posttraumatic stress disorder, in Posttraumatic Stress Disorder: Etiology, Phenomenology, and Treatment. Edited by Wolfe ME, Mosnaim AD. Washington, DC, American Psychiatric Press, 1990, pp 204–225

Friedman MJ, Southwick SM: Toward pharmacotherapy for post-traumatic stress disorder, in Neurobiological and Clinical Consequences of Stress: From Normal Adaptation to Posttraumatic Stress Disorder. Edited by Friedman MJ, Charney DS, Deutch AT. Philadelphia, PA, Lippincott-Raven Press, 1995, pp 465–481

Harmon RJ, Riggs D: Clonidine for posttraumatic stress disorder in preschool children. J Am Acad Child Adolesc Psychiatry 35(9):1247–1249, 1996 8824068

Horrigan JP, Barnhill LJ: The suppression of nightmares with guanfacine [letter]. J Clin Psychiatry 57(8):371, 1996 8752021

Horrigan JP, Barnhill LJ: Risperidone and PTSD in boys. J Neuropsychiatry Clin Neurosci 11:126–127, 1999

Kant R, Chalansani R, Chengappa KN, et al: The off-label use of clozapine in adolescents with bipolar disorder, intermittent explosive disorder, or posttraumatic stress disorder. J Child Adolesc Psychopharmacol 14(1):57–63, 2004 15142392

Keeshin BR, Strawn JR: Risperidone treatment of an adolescent with severe posttraumatic stress disorder. Ann Pharmacother 43(7):1374, 2009 19584378

Keeshin BR, Strawn JR: Psychological and pharmacologic treatment of youth with posttraumatic stress disorder: an evidence-based review. Child Adolesc Psychiatric Clin N Am 23(2):399–411, 2014 24656587

Langeland W, Olff M: Psychobiology of posttraumatic stress disorder in pediatric injury patients: a review of the literature. Neurosci Biobehav Rev 32(1):161–174, 2008 17825911

Looff D, Grimley P, Kuller F, et al: Carbamazepine for PTSD. J Am Acad Child Adolesc Psychiatry 34(6):703–704, 1995 7608041

Marshall RD, Beebe KL, Oldham M, et al: Efficacy and safety of paroxetine treatment for chronic PTSD: a fixed-dose, placebo-controlled study. Am J Psychiatry 158(12):1982–1988, 2001 11729013

Meighen KG, Hines LA, Lagges AM: Risperidone treatment of preschool children with thermal burns and acute stress disorder. J Child Adolesc Psychopharmacol 17(2):223–232, 2007 17489717

Mylle J, Maes M: Partial posttraumatic stress disorder revisited. J Affect Disord 78(1):37–48, 2004 14672795

Perry BD: Neurobiological sequelae of childhood trauma: PTSD in children, in Catecholamine Function in Posttraumatic Stress Disorder: Emerging Concepts. Edited by Murburg MM. Washington, DC, American Psychiatric Press, 1994, pp 233–255

Pfefferbaum BJ: Aspects of exposure in childhood trauma: the stressor criterion. J Trauma Dissociation 6(2):17–26, 2005 16150666

Robb AS, Cueva JE, Sporn J, et al: Sertraline treatment of children and adolescents with posttraumatic stress disorder: a double-blind, placebo-controlled trial. J Child Adolesc Psychopharmacol 20(6):463–471, 2010 21186964

Robert R, Blakeney PE, Villarreal C, et al: Imipramine treatment in pediatric burn patients with symptoms of acute stress disorder: a pilot study. J Am Acad Child Adolesc Psychiatry 38(7):873–882, 1999 10405506

Robert R, Tcheung WJ, Rosenberg L, et al: Treating thermally injured children suffering symptoms of acute stress with imipramine and fluoxetine: a randomized, double-blind study. Burns 34(7):919–928, 2008 18675519

Rothbaum BO, Price M, Jovanovic T, et al: A randomized, double-blind evaluation of D-cycloserine or alprazolam combined with virtual reality exposure therapy for posttraumatic stress disorder in Iraq and Afghanistan War veterans. Am J Psychiatry 171(6):640–648, 2014 24743802

Scheeringa MS, Myers L, Putnam FW, et al: Diagnosing PTSD in early childhood: an empirical assessment of four approaches. J Trauma Stress 25(4):359–367, 2012 22806831

Seedat S, Lockhat R, Kaminer D, et al: An open trial of citalopram in adolescents with post-traumatic stress disorder. Int Clin Psychopharmacol 16(1):21–25, 2001 11195256

Seedat S, Stein DJ, Ziervogel C, et al: Comparison of response to a selective serotonin reuptake inhibitor in children, adolescents, and adults with posttraumatic stress disorder. J Child Adolesc Psychopharmacol 12(1):37–46, 2002 12014594

Southwick SM, Yehuda R, Giller, EL Jr, et al: Use of tricyclics and monoamine oxidase inhibitors in the treatment of PTSD: a quantitative review, in Catecholamine Function in Posttraumatic Stress Disorder: Emerging Concepts. Edited by Murburg MM. Washington, DC, American Psychiatric Press, 1994, pp 293–305

Stathis S, Martin G, McKenna JG: A preliminary case series on the use of quetiapine for posttraumatic stress disorder in juveniles within a youth detention center. J Clin Psychopharmacol 25(6):539–544, 2005 16282834

Stein DJ, Ipser JC, Seedat S, et al: Pharmacotherapy for post traumatic stress disorder (PTSD). Cochrane Database Syst Rev 25(1):CD002795, 2006 16437445

Steiner H, Saxena KS, Carrion V, et al: Divalproex sodium for the treatment of PTSD and conduct disordered youth: a pilot randomized controlled clinical trial. Child Psychiatry Hum Dev 38(3):183–193, 2007 17570057

Stoddard FJ Jr, Luthra R, Sorrentino EA, et al: A randomized controlled trial of sertraline to prevent posttraumatic stress disorder in burned children. J Child Adolesc Psychopharmacol 21(5):469–477, 2011 22040192

Tucker P, Trautman RP, Wyatt DB, et al: Efficacy and safety of topiramate monotherapy in civilian posttraumatic stress disorder: a randomized, double-blind, placebo-controlled study. J Clin Psychiatry 68(2):201–206, 2007 17335317

Wheatley M, Plant J, Reader H, et al: Clozapine treatment of adolescents with posttraumatic stress disorder and psychotic symptoms. J Clin Psychopharmacol 24(2):167–173, 2004 15206664

Yeh MS, Mari JJ, Costa MCP, et al: A double-blind randomized controlled trial to study the efficacy of topiramate in a civilian sample of PTSD. CNS Neurosci Ther 17(5):305–310, 2011 21554564

Yehuda R: Recent developments in the neuroendocrinology of posttraumatic stress disorder. CNS Spectr 3(S2):22–29, 1998

CHAPTER

15

Addressing Comorbidity

Flint M. Espil, Ph.D.
Rachel L. Martin, B.A.
Brian Bauer, M.S.
Daniel W. Capron, Ph.D.

SEVERAL STUDIES have examined posttraumatic stress disorder (PTSD) and comorbid diagnoses among several groups, including survivors of natural disasters, war refugees, veterans, and individuals in outpatient and inpatient psychiatric clinics (e.g., Ginzburg et al. 2010; Kar and Bastia 2006; Mueser and Taub 2008). Many of these studies are retrospective, asking participants to report and reflect on events that occurred much earlier in life, whereas other approaches center on interviewing individuals during or shortly after crises. Results from such studies indicate that among the disorders that often co-occur with PTSD, the two most common types are mood and anxiety disorders. Major depressive disorder appears to be the single most common of these, with several authors citing between 21% and 94% of patients with PTSD also meeting clinical criteria for depression.

When these studies also consider youth exposed to traumatic events but not quite meeting full clinical criteria for PTSD, they find elevated rates of mood and anxiety problems as well. More research is needed to determine the relationship among trauma, anxiety, and mood disorders. For example, it may be that depression and anxiety increase risk for PTSD, or PTSD might place people at risk for developing mood and anxiety problems. There might also be a substantial symptom overlap between PTSD and mood and anxiety disorders, suggesting that all three stem from similar underlying factors.

From a longitudinal perspective, we know that youth who experience traumatic events are at greater risk for future problems. Individuals exposed to traumatic events during childhood are more likely to develop PTSD in adulthood than are individuals who do not report a childhood history of trauma. Additionally, those exposed to traumatic events in childhood are more likely to be exposed to traumatic events in adulthood. Childhood trauma is not a risk factor unique to PTSD but appears to be a risk factor for the development of psychiatric problems more generally. One form of traumatic event, childhood maltreatment, appears to be especially predictive of the development of PTSD. Among the subtypes of childhood maltreatment, emotional maltreatment remains a significant predictor of later PTSD development, even when controlling for other risk factors. In this chapter, we first discuss developmentally appropriate ways to assess and treat comorbid disorders among youth with trauma, review potential challenges during treatment, and then broadly discuss the sociocultural implications of intervening at younger ages.

Developmental Assessment Considerations

Given the high comorbidities among youth exposed to trauma, differential diagnosis of specific disorders can be difficult. For example, suppose a crying child approaches her teacher, frantically stating that she was just in a car accident despite sitting quietly at her desk for the past hour. Would this be considered a hallucination or even a delusion—both symptoms common in psychoses? Probably not, especially given the very low base rates of psychotic disorders in young children. Such experiences could be flashbacks to traumatic experiences or intensely intrusive thoughts of a previous experience. In this scenario, the child may have been reexperiencing the events of a past motor vehicle accident while daydreaming in class and may not have the insight or verbal repertoire to effectively communicate this experience.

Treatment providers should take care to distinguish between true psychotic hallucinations and delusions and flashbacks or intrusive thoughts associated with traumatic experiences. If symptoms of depressed mood and anxiety are present—a much more likely scenario—then providers should carefully determine whether these symptoms are secondary to the symptoms of PTSD and whether they are causing distress or impairment in addition to the symptoms of PTSD. This process involves carefully considering the timeline of symptoms, in terms of both onset and course, relative to the traumatic events. Preschool and school-age youth with symptoms of anxiety and depression may present differently from adolescents and adults. For example, children with anxiety may report chronic cases of an upset stomach, and children with depressive disorders may present as much more irritable than sad.

A variety of measures are available to help assess both PTSD and comorbid disorders. Given that the focus of this chapter is on the comorbid symptoms, we do not include a list of measures for diagnosing PTSD and its related symptoms. Educators, counselors, clinicians, and other mental health professionals should take care to use only measures shown to possess appropriate levels of reliability (i.e., consistency across measurements and items) and validity (i.e., the extent to which the measure actually assesses what it purports to assess) to determine whether comorbid problems are present. Data can be collected through a variety of means, including youth self-report, caregiver or teacher report, structured interviews administered by a trained professional, and behavioral observation. Each of these techniques has its own set of advantages and disadvantages, and implementation will depend on the time, training, and other resources available to families and professionals.

For assessment of preschool and school-age youth, several psychometrically sound measures are available. For younger children, reports from parents or other primary caregivers become paramount given the developmental limitations (e.g., verbal expression, insight) of very young children. Behavioral observation of children can also help lend insight into problems reported by caregivers or teachers, especially if there are concerns related to anxiety, inattention, or disruptive behavior.

Comorbid problems become even more salient during adolescence, the period when individuals are most at risk for the development of PTSD (Nooner et al. 2012). As children move into adolescence, many begin turning to maladaptive coping strategies for symptoms of trauma. These may include substance use, self-harm, and suicide. Accordingly, the assessment of comorbid problems should take these potential concerns into consideration. As youth enter adolescence, they become more accurate in their ability to complete self-report measures. Parent report, however, should still be used whenever possible to corroborate data obtained by adolescents, and age, grade, and developmental level of youth should always be considered when using standardized instruments. For a list of commonly used assessment measures for youth comorbidity, see Table 15–1. Although this list is by no means exhaustive, it may serve as a useful tool for parents, educators, and mental health professionals when making differential diagnoses.

Assessment for comorbid disorders has been confined largely to self-report measurements that are susceptible to a number of biases and cognitive distortions and are also hindered by stigma and underreporting. Reporter biases such as inaccurate reporting from parents and cognitive biases such as social desirability bias (i.e., the tendency for individuals to answer questions in a manner that would be viewed favorably by others) can lead to inaccurate diagnoses and poorer treatment outcomes. To overcome these challenges, research focused on biological and behavioral correlates of PTSD and other often co-occurring disorders could help identify and discern differential diagnoses. Assessments that also focus on physiological responses and processes (e.g., heart rate, galvanic skin response) and use more objective methodologies such as electroencephalography and functional magnetic resonance imaging could bolster the accuracy of diagnoses when added to self-report measures. Although self-report measurements are vital for understanding the youth's personal narrative, the development of more objective assessment techniques could help clarify other co-occurring diagnoses and lead to greater treatment fidelity.

After a thorough assessment, the youth, family, and provider typically review the findings and determine the most appropriate course of action. If the results of the assessment indicate the presence of comorbid disorders, it can be difficult to determine which disorder, or disorders, to treat first. The consensus among experts in the treatment of PTSD is that the disorder causing the most distress and impairment should typically be treated first, with careful consideration of the resources (e.g., time, money, transportation) of the youth and his or her family. If the youth also has a long history of conduct disorder, oppositional defiant disorder, or self-destructive behaviors, these may need to be addressed first given the high likelihood of interference with other treatment approaches. If families prefer the simultaneous treatment of both trauma and other disorders and resources allow it, several evidence-based approaches are available. Decisions such as these, along with other potential challenges to treating trauma and comorbid problems in youth, are discussed in the next section.

TABLE 15–1. Commonly used measures to assess comorbid disorders in youth

Measure	Reference	Developmental level		
		Pre-kindergarten	School age	Adolescent
Caregiver or teacher report				
Behavior Assessment System for Children (BASC-3)	Kamphaus and Reynolds 2015	X	X	X
Achenbach System of Empirically Based Assessment	Achenbach 2009	X	X	X
Revised Child Anxiety and Depression Scale	Ebesutani et al. 2010		X	X
Multidimensional Anxiety Scale for Children	March et al. 1997		X	X
Conners 3	Conners 2008		X	X
Spence Children's Anxiety Scale	Spence 1998	X	X	X
Screen for Child Anxiety Related Disorders	Birmaher et al. 1995		X	X
Self-Report				
Behavior Assessment System for Children (BASC-3)	Kamphaus and Reynolds 2015		X	X
Achenbach System of Empirically Based Assessment	Achenbach 2009		X	X
Revised Child Anxiety and Depression Scale	Chorpita et al. 2000		X	X
Multidimensional Anxiety Scale for Children	March et al. 1997		X	X
Conners 3	Conners 2008		X	X
Spence Children's Anxiety Scale	Spence 1998		X	X
Screen for Child Anxiety Related Disorders	Birmaher et al. 1995		X	X
Children's Depression Inventory 2	Kovacs and Staff 2003		X	X

TABLE 15–1. Commonly used measures to assess comorbid disorders in youth *(continued)*

Measure	Reference	Developmental level		
		Pre-kindergarten	School age	Adolescent
Interview				
Anxiety Disorders Interview Schedule	Silverman and Albano 1996		X	X
Kiddie Schedule for Affective Disorders and Schizo-phrenia	Puig-Antich and Ryan 1986		X	X
Mini International Neuropsychiatric Interview for Children and Adolescents	Sheehan et al. 2009		X	X
Children's Interview for Psychiatric Syndromes	Weller et al. 1999		X	X

Potential Challenges During Treatment

Comorbid disorders occurring with trauma pose unique challenges in clinical, theoretical, and logistical domains. Variables such as the intensity, type, and frequency of trauma can have a significant impact on the presentation of comorbid conditions. Using retrospective data, the evidence is clear that childhood traumatic events have serious adverse health outcomes throughout developmental stages and continuing into adulthood, with each outcome compounding the overall problems for individuals (Chapman et al. 2004; Dube et al. 2003; Felitti et al. 1998). The additional challenges that youth with trauma and comorbid disorders experience often lead to poorer long-term prognoses. For example, research suggests that comorbid symptomatology with trauma predicts worse adjustment. In a study observing youth in detention centers, 92.5% had experienced at least one trauma, and 93% of youth meeting criteria for PTSD also met criteria for one or more comorbid disorders (Abram et al. 2013).

Numerous possibilities exist for explaining why youth with trauma histories and comorbid disorders have a more complicated and severe trajectory than those with a standalone disorder. One reason is that comorbid disorders, especially those involving trauma, are more difficult to treat because of the complex interplay occurring between symptoms and disorders. Understanding the theoretical underpinnings and etiology of trauma comorbidity helps reveal why these difficulties exist. For example, PTSD is a disorder characterized principally by having witnessed, or been directly exposed to, a significant trauma (e.g., exposure to death) that later causes severe impairment within the individual because of intrusive symptoms, avoidance, negative alterations in cognitions, and increased arousal and reactivity. Major depressive disorder (MDD), on the other hand, is marked by a depressed mood most of the day, nearly every day, for at least 2 weeks. This disorder is also often characterized by anhedonia, or an inability to take pleasure in previously enjoyed activities.

One hypothesis for the common co-occurrence of these two disorders is that PTSD and MDD are two distinct disorders that have symptom overlap. Evidence for this theory can be found in the diagnostic criteria for both, which show that these two disorders share the symptoms of anhedonia, sleep disturbance, guilt, and concentration difficulties. Further evidence for this theory is suggested by the fact that despite changes in symptom criteria, PTSD and MDD comorbidity rates are largely the same.

A second argument is that PTSD-MDD comorbidity is a distinct phenotype, or trauma-related subtype, of PTSD. Much of the evidence for this is in line with a stress-diathesis model of PTSD-MDD. For instance, latent structure analyses have revealed that people with PTSD and MDD often have high negative affect, low positive affect, and low extroversion. This might indicate that having these underlying personality trait vulnerabilities increases the probabilities of having these specific diagnoses. It could be that when individuals with these personality dimensions are faced with a threat, challenge, or loss, they are more prone to anxiety and sadness and are less likely to seek help and enjoy social activities, ultimately developing PTSD-MDD.

A third hypothesis is that poor emotion regulation and coping strategies combined with the symptoms of PTSD may further increase the likelihood of developing, or exacerbating, comorbid symptoms. In an attempt to reduce symptoms of PTSD and depression, some individuals may turn to alcohol and drugs as a maladaptive coping technique (Figure 15–1). On a more granular level, research suggests that adverse childhood experiences such as exposure to traumatic events can induce biological changes. Studies have shown that several years after the abuse, patients still report that despite living in a safe home away from trauma, they continue to exhibit significantly increased stress dysregulation (De Bellis et al. 1994).

Each of these hypotheses has supporting evidence, and the three hypotheses have divergent implications for treatment. These implications are further complicated when additional issues arise, such as problems assessing the timing of symptom onset. For instance, children with attention-deficit/hyperactivity disorder (ADHD) have been found to be more likely to develop PTSD than children without ADHD, but in the majority of cases it is often unclear whether ADHD symptoms are primary or secondary to PTSD. Reports from caregivers, family members, educators, and other significant others become paramount because obtaining accurate information regarding the onset of symptomatology from youth can be difficult.

Childhood trauma is also a risk factor for the future development of psychopathological eating and eating disorders. Results from a recent meta-analysis indicated that specific types of abuse are related to eating disorders: childhood physical abuse was related to any type of eating disorder, childhood emotional abuse was associated with both bulimia nervosa and binge-eating disorder, and childhood sexual abuse was associated with binge-eating disorder (Caslini et al. 1999). Similarly, there is a known relationship between traumatic events during childhood, such as maltreatment, and obesity and severe obesity. In sum, when clinicians treat children who have experienced trauma, there should be an assessment of the child's relationship to food and eating.

In addition to these other disorders, some studies indicated a link between PTSD and dissociative disorders (Twaite and Rodriguez-Srednicki

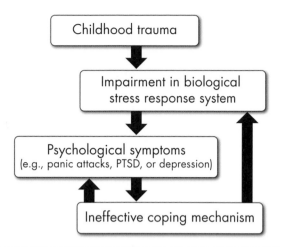

FIGURE 15–1. **The psychobiology of childhood trauma.**

2008). Dissociation may be a mechanism through which childhood trauma leads to severe cases of PTSD, or PTSD with dissociation might be a distinct subtype of PTSD. Regardless, additional research is needed to further elucidate the relationship between these trauma-related, dissociative, and other disorders that commonly occur with PTSD or among youth exposed to traumatic events.

Suicide is a major health concern that affects a wide variety of people who have either attempted suicide, have had suicidal ideation, or know someone who died by suicide. Childhood trauma is also a risk factor for lifetime suicide attempts. This relationship has been empirically and clinically supported through longitudinal research on this topic (Zatti et al. 2017). Not only do many forms of childhood trauma increase risk for suicide, but certain traumas appear to have elevated risk. For example, childhood sexual abuse, physical abuse, emotional abuse, and physical neglect appear to be more associated with lifetime suicide attempts than is emotional neglect. Within these categories, a hierarchy has emerged regarding which forms of abuse contribute most to suicide risk. Physical abuse is the highest contributor, followed by emotional abuse, sexual abuse, and physical neglect (Zatti et al. 2017). Results from Zatti and colleagues suggest that when treating individuals with previous childhood trauma, specifically physical abuse, emotional abuse, sexual abuse, and physical neglect, clinicians should be regularly evaluating suicide risk.

Many of the symptoms of PTSD (e.g., nightmares, insomnia, agitation, panic attacks) are also warning signs that a suicide attempt might be imminent. Therefore, it is important that clinicians monitor and intervene with these key risk factors, as well as check suicidal desire, plans, preparations, and means on an ongoing basis. Nightmares are a hallmark symptom of PTSD but also increase suicide risk both overall and in a time-sensitive manner. Nightmares can create avoidance of sleep, which leads to such behaviors as staying up watching television, using computers or mobile devices, or abusing substances until one passes out. Over time, these avoidance patterns lead to more dysregulated sleep, which leads to greater impairment during the daytime, greater emotion dysregulation overall, and insomnia (another imminent warning sign of a suicide attempt). The disrupted sleep pattern is also likely to lead to increased agitation, another marker of an imminent suicide attempt. Many adolescents report their suicide attempt was prompted by a need to escape extremely aversive physical or psychological states. Clients reporting agitation so severe that they want to "crawl out of their own skin" should be carefully monitored for overall suicide risk and given tools to reduce distress, such as dialectical behavior therapy distress tolerance skills, progressive muscle relaxation, and mindful breathing exercises.

A specific symptom associated with PTSD, and related disorders, worth careful monitoring is panic attacks. Panic attacks are a surge of intense arousal or fear and come on suddenly with such symptoms as increased heart rate, trembling or shaking, sweating, nausea, pounding heart, shortness of breath, feelings of choking, chest pain, feeling dizzy or unsteady, feelings of unreality or being detached from oneself, fears of losing control or going crazy, and fears of dying. It is not well known exactly why panic attacks are a sign of imminent suicide-related behaviors, but one possibility is that the extreme physiological distress causes feelings of a frantic desire to escape distress comparable to that experienced with severe agitation. The fear of future panic attacks may also drive imminent suicide risk via similar mechanisms as nightmares. Panic attacks lead to avoidance behaviors that result in a positive feedback loop that increases overall distress and impairment. Fortunately, panic attacks are highly responsive to behavioral and cognitive-behavioral interventions. The most effective technique is interoceptive exposure to panic cues such as elevated heart rate, shortness of breath, and dizziness. The clinician can have the client bring on these cues in session through running in place, hyperventilation, and spinning in a chair, respectively. Clinicians should educate the client about subjective units of distress (SUD) and have the client report their SUD level as they engage in these exercises. When the client identifies an exercise that leads to elevated SUD, the clinician can develop a plan for exposure treatment around the exercise.

Eliminating panic attacks can be done in as little as 4–8 weeks with consistent exposure exercises.

Because of the complex interplays between trauma and other co-occurring disorders, there are often no standard guidelines for how to treat an individual with these disorders, especially among youth. For adolescents with trauma, first-line treatment consists of trauma-focused cognitive-behavioral therapies, such as cognitive processing therapy and prolonged exposure therapy. Given the additional burden of comorbid disorders, treatment providers should spend ample time ensuring youth do not become overwhelmed and drop out of treatment. Treatment providers should be especially vigilant for signs of treatment disengagement and drop-out at the point in the cognitive-behavioral therapies where exposure exercises begin. Imaginal exposure is a behavioral treatment component that involves repeatedly imagining the trauma. Youth will often tell their parents that the treatment is not working or that they do not like going to therapy right before exposure begins. Therapists and parents must work together to determine whether treatment disengagement is something truly related to the therapist or therapy or is a sign of avoidance. It is crucial to recognize avoidance and make all possible attempts to stop it from interfering with treatment.

Although no pharmacotherapies are specifically used to treat PTSD, antidepressants (e.g., selective serotonin reuptake inhibitors, serotonin-norepinephrine reuptake inhibitors) are routinely prescribed. This can be problematic because some research indicates people with co-occurring disorders may respond more poorly to these medications than do people with PTSD alone. In some studies, children and adolescents who take antidepressants report little to no improvement in overall well-being. Benzodiazepines are often prescribed for adults with anxiety disorders, but they cannot be recommended for youth because of a lack of studies on treatment outcomes and the possibility of addiction. In addition, benzodiazepines for PTSD are not an optimal treatment, regardless of addiction concerns, because of their ability to interfere with exposure-based elements of therapy. An essential component in the treatment success of exposure-based approaches is to have a patient experience the rise and fall of anxiety during fearful situations. However, if a patient is taking benzodiazepines, he or she is unable to experience the full anxiety from the exercise and will not experience the maximum benefits from treatment. The patient may continue to experience PTSD symptoms and maintain avoidance when not taking benzodiazepines because he or she was not able to experience the maximum possible potency of treatment.

Psychopharmacology and psychotherapy are particularly challenging in the treatment of co-occurring substance use. Individuals with trauma are at a higher risk of abusing substances because of a need to cope with their symptoms of PTSD (Bensley et al. 1999). Substance use often serves an avoidance function, allowing individuals to prevent or blunt the symptoms of reexperiencing, hyperarousal, and negative mood (similar to benzodiazepines, as described in the previous paragraph). This pattern of avoidance ultimately prevents individuals from facing the memories of their trauma—a primary focus of treatment. For these reasons, treatment providers may elect to deal with substance use issues before focusing on the trauma. In these instances, providers should coordinate care with medical professionals to prepare for detoxification and withdrawal and should discuss the potential increase in severity of trauma symptoms. Failing to do so may increase the likelihood of substance use relapse. Approaches in adults have successfully integrated substance use and trauma treatment simultaneously, but these approaches have not been tested to the same extent among youth.

Comorbid disorders also bring several logistical considerations. For example, youth presenting with substance use disorder or a history in the juvenile justice system may require greater case management and coordination of community resources and are often perceived by clinicians to have more self-destructive behaviors (Back et al. 2009). In addition, dual-diagnosis clients require the clinician to have a higher level of education and training; therefore, practitioners may limit openings in their caseloads for such clients and make treatment harder to attain. Further, if youth have a history of trauma and extensive legal trouble, trauma-sensitive procedures (e.g., parole officer check-ins, procedures, arrests) should be considered and communicated with other personnel responsible for care when devising a treatment plan. The myriad complicating factors in such cases have contributed to a glaring lack of standardized guidelines for assisting youth with trauma and comorbid problems.

Geographical treatment barriers are another area of concern for youth with a comorbid PTSD disorder. As mentioned previously, these youth will likely require clinicians who have specific areas of expertise in order to optimize treatment outcomes. This is problematic because the extended list of expertise requirements (e.g., child and adolescent focus, dual diagnosis, PTSD treatment) could limit the number of available clinicians in any given area. Therefore, other treatment modalities could be useful to fully reach and give appropriate services to this population. With the proliferation of smartphone usage and other mobile technologies, computer-delivered treatments could be one way of overcoming the shortage of available clinicians in a geographic area. There is some initial evidence for the effectiveness of PTSD and health coaching through mobile application technology in reducing PTSD symptoms. In addition, performing exposure-based therapies via telehealth could disseminate treatments more widely. Exposure therapies delivered via telehealth have been effective in reducing symptoms of PTSD, depression, and anxiety, although with slightly less effectiveness compared with in-person exposure therapy (Gros et al. 2011). These delivery modalities need more studies focused on the youth population to determine whether they can be comparatively efficacious for younger individuals, but they still represent a promising new avenue for reaching and treating this specific population.

In sum, the added complexity of comorbid disorders presents additional challenges for both the treatment providers and youth. Many young individuals with a history of trauma also have a co-occurring mental disorder, which is linked with poorer outcomes (e.g., legal trouble) and greater symptom severity. Although psychotherapies and psychopharmacology appear to be effective in treating trauma and co-occurring disorders, it is essential that providers have the knowledge and experience for accurate assessment and treatment. The requirement to possess this knowledge and experience, combined with the fact that many mental health practitioners perceive this population to be more difficult, could impact treatment availability in some areas. Future research addressing these unique challenges among youth is needed to further develop and refine treatment recommendations.

Sociocultural Implications of Early Intervention

Trauma-exposed youth are susceptible to and affected by many sociocultural issues. Children exposed to traumatic events who also meet criteria for comorbid disorders are more likely to drop out of school. School problems may lead to a negative ripple effect that reduces college aspirations, employment opportunities, and overall financial stability. Poor adjustment or performance in school and lower employment opportunities are risk factors for criminal and legal problems.

One mechanism through which trauma confers risk for adverse school and legal outcomes is aggression. Aggression and/or behavior outbursts are a common symptom of children with a history of trauma. These outbursts, when severe, may result in school problems and eventually in incarceration. In fact, one in six male inmates reports being physically or sexually abused prior to age 18, with physical abuse (56%) more common than sexual abuse (10%; Harlow 1999). Childhood trauma has also been shown to significantly predict arrests for alcohol and/or drug-related offenses.

Incarcerated youth who have experienced trauma are also at risk for comorbid disorders. Childhood trauma has been shown to have strong negative associations with adulthood psychological wellness. When compared with children who have not experienced childhood trauma, those who were traumatized were found to have an increased likelihood of antisocial personality disorder. Among incarcerated men with a history of trauma, those who were sexually abused were twice as likely to be in treatment for comorbid depression disorder and one and a half times more likely to be in treatment for comorbid anxiety disorder or substance use disorder (Wolff and Shi 2012).

In addition to physical and sexual abuse, childhood abandonment is another type of traumatic event prevalent in prisoners. More than 25% of incarcerated men report having been abandoned during childhood or adolescence (Wolff and Shi 2012). Similar to physical and sexual abuse, abandonment has been linked to psychological problems in adulthood. Incarcerated men with a history of abandonment are more likely to be in treatment for comorbid depression and anxiety.

In addition to affecting individuals' aggression, childhood traumas can also play a role in the development of sexual behavior problems. For example, childhood traumas, such as sexual abuse, are a risk factor for increased risky sexual behaviors (e.g., unprotected sex, multiple sexual partners, sex with a stranger). Children who suffered trauma during childhood, especially sexual abuse, often have difficulties with creating strong and healthy interpersonal relationships and social support. These cognitive developmental issues could lead to one of two major outcomes: 1) isolation and distrust of others or 2) extreme need for closeness and inappropriate disclosures. Childhood sexual abuse appears to significantly impact future sexual behaviors: compared with peers who were not abused, abused adolescents are more likely to engage in unprotected sexual intercourse, have multiple sexual partners, and be involved in a pregnancy. Treatment of children who are sexually abused should increase focus on sexual health education and appropriate attachment.

One potential risk for experiencing childhood trauma is geographical location. Children from low socioeconomic status neighborhoods are more likely to be exposed to crime and traumatic events. Within these settings, trauma does not necessarily imply physical abuse, sexual abuse, or maltreatment directed at the child but also includes bearing witness to acts of violence. Through witnessing violence and associated stimuli such as guns, drugs, and knives, children can manifest PTSD symptoms. Additionally, these experiences with violence can disturb children's developing ability to problem solve and think logically.

In addition to witnessing violence, living in a low socioeconomic neighborhood may increase the risk of victimization for youth. Affiliations with deviant peers, participation in risky sexual behaviors, and peer-involved drug and/or alcohol use all increase the risk of victimization. A study of homeless young women within low socioeconomic neighborhoods indicated that physical and sexual abuse were associated with greater participation in deviant peer groups as well as being victimized (Whitbeck et al. 1999). Furthermore, a history of victimization while living on the streets was also significantly associated with comorbid depressive symptoms. Several young women reported running away from home to escape family abuse, and these women were more likely to also report both subsequent victimization while homeless and comorbid depressive symptoms (Whitbeck et al. 1999).

Individuals from gender and ethnic minorities are even more at especially high risk of experiencing multiple traumas and hardships (e.g., racism, family adversities, chronic stressors) that can compound and lead to more severe mental health presentations. In a large study of African American and Latino and Latina men and women from low socioeconomic neighborhoods, researchers found that although these populations were relatively resilient, their high cumulative traumas (which, in addition to adult traumas, included childhood traumas such as sexual abuse, physical abuse, disasters, accidents, and exposure to community violence), were associated with a higher prevalence of PTSD, anxiety, and depressive symptoms (Myers et al. 2015).

Although childhood trauma can lead to significant negative outcomes, not all children who are exposed to trauma experience these negative life events. As such, there must be some protective factors that can help individuals cope with these traumatic events. One protective factor against developing psychopathologies could be resilience. Resilience is the individual's ability to successfully adapt to change and is a measure of stress coping ability or emotional stamina. Children with higher resilience who were exposed to trauma appear to have significantly better outcomes than do those with low resilience. Thus, resilience may be a key factor in helping children who have been exposed to trauma cope with their experiences and preventing future maladaptive coping techniques or psychopathologies. Clinicians treating individuals who were exposed to childhood trauma should consider incorporating resilience training techniques into their treatment plan to give their patients more skills to cope with their experiences.

Conclusion

Comorbid trauma in youth is often accompanied by difficult symptoms and disorders such as substance use disorders, depression, anxiety, and oppositional disorders. Each of these disorders and symptoms on its own is the subject of substantial scientific inquiry, with significant training and understanding required to adequately treat the individual. The interactions between comorbid disorders present unique challenges, especially in youth. These challenges include difficulties with legal and educational systems, trouble with home life, and difficulty finding qualified professionals to treat such individuals.

KEY CONCEPTS

- Comorbidity plays an important role in the assessment and treatment of youth exposed to traumatic stress.
- A number of developmentally appropriate assessment strategies exist for treatment of comorbid disorders in trauma-exposed youth.
- Clinicians should identify potential confounding factors of comorbid disorders when treating trauma.
- Early intervention is critical in dealing with the long-term effects of traumatic stress.

Discussion Questions

1. Can early intervention assuage the psychological factors that result from childhood trauma?

2. What can be done to help decrease the trauma exposure some youth face in low socioeconomic neighborhoods?

3. How might future studies begin examining the effects of comorbidity on PTSD treatment and incorporate these into evidence-based treatment protocols?

Suggested Readings

Cohen JA, Berliner L, Mannarino A: Trauma focused CBT for children with co-occurring trauma and behavior problems. Child Abuse Negl 34(4):215–224, 2010 20304489

De Bellis MD: Developmental traumatology: a contributory mechanism for alcohol and substance use disorders. Psychoneuroendocrinology 27(1–2):155–170, 2002 11750776

Nooner KB, Linares LO, Batinjane J, et al: Factors related to posttraumatic stress disorder in adolescence. Trauma Violence Abuse 13(3):153–166, 2012 22665437

References

Abram KM, Teplin LA, King DC, et al: PTSD, trauma, and comorbid psychiatric disorders in detained youth. Juvenile Justice Bulletin 1:13, 2013

Achenbach TM: Achenbach System of Empirically Based Assessment (ASEBA): Development, Findings, Theory, and Applications. Burlington, University of Vermont Research Center on Children, Youth and Families, 2009

Back SE, Waldrop AE, Brady KT: Treatment challenges associated with comorbid substance use and posttraumatic stress disorder: clinicians' perspectives. Am J Addict 18(1):15–20, 2009 19219661

Bensley LS, Spieker SJ, Van Eenwyk J, et al: Self-reported abuse history and adolescent problem behaviors II: alcohol and drug use. J Adolesc Health 24(3):173–180, 1999 10195800

Birmaher B, Khetarpal S, Cully M, et al: Screen for Child Anxiety Related Disorders (SCARED). Pittsburgh, PA, Western Psychiatric Institute and Clinic, University of Pittsburgh, 1995

Caslini M, Bartoli F, Crocamo C, et al: Disentangling the associations between child abuse and eating disorders: a systematic review and meta-analysis. Psychosom Med 78(1):79–90, 1999 26461853

Chapman DP, Whitfield CL, Felitti VJ, et al: Adverse childhood experiences and the risk of depressive disorders in adulthood. J Affect Disord 82(2):217–225, 2004 15488250

Chorpita BF, Yim L, Moffitt C, et al: Assessment of symptoms of DSM-IV anxiety and depression in children: a revised child anxiety and depression scale. Behav Res Ther 38(8):835–855, 2000 10937431

Conners CK: Conners 3. North Tonawanda, NY, MHS Assessments, 2008

De Bellis MD, Chrousos GP, Dorn LD, et al: Hypothalamic-pituitary-adrenal axis dysregulation in sexually abused girls. J Clin Endocrinol Metab 78(2):249–255, 1994 8106608

Dube SR, Felitti VJ, Dong M, et al: Childhood abuse, neglect, and household dysfunction and the risk of illicit drug use: the Adverse Childhood Experiences study. Pediatrics 111(3):564–572, 2003 12612237

Ebesutani C, Bernstein A, Nakamura BJ, et al; Research Network on Youth Mental Health: A psychometric analysis of the revised child anxiety and depression scale—parent version in a clinical sample. J Abnorm Child Psychol 38(2):249–260, 2010 19830545

Felitti VJ, Anda RF, Nordenberg D, et al: Relationship of childhood abuse and household dysfunction to many of the leading causes of death in adults: the Adverse Childhood Experiences (ACE) study. Am J Prev Med 14(4):245–258, 1998 9635069

Ginzburg K, Ein-Dor T, Solomon Z: Comorbidity of posttraumatic stress disorder, anxiety and depression: a 20-year longitudinal study of war veterans. J Affect Disord 123(1)249–257, 2010 19765828

Gros DF, Yoder M, Tuerk PW, et al: Exposure therapy for PTSD delivered to veterans via telehealth: predictors of treatment completion and outcome and comparison to treatment delivered in person. Behav Ther 42(2):276–283, 2011 21496512

Harlow CW: Bureau of Justice Statistics Selected Findings (Rep No NCJ 172879). Washington, DC, U.S. Department of Justice, Bureau of Justice Statistics, 1999

Kamphaus RW, Reynolds CR: Behavior Assessment System for Children—Third Edition (BASC-3): Behavioral and Emotional Screening System (BESS). Bloomington, MN, Pearson, 2015

Kar N, Bastia BK: Post-traumatic stress disorder, depression and generalised anxiety disorder in adolescents after a natural disaster: a study of comorbidity. Clin Pract Epidemiol Ment Health 2(1):17, 2006 16869979

Kovacs M, Staff MHS: Children's Depression Inventory 2 (CDI2). North Tonawanda, NY, MHS Assessments, 2003

March JS, Parker JD, Sullivan K, et al: The Multidimensional Anxiety Scale for Children (MASC): factor structure, reliability, and validity. J Am Acad Child Adolesc Psychiatry 36(4):554–565, 1997 9100431

Mueser KT, Taub J: Trauma and PTSD among adolescents with severe emotional disorders involved in multiple service systems. Psychiatr Serv 59(6):627–634, 2008 18511582

Myers HF, Wyatt GE, Ullman JB, et al: Cumulative burden of lifetime adversities: trauma and mental health in low-SES African Americans and Latino/as. Psychol Trauma 7(3):243–251, 2015 25961869

Nooner KB, Linares LO, Batinjane J, et al: Factors related to posttraumatic stress disorder in adolescence. Trauma Violence Abuse 13(3):153–166, 2012 22665437

Puig-Antich J, Ryan N: Kiddie Schedule for Affective Disorders and Schizophrenia. Pittsburgh, PA, Western Psychiatric Institute, 1986

Sheehan D, Shytle D, Milo K, et al: Mini International Neuropsychiatric Interview for Children and Adolescents English Version 6. Boston, MA, Mapi Research Trust, 2009

Silverman WK, Albano AM: Anxiety Disorders Interview Schedule for DSM-IV: Child Interview Schedule, Vol 2. Boulder, CO, Graywind, 1996

Spence SH: A measure of anxiety symptoms among children. Behav Res Ther 36(5):545–566, 1998 9648330

Twaite JA, Rodriguez-Srednicki O: Childhood sexual and physical abuse and adult vulnerability to PTSD: the mediating effects of attachment and dissociation. J Child Sex Abuse 13(1):17–38, 2008 15353375

Weller EB, Fristad MA, Weller RA, Rooney MT: Children's Interview for Psychiatric Syndromes: ChIPS. Washington, DC, American Psychiatric Press, 1999

Whitbeck LB, Hoyt DR, Yoder KA: A risk-amplification model of victimization and depressive symptoms among runaway and homeless adolescents. Am J Community Psychol 27(2):273–296, 1999 10425702

Wolff N, Shi J: Childhood and adult trauma experiences of incarcerated persons and their relationship to adult behavioral health problems and treatment. Int J Environ Res Public Health 9(5):1908–1926, 2012 22754481

Zatti C, Rosa V, Barros A, et al: Childhood trauma and suicide attempt: a meta-analysis of longitudinal studies from the last decade. Psychiatry Res 256:353–358, 2017 28683433

PART III
Associated Clinical Issues

16

Dissociation

Chelsea N. Grefe, Psy.D.
Elizabeth Weiss, Psy.D.

Eva was placed with her grandparents at age 4 after her single-parent father went to prison. She was typically warm and affectionate with her grandparents but at times would become aggressive, hitting her grandfather unexpectedly or suddenly thrusting her pelvis against her grandmother while making sexually explicit comments. Despite being able to solve problems above her age level at home, she did not progress in preschool tasks. Eva was extremely shy, often not recognizing her peers, even when they greeted her by name. When she felt distressed, her face would become blank and she would urgently request screen time, showing increased signs of stress until she could play games on a phone or tablet.

The child in this vignette displayed some of the classic patterns of dissociation, which has been defined as "a neurological state that is recognized as an acute disconnection with the reality of a situation or the self" (Carrion and Weems 2017, p. 69). Dissociative patterns that reflect a lack of coherence in mental functioning include perplexing shifts of consciousness, such as not recognizing well-known peers; marked shifts in knowledge, such as a discrepancy in skills in different environments; and shifts in patterns of behavior, such as sudden aggressive or sexualized behaviors.

Current theories on the development and trajectory of dissociation in children and adolescents highlight the impact of disorganized attachment and trauma on structural changes in the brain and subsequent development. Lotti (1999), an attachment theorist, described how disorganized attachment in the parent-infant relationship can lead to dissociation. When caregivers display fearful and frightening behaviors, this can lead to internal and competing working models during infant development. Infants who vacillate by reacting with avoidance and fear and attention and expectation experience competing schemas. These schemas lead to confusion, impaired integration, and dissociation in infants and young children. If a child experiences a traumatic event, seeking comfort is difficult because of his or her disorganized attachment to the caregiver. Lotti (1999) described how a child may create a feedback loop of increasing fear as he or she seeks comfort, which is unavailable to the child. Children with insecure attachments have difficulty relying on caregivers and cannot regulate emotions by themselves, resulting in anger, anxiety, and self-defeating aggression or dissociative states (van der Kolk 2005). Dissociative reactions may result in the child's failure to develop a typical response to a stressor because of inconsistent soothing from his or her caregiver.

Ogawa et al. (1997) and Dutra et al. (2009) also showed support for the association between disorganized attachment and pathological dissociation in early adulthood. In their longitudinal study, Ogawa and colleagues (1997) concluded that the quality of the parent-infant relationship accounted for one quarter of variance in young adult dissociative symptoms, and within this group, later trauma predicted significantly higher dissociative symptoms. More specifically, Dutra and colleagues (2009) found that a mother's lack of positive affective involvement, flatness of affect, and disrupted affective communication were significant precursors to dissociative symptoms in 19-year-old study subjects.

In addition to attachment theories on dissociation, Frank Putnam argued that dissociation can occur when the development of normal states is disrupted by exposure to trauma. Putnam's (1997) discrete behavioral state model describes how infants display discrete behavioral states (drowsy, irregular sleep, regular sleep, fussy, crying, feeding, alter-inactive). As the infant grows, these states gradually become self-organizing and self-stabilizing until the child begins to experience an integrated sense of self. Children exposed to trauma experience a disruption of the development and creation of bridging states. Instead, trauma behavioral states develop, impacting the cellular and synaptic firing of normal brain development. In the absence of positive attachment and caregiving, these children do not develop healthy metacognitive linkages between states. Thus, children do not achieve an integrated sense of self, resulting in trauma-related and dissected states, or dissociation. Maltreated children create dissociative adaptations in their experience and awareness of self, including automatization of behavior, compartmentalization of painful memories and feelings, and detachment from awareness of self and emotions. Thus, dissociation is created as a deviation from normal development. On the basis of current theoretical perspectives, children are more likely to develop dissociative symptoms if they lack positive child-caregiver attachments and/or experience trauma.

Developmental Approaches: Neurobiology, Symptoms, Assessments, and Treatment

Neurobiological Considerations

During the past two decades, neurobiological research has begun to explain the underlying cerebral basis for trauma-related dissociation and its impact on a child's behavioral, cognitive, social, and emotional functioning (Diseth 2005). Early stressful life experiences can impact the secretion of neurotransmitters as well as the development and growth of both structural and functional abnormalities in the brain associated with memory, cognition, and emotion. It is important to discuss these neurological underpinnings to better understand dissociation symptomatology in youth.

Diseth (2005) summarized neurobiological research describing how alterations in a child's stress response may lead to dissociative symptoms. Exposure to a traumatic event or chronic stress can lead to hormonal imbalances in children's brains, causing an excess production of stress hormones and neurotransmitters, which impact a child's ability to self-regulate. Behaviorally, children and adolescents demonstrate increased startle responses, irritability, and anxiety (Diseth 2005; Silberg 2013). Children who experience exposure to multiple traumas may demonstrate a habituated response to chronic stress, resulting in atypical reactions to dangerous situations (Diseth 2005). Koopman and colleagues (2004) revealed that greater dissociative symptoms were associated with lower heart rates during stressful interviews of incarcerated adolescents. More specifically, lower heart rates were associated with two specific types of dissociation: derealization and identity alternation (Koopman et al. 2004).

Exposure to traumatic stress can also lead to differentiated activity between brain hemispheres and a reduction in the size of the corpus callosum, the nerve fiber connecting the right and left hemispheres. Traumatized youth and young adults may demonstrate increased activity in the right side of the brain, which is associated with nonverbal emotional communication, and decreased activity in the left side of the brain, which is associated with language. Right-side lateralization and a smaller corpus callosum can impact the brain's ability to integrate visual information (right side) with verbal encoding (left side) across the corpus callosum, leading to an emotion-based style response to distress (Diseth 2005; Silberg 2013). If the child is unable to process information verbally, he or she may experience recurrent reexperiencing of traumatic sights and sounds, often found during flashbacks.

Traumatic stress can also lead to dysfunction in the limbic system (memory, emotion, learning) due to changes in amygdala functioning and reduced hippocampal size. According to Silberg (2013), the overwhelming affect due to early trauma disrupts the development of the affect regulation system. The amygdala controls emotional responses by regulating hormonal and automatic response systems. When the amygdala is overstimulated by repeated trauma, it can lead to changes in behavioral control, such as increased hyperarousal related to anxiety, aggression, impulsivity, and sexual activity (Diseth 2005). The hippocampus, which is responsible for learning and memory, contextualizes information and regulates the individual's reaction to stress.

Last, the maturation of the prefrontal cortex is altered by exposure to prolonged stress. The prefrontal cortex helps evaluate current experiences and determines their relationship to past experiences. Early maturation of the prefrontal cortex, when the cortex develops too quickly and does not reach adult capacity, impacts the main functions of this area, including regulating behavior, impulsivity, attention, and cognition. If the prefrontal cortex is unable to provide input to the amygdala, the region cannot easily calm the fear response, leading to hyperarousal symptoms (Silberg 2013).

The experience of overwhelming trauma in children and adolescents can impact their developmental trajectory, resulting in dysregulation of their consciousness, behavior, and memory. The brain's hormonal imbalances and changes in structure and function cause children and adolescents difficulty in interpreting and responding to their environment, regulating their mood, and managing their behavior. These specific neurobiological changes explain how dissociative symptoms originate, arguing that dissociation may be viewed as a developmental disruption in integrating a child's adaptive memory, sense of identity, and emotional self-regulation (International Society for the Study of Dissociation 2004).

Symptomatology

Developmentally, children and adolescents display unique symptoms of dissociation compared with adults. Youth who demonstrate dissociative symptoms have developed an elaborate system of affect avoidance, resulting in "aberrations in consciousness, perceptions, and body experiences, along with fluctuations of behavior, associated affects, and memory" (Silberg 2013, p. 35). Children and adolescents can demonstrate dazed states; confusion in identity; and dysregulations in mood, behavior, cognitions, somatic experiences, and relationships. DSM-5 describes the diagnostic criteria for dissociative disorders in adults and how these symptoms may present in youth (American Psychiatric Association 2013); however, the current criteria do not capture the extent to which symptoms are behaviorally manifested in children and adolescents.

Because symptoms differ between child and adult populations, it is important to understand how symptoms manifest in children and adolescents in order to best inform treatment. Research has shown that dissociative symptoms often serve as protective factors for traumatized youth. Dissociative experiences can protect the child or adolescent from the traumatic experience as a way to self-regulate or self-soothe (Cook et al. 2005; Putnam 1993). Many traumatized youth display dissociative symptoms when triggered by stress, trauma, or trauma-related stimuli, which can become a habitual form of regulating emotional information because they often detach from themselves or their environments (Putnam 1993; Vermetten and Spiegel 2014).

Despite dissociation serving as a protective factor, it can lead to difficulties with behavioral management, emotion regulation, and self-concept (Cook et al. 2005). Because traumatized children are unable to integrate and develop a normal sense of self, their thoughts and emotions are disconnected. They may experience somatic sensations outside their conscious awareness and engage in behavioral repetitions that occur without awareness or planning. Thus, Cook and colleagues (2005) argue that children and adolescents who display dissociative symptoms are at risk for further victimization or exposure to other forms of trauma and learning difficulties.

Dissociation is often associated with sexual behavior problems, post-traumatic stress disorder (PTSD), depression, aggression, delinquency, and conduct problems in youth (Gerson and Rappaport 2013; Putnam 1993). In addition, youth who experience dissociative symptoms are more likely to display future neglectful parenting behavior, leading to increased generational trauma, and display difficulty with emotional regulation and attachment (Cook et al. 2005; Gerson and Rappaport 2013). In a study by Kisiel and Lyons (2001), dissociation was found to correlate with risk-taking behaviors, poor school performance, less involvement in extracurricular activities, and poor social relationships. In addition, dissociation plays a mediating role between sexual abuse and mental health outcomes, both internalizing and externalizing problems (Kisiel and Lyons 2001). Dissociation is related to impairment of executive functioning exhibited by poor inhibition skills, which can further mediate a child's ability to sustain auditory attention (Cromer et al. 2006).

Dissociative symptoms in youth can be classified into five categories that outline common behavioral experiences in children and adolescents: shifts in consciousness; hallucinatory experiences; fluctuations in knowledge, mood, or patterns of behavior; memory lapses; and abnormal somatic experiences (Putnam 1993; Silberg 2013) (see Table 16–1). Notably, as children enter adolescence and young adulthood, the frequency of dissociative identity disorder (DID)-like symptoms increases with age, and these dissociative symptoms appear more rigid and resemble adult symptomatology (Silberg and Dallam 2009). Preschool and school-age youth may present similarly with these symptoms, whereas adolescents and young adults may present more similarly to adults. In the subsequent sections of this chapter, we focus on the presentation of dissociative symptoms in preschool-age and elementary-age children and adolescents.

Shifts in Consciousness

Preschool, school-age, and adolescent children can experience lapses in consciousness, awareness, or attention known as *depersonalization* that can last from minutes to hours at a time. Youth may feel detached from their current environment or feel as if they are an outside observer of their feelings, thoughts, or actions (American Psychiatric Association 2013). During these moments, children may not respond to their name or may appear to be involved in their own fantasy world. These episodes occur out of context relative to the child's current environment. Behaviorally, children can demonstrate a trance-like state and a look of nonrecognition of familiar people and surroundings; they may freeze in the middle of play or a conversation and later become distraught by the lapse in consciousness (Putnam 1993; Silberg 2013). Adolescents who experience depersonalization may feel that their bodies do not belong to them or feel that they are not themselves when looking in a mirror. Additionally, children and adolescents may enter into a flashback state, confusing the past and present. During these moments, children and adolescents can engage in reenactment of past events and seem caught in a bad dream. Additionally, children and adolescents may also display sleep abnormalities, such as sleepwalking and sleeplessness. They may have difficulty awakening from sleep, may be difficult to arouse, or may show aggressive behavior with little awareness (Silberg 2013, 2014).

TABLE 16–1. Classes of dissociative symptoms in children and adolescents

	Symptoms
Class 1	Shifts in consciousness
Class 2	Hallucinatory experiences
Class 3	Marked fluctuations in knowledge, mood, or patterns of behavior
Class 4	Memory lapses
Class 5	Abnormal somatic experiences

Carrion and Steiner (2000) revealed high rates of dissociation symptoms among juvenile delinquents, with depersonalization being the most common experience. In this study, 96.8% of juveniles endorsed a history of trauma, and 28.3% met the criteria for a dissociative disorder, further documenting that exposure to multiple traumatic events can lead to dissociation (Carrion and Steiner 2000). In addition, research has shown that pathological dissociation is significantly associated with intrafamilial childhood trauma and with the perpetrator being a family member, providing further evidence linking early traumatic experiences with dissociative symptoms (Plattner et al. 2003).

Children and adolescents may also experience changes in their identity, disturbances in their sense of self, or detachment from reality, also known as *derealization* (American Psychiatric Association 2013; Putnam 1993). Because young children developmentally lack a sense of autonomy, preschool-age youth may use their own body parts as transitional objects that have imaginary self-states, for example, calling them "handy" or "footy" (Silberg and Dallam 2009). In these moments, children's body parts appear autonomous from their body. School-age children and adolescents may feel that they are not themselves when feeling angry and upset.

Hallucinatory Experiences

Children and adolescents can experience vivid hallucinatory experiences, which include hearing voices, seeing ghosts, having vivid imaginary friends, or feeling either younger or older than their current age. Preschool-age children can engage in fantasy play with stuffed animals, dolls, or other toys by talking to the toys, hearing their answers, and consulting them for advice. During this vivid imaginary companionship, children may assume different roles in play by differentiating their behavior and voices (Putnam 1993). This imaginary play differs from typical developmental play and may include posttraumatic symptomatology and involve elements of conflict, destruction, and malevolence (Silberg and Dallam 2009). Young children may report seeing imaginary friends, which may play a role in dictating their behavior, or other forms of hallucinations, such as ghosts or odd shapes. In order to differentiate imaginary friends in nontraumatized versus traumatized children, Silberg (2013) hypothesized the following: dissociative children 1) are more confused about whether the friend is only pretend, 2) feel bossed or bothered by the friend, 3) feel that the friend can take over their body, and 4) believe that there are conflicting imaginary friends who make them feel conflicted about how to behave. Dissociative children may perceive having less control over imaginary friends than do nondissociative children and report that imaginary friends argue with them, boss them around, and cause difficulties (Silberg 2013).

School-age children and adolescents may report hearing voices. Children who have experienced traumatic death may hear the sound of a loved one; children with a history of abuse may hear the voice of their perpetrator. Children and adolescents who hear the voices of past perpetrators may respond by becoming aggressive or agitated or may speak in an uncharacteristic voice tone. For clinicians, it is important to differentiate children's reports of hearing voices as being dissociative versus being psychotic symptoms. Often, children and adolescents who are experiencing psychotic symptoms report disorganized information about the voices, such that the personality traits and/or identities are constantly shifting, whereas children who are experiencing dissociative symptoms can have a connection to the voice(s) and experience information in a more organized and consistent manner (Silberg 2013, 2014).

Fluctuations in Knowledge, Mood, or Patterns of Behavior

Preschool, school-age, and adolescent youth can experience fluctuations in mood or patterns of behavior exhibited by changes in relationships with family members, inconsistent skills and abilities, unpredictable mood shifts, and uncharacteristic behaviors. Preschool children may exhibit unpredictable and intense tantrums that appear out of context from the current environment (Silberg and Dallam 2009). At times, children and adolescents may experience an internal or external trigger associated with a traumatic reminder that may instigate a rapid change in behavior or mood; at other times, youth experience fluctuating moods as "happening to them" without a known trigger or onset (Silberg 2013, 2014).

Often, younger children lack the language to describe their internal states and instead may communicate through aggressive behaviors or fantasy play by reenacting trauma (van der Kolk 2005). Young children and adolescents can display changes in their relationships and levels of attachment toward caregivers from loving and affectionate to hostile and aggressive. Sudden regression in behavior (i.e., acting younger than one's chronological age), rageful behavior, or talking about oneself in the third person highlight the difficulty youth experience in integrating affect, consciousness, and identity (International Society for the Study of Dissociation 2004).

In school settings, children and adolescents can experience changes in their cognitive skills from day to day in which behavior is often interpreted as willful, avoidant, or oppositional (Putnam 1993). When faced with stressful or trauma-associated stimuli, children and adolescents may become confused and disoriented (van der Kolk 2005). In addition, adolescents tend to exhibit an increased frequency in acting out, shifting patterns of relatedness, and unstable relationships, symptoms that are similar to adults with DID (Cook et al. 2005; Kisiel and Lyons 2001). Notably, comorbid and nondissociative symptoms may also increase during adolescence, including conduct problems, mood and eating disorders, self-mutilation, substance abuse, and suicidal ideations or attempts (Cook et al. 2005; Gerson and Rappaport 2013). These symptoms, combined with the lack of research in diagnosing dissociative symptoms in adolescence, place teens at increased risk for being diagnosed as psychotic or as having another comorbid diagnosis (Silberg and Dallam 2009; Silberg 2014).

Memory Lapses

Children and adolescents can experience amnesic episodes, exhibiting failure to remember their behavior during an angry episode, the early years of their life, recently completed assignments, or experiences with family or friends. It is common for children to experience amnesia related to past traumatic events or to experience transient forgetting, responding, "I forgot," when asked about their trauma. This response can serve as either a distraction or avoidant behavior due to guilt or shame for a recent event (International Society for the Study of Dissociation 2004). Behaviorally, in preschool and school-age children, amnesia can be perceived as lying, forgetfulness, or denial of the event; however, gentle focusing of attention can promote access to dissociated memory (Silberg and Dallam 2009). In adolescents, amnesia can appear more rigid. Similar to adults, adolescents can display symptoms of dissociative amnesia, forgetting their names and life circumstances.

Abnormal Somatic Experiences

Dissociative youth may experience abnormal somatic symptoms, including shifting somatic complaints, self-harming behaviors, conversion symptoms, pseudoseizures, pain insensitivity, and bowel or bladder incontinence (Silberg 2013, 2014). Young children and adolescents may complain of pain at the site of previous abuse or injuries or complain about a lack of sensitivity to pain. Youth may also exhibit self-injurious behavior, such as skin picking, nail tearing, or head banging to silence internal voices of perpetrators. Preadolescents and adolescents can also engage in cutting behavior, using such objects as razor blades or pencils. Young children and adolescents also self-report shifting abilities related to strength, such as experiencing increased strength when angry. Additionally, it is not uncommon for traumatized youth to experience pain or conversion disorders without an organic cause as well as daytime or nighttime enuresis or encopresis (Silberg 2013, 2014).

Assessing Dissociation in Traumatized Children and Adolescents

Identifying and assessing dissociation in traumatized children and adolescents is essential in order for them to receive the most effective treatments. Assessment may include the following components:

1. Clinical interviews—Clinical interviews seek to obtain complete histories of events and symptom development from reliable informants, with children and adolescents providing information in ways that are appropriate for the individual. Silberg (2013, pp. 250–251) provides an *Interview Guide for Dissociative Symptoms in Children* with questions for each major type of dissociative symptom. Examples include "Where are you when you are not paying attention?" and "Do your friends say you have done things that you cannot remember doing?"
2. Comorbid conditions—Dissociative symptoms are often first identified and assessed when comorbid conditions are being assessed. Common comorbid conditions include PTSD, obsessive-compulsive disorder, eating disorders, reactive attachment disorder, disinhibited social engagement disorder, conduct disorder, oppositional defiant disorder, attention-deficit/hyperactivity disorder, affective disorders, and substance use disorders. Current diagnostic criteria for PTSD include dissociative symptoms such as flashbacks (children may reenact the event in play), numbness or alienation from self, and forgetfulness about aspects of the event (dissociative amnesia). When symptoms of depersonalization (the experience of being an outside observer) or derealization (experience of unreality, distance, or distortion) are present, a person may meet criteria for the dissociative subtype.

3. Screening tests—Screening tests may be used in both initial and ongoing assessment. Table 16–2 provides an overview of self-report and caregiver report tools that range from trauma focused to dissociation specific.
4. Structured clinical interviews—The two structured clinical interviews that address dissociation in children and adolescents are the Child and Adolescent Needs and Strengths-Trauma Comprehensive and the Adolescent Multidimensional Inventory of Dissociation. Refer to Table 16–2 for additional information.
5. Medical evaluation—General medical disorders that can mimic dissociative symptoms include neurological and endocrinal disorders.

Treatment

For traumatized children and adolescents, engaging in dissociative avoidance strategies has become a habitual way of life, in which they learn to avoid overwhelming or painful levels of affect in their environments (Vermetten and Spiegel 2014). Over time, these affect avoidance strategies become well organized and form their own behavioral, emotional, and identity features. Therefore, treatment strategies for dissociative symptoms require a level of commitment and optimism from the therapist, a focus on teaching skills and processing the underlying trauma, involvement of family, and a multisystemic approach (Putnam 1993; Silberg 2013).

The *Guidelines for the Assessment and Treatment of Dissociative Symptoms in Children and Adolescents* (International Society for the Study of Dissociation 2004) incorporate cognitive-behavioral therapy techniques, exposure, and family work to target specific dissociation symptomatology in youth. Prior to implementing treatment interventions, the physical and emotional safety of the child is paramount (International Society for the Study of Dissociation 2004). In addition, the role of the therapist is important in reinforcing and shaping the child's behavior. The therapeutic relationship can model a relationship on the basis of respect and nurturing while providing trust, reciprocity, and an empathetic connection. Additionally, the attitude of the therapist can help empower the child or adolescent throughout treatment. While building the therapeutic relationship, therapists should be mindful of their own attitudes and behavior when working with traumatized children. Suggested treatment principles include conveying an attitude of respect for individual coping techniques and a belief in healing and future thriving, using a practical approach to symptom management, creating a relationship of validation

TABLE 16–2.   Standardized measures to assess dissociation

Measure	Reference	Ages	Description
Clinician-administered measures			
Child and Adolescent Needs and Strengths (CANS)–Trauma Comprehensive	Kisiel et al. 2010	0–18 years	CANS is a 110-item integrated assessment of clinical and psychosocial factors, including trauma exposure/reminders, traumatic stress, grief/loss, anxiety/mood, externalizing symptoms, relationships and attachment, psychosocial functioning, cognition and development, health, parenting and parent, caregiver, family mental health and functioning. Dissociation is measured within the overall context of the child or adolescent's life.
Adolescent Multidimensional Inventory of Dissociation (A-MID)	Dell 2006	12–18 years	A-MID is a 218-item scale designed to comprehensively assess and diagnose dissociative phenomena. It measures dissociative symptoms, including self-confusion, angry intrusions, dissociative disorientation, amnesia, distress about memory problems, subjective experience of the presence of alternate personalities, derealization/depersonalization, persecutory intrusions, trance, flashbacks, body symptoms, and circumscribed loss of remote autobiographical memory. Response sets serve as validity scales and include defensiveness, emotional suffering, rare symptoms, attention-seeking behavior, factitious behavior, and a severe borderline personality disorder index.

TABLE 16–2. **Standardized measures to assess dissociation** *(continued)*

Measure	Reference	Ages	Description
Self-report/caregiver report			
Trauma Symptom Checklist for Young Children (TSCYC)	Briere 2005	3–12 years	The TSCYC is a 90-item caretaker-report scale to assess PTSD symptoms in young children. The eight clinical scales are Anxiety, Depression, Anger/Aggression, Posttraumatic Stress—Intrusion, Posttraumatic Stress—Avoidance, Posttraumatic Stress—Arousal, Dissociation, and Sexual Concerns.
Child Dissociative Checklist (CDC)	Putnam et al. 1993	5–12 years	The CDC is a 20-item scale given to parents or caregivers to screen for dissociative symptoms in their child.
Child Dissociative Experience Scale and Post-Traumatic Stress Inventory (CDES/PTSI)	Stolbach 1997	6–12 years	The CDES is a 37-item scale that asks children to rate the extent to which they are like or unlike children with described dissociative or posttraumatic traits.
Children's Perceptual Alterations Scale (CPAS)	Evers-Szostak and Sanders 1992	8–12 years	CPAS includes 28 items designed to identify symptoms of dissociation in children. Areas include automatic experiences, imaginary playmates, amnesia, loss of time, heightened monitoring, and loss of control over behaviors and emotions.

the child or adolescent because certain youth may need to spend additional time on certain phases of treatment to solidify specific skills. When children or adolescents experience hypoarousal and dissociative shutdowns, it is important to determine the specific triggers that lead to lapses of consciousness, length of the episode(s), interruptions for the child, consequences of these states, and what experience the child or adolescent has during these states (International Society for the Study of Dissociation 2004).

Current evidence-based treatments for trauma-associated symptomatology in youth include, but are not limited to, Attachment, Self-Regulation, and Competence (ARC), trauma-focused cognitive-behavioral therapy (TF-CBT), and child-parent psychotherapy (CPP; National Child Traumatic Stress Network 2018). These treatments focus on establishing safety and incorporating both attachment and affect regulation skills, the theoretical underpinnings of dissociation.

ARC targets children and young adults, ages 2–21, who have a history of complex trauma. It is grounded in attachment theory, early childhood development, the impact of traumatic stress, and factors promoting resilience. This treatment can be delivered in multiple modalities (group, individual, or family based) and focuses on specific targets and skills based on four domains: attachment, self-regulation, competency, and trauma experience integration.

TF-CBT focuses on incorporating cognitive-behavioral therapy, family work, therapeutic relationship, and gradual exposure to reduce PTSD, depressive, and behavioral symptoms in youth with a history of trauma and complex trauma. Similarly to ARC, TF-CBT is grounded in eight treatment components outlined by the acronym PRACTICE: psychoeducation and parenting skills, relaxation training, affect expression and modulation/regulation, cognitive coping, trauma narrative and cognitive processing of the trauma narrative, in vivo exposure, conjoint (parent-child) sessions, and enhancing safety and future development.

CPP targets children ages 0–6 who have a history of maltreatment and domestic violence. CPP has a theoretical basis in attachment theory and integrates psychodynamic, developmental, trauma, social learning, and cognitive-behavioral theories. Key components of CPP include safety, affect regulation, improving the child-caregiver relationship, normalization of trauma-related response, and development of a trauma narrative to allow the child to return to a typical developmental trajectory.

Dissociation-Focused Interventions

Silberg (2013) proposed a treatment model of dissociative-focused intervention (DFI), which focuses on the overarching treatment goals of self-determination and self-regulation to target specific dissociative symptomatology in children and adolescents. DFI is also a components-based model described by the acronym EDUCATE:

- Education about trauma, dissociation, and associated symptomatology
- Dissociative motivation (assessing the child's motivation to change)
- Understanding the hidden parts of the self and exploring alternate identities
- Claiming what is hidden as one's own and learning to embrace the affective experiences and memories associated with the dissociative states in order to develop awareness and mastery over one's behavior
- Arousal, affect, attachment, and teaching emotion regulation skills
- Traumatic processing and understanding triggers, with exposure through creation of a trauma narrative
- Ending state of therapy, having the child fully accept himself or herself and understand and appreciate how his or her new life differs from the past

In contrast to treatment for adults with DID, Silberg (2013) argues that speaking directly to a child's alternate self or voice during treatment is countertherapeutic. Asking a child to switch identity states or speaking directly to a child's alternate identity reinforces that this hidden self is a helpful way to cope, thereby also reinforcing affect avoidance. In this treatment model, hidden internal states are instead described in pictures, words, or symbolic play. By gaining the ability to identify triggers that lead to dissociation avoidance strategies and learning to regulate state shifts, youth begin to build new neural pathways in their brain to cope in a healthier and more adaptive way (Silberg 2013).

In the following clinical vignette, a patient used learned skills, such as understanding the hidden parts of herself and affect regulation skills, to better manage and respond to dissociative symptoms.

Clinical Vignette: School-Age Patient

Abby, an 8-year-old girl, was referred for treatment because of a history of repeated physical abuse and witnessing domestic violence. At intake, Abby reported often hearing her father's voice telling her to harm her 1-year-old cousin and run away from her mother. At home and in school, Abby experienced emotional outbursts, exhibited by crying, yelling, and throwing items. Treatment goals included reframing Abby's negative inner voices and teaching affect regulation skills. Abby learned to journal each time she heard her father's voice and slowly began to reframe its purpose. Abby learned that she heard her father's voice often when she became angry at home, when given limits, or when she perceived her niece was being given more attention than she was. She began to reframe her father's voice as her anger speaking to her, not her father. After learning affect regulation skills, Abby was able to identify specific triggers and events that preceded her emotional reactions. By understanding her triggers, Abby felt more in control of how to manage her responses. Diaphragmatic breathing and positive self-talk (e.g., "I can handle this") assisted in decreasing Abby's level of arousal. She also learned to better communicate her feelings with her teachers and mother and self-advocated when she needed a break in school or from a community-based activity if she felt emotionally overwhelmed.

Adjunctive Treatments

In addition to individual therapy for dissociative youth, adjunctive treatments are recommended by the International Society for the Study of Dissociation (2004). Psychopharmacology may assist in managing other presenting symptoms such as anxiety, inattention, depression, or behavioral dysregulation. Many dissociative youth benefit from educational interventions. A multisystemic approach between the school, parent, and therapist can increase understanding of the child's behavior, establish behavioral support plans, identify stable attachment figures in the school settings, and ensure that the youth's academic needs are being met through specialized instruction, if warranted. Art and play therapy can serve as an additional outlet for children to help express their emotions, and hypnotherapy may be helpful if a child or adolescent is experiencing a traumatic flashback.

Family therapy is often essential because many patterns in family functioning and environment may serve to reinforce current dissociative symptomatology. Involving parents and caregivers in therapy can provide opportunities for sharing psychoeducation about trauma, improve child-parent attachment and communication, and teach parents how to respond to and manage their child's behavior and understand the underlying functions of the dissociative symptoms. Parents and caregivers can also reinforce and help apply learned affect regulation skills in vivo.

Group therapy can promote positive peer interactions, increase social support, and build long-term resiliency in youth, especially adolescents. Evidence-based group therapy treatments for adolescents with complex trauma that emphasize affect regulation skills include Skills Training in Affective and Interpersonal Regulation/Narrative Story Telling (STAIR/NT), Structured Psychotherapy for Adolescents Responding to Chronic Stress (SPARCS), and Trauma Affect Regulation: Guide for Education and Therapy (TARGET) (National Child Traumatic Stress Network 2018).

Eye movement desensitization and reprocessing (EMDR) can aid in the processing of traumatic memories (International Society for the Study of Dissociation 2004). Some EMDR techniques have been adapted for children to involve a cross-modal stimulation that involves tapping or coloring while the trauma story is shared. These movements can create bilateral stimulation, an important component of the EMDR approach (see Chapter 12, "Eye Movement Desensitization and Reprocessing and Dialectical Behavior Therapy"). During EMDR, youth can engage in calming behaviors, such as tapping their knees, as they recite empowering and safety statements such as "I am safe" (Silberg 2013).

The following clinical vignette illustrates how a patient used EMDR to assist with confronting and understanding the hidden parts of himself and to process his traumatic experience.

Clinical Vignette: Adolescent Patient

Jacob, an 18-year-old male, was referred for treatment of bipolar II disorder and complaints of recurring intense panic symptoms without identifiable cause followed by "lost time." He had started college but spent many days hiding in his bathroom, unable to attend classes. His history revealed severe trauma and neglect. Most significantly, at age 7, he found his father bleeding on the floor after a suicide attempt. The bipolar diagnosis caused him significant distress, in part because he understood it to mean he would follow in his father's footsteps. Assessments confirmed diagnoses of PTSD, major depressive disorder, and significant dissociation.

The first stage of treatment was psychoeducation about the psychological effects of traumatic experience and normalization of Jacob's symptoms in the context of his life experience. He was comforted by the model yet continued to believe he was genetically flawed and that healing was not possible. The next stage included affect regulation skills for both the panic and the depression symptoms and cognitive restructuring for the traumagenic cognitions. EMDR techniques were used to increase safety and access to emotional resources. During this phase, Jacob was able to return to school and social activities most days.

The dissociated panic continued, and Jacob reported that breathing techniques and other coping tools were ineffective. Symptom tracking helped him identify possible environmental triggers for the panic, but he stated he had no emotional connection to the memories or triggers. By using EMDR tools for dissociation, Jacob identified two younger selves—the 7-year-old and an 11-year-old. He related to them as an older brother and was able to establish nurturing relationships with each. During the next phase, which involved trauma-focused EMDR with dissociative components, Jacob was able to process finding his father near death. Following several sessions focusing on the traumatic experience, the dissociative panic symptoms abated.

Case studies illustrate that dissociative children and adolescents respond well to appropriate treatment and achieve positive outcomes (Silberg and Dallam 2009). Many trauma-informed treatments, including the DFI model, incorporate the current International Society for the Study of Dissociation (2004) guidelines, highlighting the efficacy of evidence-based treatment components such as affect regulation, cognitive restructuring, family work, exposure, and understanding dissociated identities; however, additional treatment outcome research is warranted to better understanding the impact of certain treatment components on dissociative symptomatology. Although the DFI model incorporates evidence-based treatment components, there is a lack of research regarding the efficacious of this model. Further research and controlled studies are essential, not only to validate the DFI model but also to better understand treatment across developmental phases, including the impact of familial involvement and the efficacy of specific interventions in targeting symptomatology as youth age. Adolescents and young adults are particularly at risk for being misdiagnosed as psychotic. As youth age, they are susceptible to a higher level of morbidity and resistance to treatment (Silberg and Dallam 2009). Research is needed not only on how to better detect and understand the presentation of these symptoms but also how to flexibly incorporate current evidence-based treatments, such as DBT, to better target the needs of these age groups.

Sociocultural and Policy Implications and Resources

> In order to investigate a case of suspected child abuse or litigate that case, you have to not only understand the legal issues, which are complex enough, but one really has to understand something about child development, about the impact of traumatic experiences on children, in order to understand how they react to it and to understand how we react to them.
> —John E.B. Myers, J.D.

The impact of trauma and neglect significant enough to produce dissociation has broad implications for our communities, institutions, and policies. Like most children, those who develop dissociative symptoms interact with adults at school and in the health care system while also having an increased likelihood of interacting with child protective services and the law enforcement and court systems. The emotional and behavioral patterns of children with dissociation may be confusing to service providers who have not been trained in how trauma and neglect may impact a child and how to help them. There are several agencies and organizations whose mission it is to address these issues.

International Society for Study of Trauma and Dissociation

The International Society for the Study of Trauma and Dissociation is a nonprofit international association for professionals whose purpose is to develop and help make available evidence-based, clinically effective treatments and resources for addressing the impacts of trauma and dissociation. In addition to providing information on the assessment and treatment of dissociative symptoms for mental health professionals and producing the *Journal of Trauma and Dissociation*, the society provides information for educational professionals. Through the *Guidelines for the Assessment and Treatment of Dissociative Symptoms in Children and Adolescents* (International Society for the Study of Dissociation 2004), the society recommends the following educational interventions.

1. Ensure availability of supportive staff: Staff who support children and adolescents with dissociative symptoms can help reduce the extent to which disruptive behavior, mood instability, and poor attention interfere with academic functioning.
2. Set expectations and provide assistance with focus: School staff should help encourage the child or adolescent to stay focused even when mood and attention fluctuate. Setting an expectation that the child or adolescent will bring his or her full potential to the school environment can be stabilizing and can encourage the child to succeed.
3. Encourage self-monitoring: The staff should encourage children and adolescents to monitor themselves for signs of distress and to reach out for support.
4. Monitor peer interaction: Without guidance, peers may react in unsupportive ways to extreme shifts in behavior or mood. Designating one member of the staff to deal with any dramatic shifts can help.
5. Encourage use of expressive arts: Inclusion of expressive arts in the curriculum can facilitate expression of emotions in appropriate ways.
6. Ensure interactions with stable attachment figures: Children with trauma and dissociation often need stable adults in the school setting such as counselors, coaches, or teachers with whom they can build a strong attachment. Structures that support frequent interaction with these figures are beneficial.

References

American Psychiatric Association: Diagnostic and Statistical Manual of Mental Disorders, 5th Edition. Arlington, VA, American Psychiatric Association, 2013

Armstrong JG, Putnam FW, Carlson EB, et al: Development and validation of a measure of adolescent dissociation: the Adolescent Dissociative Experiences Scale. J Nerv Ment Dis 185(8):491-497, 1997 9284862

Azeem MW, Aujla A, Rammerth M, et al: Effectiveness of six core strategies based on trauma informed care in reducing seclusions and restraints at a child and adolescent psychiatric hospital. J Child Adolesc Psychiatr Nurs 24(1):11–15, 2011 21272110

Briere J: Trauma Symptom Checklist for Children. Lutz, FL: Psychological Assessment Resources, 1996

Briere J: Trauma Symptom Checklist for Young Children (TSCYC). Odessa, FL, Psychological Assessment Resources, 2005

Briere J, Johnson K, Bissada A, et al: The Trauma Symptom Checklist for Young Children (TSCYC): reliability and association with abuse exposure in a multi-site study. Child Abuse Negl 25(8):1001–1014, 2001 11601594

Carrion VG, Steiner H: Trauma and dissociation in delinquent adolescents. J Am Acad Child Adolesc Psychiatry 39(3):353–359, 2000 10714056

Carrion VG, Weems CF: Neuroscience of Pediatric PTSD. New York, Oxford University Press, 2017

Cook A, Spinazzola J, Ford J, et al: Complex trauma in children and adolescents. Psychiatr Ann 35(5):390–398, 2005

Cromer LD, Stevens C, DePrince AP, et al: The relationship between executive attention and dissociation in children. J Trauma Dissociation 7(4):135–153, 2006 17182497

Dell PF: The Multidimensional Inventory of Dissociation (MID): a comprehensive measure of pathological dissociation. J Trauma Dissociation 7(2):77–106, 2006 16769667

Diseth TH: Dissociation in children and adolescents as reaction to trauma—an overview of conceptual issues and neurobiological factors. Nord J Psychiatry 59(2):79–91, 2005 16195104

Dutra L, Bureau JF, Holmes B, et al: Quality of early care and childhood trauma: a prospective study of developmental pathways to dissociation. J Nerv Ment Dis 197(6):383–390, 2009 19525736

Evers-Szostak M, Sanders S: The Children's Perceptual Alteration Scale (CPAS): A measure of children's dissociation. Dissociation: Progress in the Dissociative Disorders 5(2):91–97, 1992

Gerson R, Rappaport N: Traumatic stress and posttraumatic stress disorder in youth: recent research findings on clinical impact, assessment, and treatment. J Adolesc Health 52(2):137–143, 2013 23332476

International Society for the Study of Dissociation: Guidelines for the evaluation and treatment of dissociative symptoms in children and adolescents. J Trauma Dissociation 5(3):119–150, 2004

Kisiel CL, Lyons JS: Dissociation as a mediator of psychopathology among sexually abused children and adolescents. Am J Psychiatry 158(7):1034–1039, 2001 11431224

Kisiel C, Lyons JS, Blaustein M, et al: Child and Adolescent Needs and Strengths (CANS) Manual: the NCTSN CANS Comprehensive--Trauma Version: A Comprehensive Information Integration Tool for Children and Adolescents Exposed to Traumatic Events. Chicago, IL, Praed Foundation, 2010

Koopman C, Carrion V, Butler LD, et al: Relationships of dissociation and childhood abuse and neglect with heart rate in delinquent adolescents. J Trauma Stress 17(1):47–54, 2004 15027793

Lotti G: Disorganized attachment as a model for the understanding of dissociative psychopathology, in Attachment Disorganization. Edited by Solomon J, George C. New York, Guilford, 1999, pp 291–317

National Child Traumatic Stress Network: Treatments that Work. 2018. Available at: www.nctsn.org/resources/topics/treatments-that-work/promising-practices. Accessed March 22, 2018.

Ogawa JR, Sroufe LA, Weinfield NS, et al: Development and the fragmented self: longitudinal study of dissociative symptomatology in a nonclinical sample. Dev Psychopathol 9(4):855–879, 1997 9449009

Plattner B, Silvermann MA, Redlich AD, et al: Pathways to dissociation: intrafamilial versus extrafamilial trauma in juvenile delinquents. J Nerv Ment Dis 191(12):781–788, 2003 14671454

Putnam FW: Dissociative disorders in children: behavioral profiles and problems. Child Abuse Negl 17(1):39–45, 1993 8435785

Putnam FW: Dissociation in Children and Adolescents. New York, Guilford, 1997

Putnam FW, Helmers K, Trickett PK: Development, reliability, and validity of a child dissociation scale. Child Abuse Negl 17(6):731–741, 1993 8287286

Silberg JL: The Child Survivor: Healing Developmental Trauma and Dissociation. New York, Routledge, 2013

Silberg JL: Dissociative disorders in children and adolescents, in The Handbook of Developmental Psychopathology. Edited by Lewis M, Rudolph KD. New York, Springer, 2014, pp 761–775

Silberg JL, Dallam S: Dissociation in children and adolescents: at the crossroads, in Dissociation and the Dissociative Disorders: DSM-V and Beyond. Edited by Dell PF, O'Neil JA. New York, Routledge, 2009, pp 67–81

Steiner H, Araujo KB, Koopman C: The Response Evaluation Measure (REM-71): a new instrument for the measurement of defenses in adults and adolescents. Am J Psychiatry, 158(3):467–473, 2001 11229990

Stolbach BC: The Children's Dissociative Experiences Scale and Posttraumatic Symptom Inventory: rationale, development, and validation of a self-report measure. Dissertation Abstracts International 58(3):1548B, 1997

related to trauma exposure and can induce additional effects, including excessive daytime sleepiness, inattentiveness and trouble focusing, and agitation. It is now recognized that sleep disorders are separate conditions that coexist with other medical and psychiatric diagnoses. DSM-5 (American Psychiatric Association 2013) and the International Classification of Sleep Disorders (American Academy of Sleep Medicine 2014) both have changed the diagnostic criteria of several conditions to indicate the independent standing of sleep disorders and to highlight that they require separate specific treatment.

Disruption of rapid eye movement (REM) sleep in the aftermath of trauma can compromise the adaptive functions of REM sleep. There is evidence that REM sleep plays a role in the consolidation of recent learning and processing emotional memory, as well as providing the conditions for the brain to recover from or develop resilience toward emotional challenges experienced while awake (Germain 2013). In adult patients with PTSD, studies have observed a negative correlation between PTSD severity and REM sleep continuity. This would seem logical because nightmares are experienced during REM sleep and, generally, thematically relate to daytime experiences and the emotions associated with them (Germain 2013). Nightmares are also characteristic of PTSD, and individuals who have experienced trauma are likely to be affected by an increased number of awakenings due to trauma-related nightmares, which leads to increased WASO and decreased quality of sleep.

Obstructive sleep apnea is a widely experienced sleep disturbance among adults with PTSD (Yesavage et al. 2012). Daytime symptoms of obstructive sleep apnea include daytime sleepiness; difficulty concentrating during wake hours; and, in severe cases, development of affective disorders, namely, depression and anxiety. Notably, obstructive sleep apnea tends to worsen in REM sleep because of the normal atonia associated with the stage of REM, which in some instances can manifest as more frequent nightmares. Therefore, treatment of obstructive sleep apnea may be a successful method of combating daytime PTSD symptoms; some studies have indicated that consistent use of a continuous positive air pressure (CPAP) device may reduce PTSD-related nightmares, but this is not conclusive (Tamanna et al. 2014).

The cognitive-behavioral interventions to improve sleep quality may also alleviate the symptoms of comorbid affective psychiatric disorders and improve daytime energy levels and functioning (Talbot et al. 2014). Use of cognitive-behavioral therapy for insomnia (CBT-I) also serves to reduce any anxiety or fear associated with the process of going to sleep; SOL is often overestimated in subjective measures of sleep (i.e., sleep diaries). About half of all PTSD patients who undergo standard treatments for the PTSD continue to struggle with insomnia. (Talbot et al. 2014). However, studies of adults with PTSD suggest that treating insomnia first with CBT-I achieves both improved objective quality and subjective satisfaction with sleep, as well as the reduction of daytime PTSD symptoms. Moreover, the effects of CBT-I treatment have been observed to endure months after the completion of treatment (Talbot et al. 2014).

The sleep of adults with PTSD has been explored extensively; however, less is known about the sleep of children exposed to traumatic experiences. In this chapter, we discuss the different approaches that may be used to assess the sleep of children exposed to trauma, summarize briefly the extant literature for each method, and touch on the pros and cons of each to assist in determining which tool would be appropriate for implementation by the reader. We finish with a summary of the treatment of sleep disorders in pediatric populations, tailored to the posttrauma population.

Subjective Evaluation of Sleep: Interview and Questionnaires

Description

The assessment of sleep in children exposed to trauma usually begins with exploring the subjective experience of sleep. Because sleep disruptions are part of the diagnostic criteria of PTSD, a clinical interview may uncover the presence of nightmares or subjective sleep disturbances. However, one difficulty when interviewing children is that the identified patient and caregiver may provide different answers about sleep symptoms. Caregivers are aware of sleep symptoms only if the child has let them know. For example, in a series of pediatric burn patients in which both the affected child and caregiver were interviewed about sleep symptoms, the patient report of nightmares was 37%, and caregiver report of nightmares was 27% (Kravitz et al. 1993). Other limitations of the use of clinical interview for research are the nonstandardized nature of an interview and that it can be time consuming, which is why questionnaires may be favored in a research setting (Chimienti et al. 1989).

Research on the presence of subjective sleep disturbance in children exposed to trauma most commonly uses caregiver report or child report standardized questionnaires. The questionnaires may be PTSD-specific, general behavioral/psychiatric, or sleep-specific scales.

for determining when the individual is asleep or awake. For normal sleep and for certain sleep disorders (i.e., insomnia, circadian rhythm disorders), actigraphy correlates strongly with polysomnography (PSG), the gold standard for sleep assessment (Morgenthaler et al. 2007). The correlation is stronger than that between PSG and sleep diaries, suggesting that actigraphy can be a reliable tool for assessing certain aspects of sleep, such as patterning, total sleep time, and sleep efficiency. Three studies have used actigraphy to assess the sleep of abused children, and all three demonstrated increased sleep latency and sleep fragmentation (Kovachy et al. 2013).

Developmental Considerations and Limitations

Actigraphy has been used in all age ranges, from infants to the elderly. The tracking device is typically worn on the wrist but may be worn on the ankle in very young populations or those sensitive to any type of monitor. Actigraphy mattresses and other modified limited-contact devices have been made commercially available. Because of the unobtrusive nature of the monitoring equipment, actigraphy is useful for the assessment of items requiring more longitudinal data around sleep, such as the assessment of insomnia or circadian rhythm disorders. However, it is not an exact measurement of the sleep state or stages, and it cannot be used to diagnose certain sleep disorders, such as sleep-related breathing disorders, periodic limb movement disorder, or narcolepsy. The data obtained from actigraphy monitoring are limited to activity or movement, the total sleep time, sleep latency, WASO, sleep-wake timing, and sleep efficiency. Although the agreement of actigraphy with PSG outperforms agreement with subjective sleep logs, the correlation of actigraphy ranges from 0.15 to 0.92 (Morgenthaler et al. 2007) and tends to be limited in the presence of other sleep disorders such as sleep-disordered breathing.

Objective Evaluation of Sleep: Polysomnography

Description

PSG is the gold standard for the assessment of sleep. The PSG procedure involves electroencephalography, electrooculography, and electromyography for the definition of sleep-wake states, as well as other monitors for the assessment of breathing at the nose and mouth; thoracic and abdominal belts for measuring the effort of breathing; pulse oximetry; and electrocardiography. Extensive research using PSG has been performed in adults exposed to traumatic experiences. Adults with PTSD have been found to have altered sleep architecture (increased stage 1 sleep, reduced slow-wave sleep, and increased REM density) (Kobayashi et al. 2007), as well as a high prevalence of other sleep disorders, such as sleep-disordered breathing (Yesavage et al. 2012). To date, we are aware of only one study using PSG to evaluate sleep in children who have been exposed to abuse. The children exposed to abuse demonstrated reduced total sleep time, sleep efficiency, and REM sleep and increased WASO (Collado-Corona et al. 2005).

Developmental Considerations and Limitations

Polysomnography has been used in all ages, from infants to the elderly. PSG provides the most thorough assessment of sleep physiology. Only PSG is able to determine the stages of sleep and the sleep architecture and microarchitecture, and it is necessary for the diagnosis of certain sleep disorders (e.g., sleep-disordered breathing, narcolepsy). However, polysomnography requires significant equipment for monitoring and extensive expertise for the application of the monitoring equipment and interpretation of the results. It is more labor intensive and costly, so it does not lend itself as readily to longitudinal assessment of sleep. Further, the extensive equipment required can be overwhelming for some children, who may not understand the utility of the monitoring equipment or may become anxious with the sleep laboratory environment. However, systematic desensitization to the equipment has been shown to help children with neuropsychiatric conditions effectively complete polysomnography (Primeau et al. 2016).

Treatment

Although behavioral interventions for PTSD in pediatric populations are established, change in sleep symptoms after improvement in PTSD symptoms has not been described. In adults, even after successful completion of PTSD treatment, sleep symptoms persist and are the most common residual symptom seen (Zayfert and DeViva 2004). Because sleep symptoms represent disorders that impair daytime functioning, increase the risk for development of physical and psychiatric disease, and reduce quality of life, they deserve independent treatment.

Behavioral interventions for improving insomnia symptoms are the cornerstone for treating insomnia-related sleep disruption in children. Among other things, pediatric behavioral sleep medicine includes appropriate sleep hygiene, such as keeping consistent sleep-wake timing, allowing an age-appropriate amount of time for sleep, and having a good wind-down routine. Children with high anxiety may benefit from relaxation tools, such as guided imagery, or alternative responses, such as getting up to read a book, when they are unable to sleep. Medications, if prescribed, should be considered as an adjunct for the short term while addressing behavioral modification (Owens et al. 2005). Case reports indicate improvement in nightmares with the use of prazosin, clonidine, and guanfacine (Kovachy et al. 2013). A behavioral intervention for nightmares, imagery rehearsal therapy (IRT), has also been developed and used in younger children (ages 6–11) (Simard and Nielsen 2009), older children (ages 9–11) (St-Onge et al. 2009), and adolescents with posttraumatic stress symptoms (Krakow et al. 2001). IRT involves selection of a specific stress dream, modification of the ending of the dream, and rehearsal of the alternative outcome to improve mastery over the fearful dream. IRT is effective for decreasing nightmare frequency and distress, although it tends not to improve daytime symptoms. In adults with PTSD, the treatment of sleep disorders has been shown to improve daytime functioning (Talbot et al. 2014) and to be effective to help prepare a patient for prolonged exposure therapy (Baddeley and Gros 2013).

Selecting appropriate assessment tools for investigating sleep is essential for treating sleep disorders in children exposed to trauma or experiencing posttraumatic stress symptoms, because the treatment of sleep disruption will vary significantly by the condition being addressed. For example, if only medications or behavioral interventions for insomnia are prescribed for a child who awakens frequently and is very sleepy during the daytime, perhaps another condition that causes frequent awakenings, such as sleep-disordered breathing, might be missed, and the child's condition might fail to improve or may respond only partially. It is also possible that more than one sleep problem will exist in a child exposed to stressful experiences. Children may report both nightmares and difficulty staying asleep or returning to sleep on their own. A thorough assessment will allow both symptoms to be explored so treatment planning can address all disruptive symptoms. If a child demonstrates sleep symptoms resistant to behavioral modification or medication treatment, a coexisting sleep disorder might be present, and referral to a sleep medicine specialist for further evaluation may be considered.

Conclusion

Sleep problems are prevalent in children exposed to trauma and can be investigated by caregiver and child report, as well as through objective measurement of sleep. The sleep symptoms reported and the clinical setting help determine the tools appropriate for assessing sleep; some children may require referral to a sleep center for more focused evaluation and treatment of sleep disorders. Sleep symptoms of PTSD are not usually improved through treatment of PTSD alone; however, focused treatment of sleep disorders can help to improve quality of life and reduce daytime psychiatric symptoms.

KEY CONCEPTS

- Sleep disruption is common in children exposed to trauma, and sleep disruption may represent a treatable sleep disorder.
- Sleep may be assessed by child and caregiver report or monitored by actigraphy or polysomnography. Each tool has limitations and relative merits.
- Treatment of sleep disorders can help improve daytime functioning and quality of life for children exposed to trauma.

Discussion Questions

1. What is the importance of assessing sleep in children who have been exposed to traumatic experiences?

2. What are the relative merits of a clinical interview or questionnaires versus more objective sleep monitoring? What are the drawbacks to the clinical interview and questionnaires?

3. What treatments have been used for the treatment of nightmares in children with exposure to stressful experiences?

Suggested Readings

Kobayashi I, Boarts JM, Delahanty DL: Polysomnographically measured sleep abnormalities in PTSD: a meta-analytic review. Psychophysiology 44(4):660–669, 2007 17521374

Kovachy B, O'Hara R, Hawkins N, et al: Sleep disturbance in pediatric PTSD: current findings and future directions. J Clin Sleep Med 9(5):501–510, 2013 23674943

Simard V, Nielsen T: Adaptation of imagery rehearsal therapy for nightmares in children: a brief report. Psychotherapy (Chic) 46(4):492–497, 2009 22121846

References

Achenbach TM, Rescorla LA: Manual for the ASEBA School-Age Forms and Profiles. Burlington, VT, University of Vermont Research Center for Children, Youth, and Families, 2001

American Academy of Sleep Medicine: International Classification of Sleep Disorders, 3rd edition. Darien, IL, American Academy of Sleep Medicine, 2014

American Psychiatric Association: Diagnostic and Statistical Manual of Mental Disorders, 5th Edition. Arlington, VA, American Psychiatric Association, 2013

Baddeley JL, Gros DF: Cognitive behavioral therapy for insomnia as a preparatory treatment for exposure therapy for posttraumatic stress disorder. Am J Psychother 67(2):203–214, 2013 23909060

Chemtob CM, Nomura Y, Abramovitz RA: Impact of conjoined exposure to the World Trade Center attacks and to other traumatic events on the behavioral problems of preschool children. Arch Pediatr Adolesc Med 162(2):126–133, 2008 18250236

Chimienti G, Nasr JA, Khalifeh I: Children's reactions to war-related stress: affective symptoms and behaviour problems. Soc Psychiatry Psychiatr Epidemiol 24(6):282–287, 1989 2512645

Chorpita BF, Yim LM, Moffitt CE, et al: Assessment of symptoms of DSM-IV anxiety and depression in children: a Revised Child Anxiety and Depression Scale. Behav Res Ther 38(8):835–855, 2000 10937431

Collado-Corona MA, Loredo-Abdalá A, Serrano-Morales JL, et al: Sleep alterations in childhood victims of sexual and physical abuse [in Spanish]. Cir Cir 73(4):297–301, 2005 16283961

Frederick C, Pynoos R, Nader R: Childhood Posttraumatic Stress Reaction Index (CPTS-RI). Los Angeles, University of California at Los Angeles, 1992

Germain A: Sleep disturbances as the hallmark of PTSD: where are we now? Am J Psychiatry 170(4):372–382, 2013 23223954

Kobayashi I, Boarts JM, Delahanty DL: Polysomnographically measured sleep abnormalities in PTSD: a meta-analytic review. Psychophysiology 44(4):660–669, 2007 17521374

Koren D, Arnon I, Lavie P, et al: Sleep complaints as early predictors of posttraumatic stress disorder: a 1-year prospective study of injured survivors of motor vehicle accidents. Am J Psychiatry 159(5):855–857, 2002 11986142

Kovachy B, O'Hara R, Hawkins N, et al: Sleep disturbance in pediatric PTSD: current findings and future directions. J Clin Sleep Med 9(5):501–510, 2013 23674943

Krakow B, Sandoval D, Schrader R, et al: Treatment of chronic nightmares in adjudicated adolescent girls in a residential facility. J Adolesc Health 29(2):94–100, 2001 11472867

Kravitz M, McCoy BJ, Tompkins DM, et al: Sleep disorders in children after burn injury. J Burn Care Rehabil 14(1):83–90, 1993 8454673

Llabre MM, Hadi F: War-related exposure and psychological distress as predictors of health and sleep: a longitudinal study of Kuwaiti children. Psychosom Med 71(7):776–783, 2009 19592513

Morgenthaler T, Alessi C, Friedman L, et al; Standards of Practice Committee; American Academy of Sleep Medicine: Practice parameters for the use of actigraphy in the assessment of sleep and sleep disorders: an update for 2007. Sleep 30(4):519–529, 2007 17520797

Owens JA, Spirito A, McGuinn M: The Children's Sleep Habits Questionnaire (CSHQ): psychometric properties of a survey instrument for school-aged children. Sleep 23(8):1043–1051, 2000 11145319

Owens JA, Babcock D, Blumer J, et al: The use of pharmacotherapy in the treatment of pediatric insomnia in primary care: rational approaches. A consensus meeting summary. J Clin Sleep Med 1(1):49–59, 2005 17561616

Primeau M, Gershon A, Talbot L, et al: Individuals with autism spectrum disorders have equal success rate but require longer periods of systematic desensitization than control patients to complete ambulatory polysomnography. J Clin Sleep Med 12(3):357–362, 2016 26564388

Pynoos RS, Steinberg AM: The UCLA PTSD Reaction Index for DSM-5. Los Angeles, CA, Behavioral Health Innovations, 2013

Rofe Y, Lewin I: The effect of war environment on dreams and sleep habits. Series in Clinical and Community Psychology: Stress and Anxiety 8:67–79, 1982

Simard V, Nielsen T: Adaptation of imagery rehearsal therapy for nightmares in children: a brief report. Psychotherapy (Chic) 46(4):492–497, 2009 22121846

St-Onge M, Mercier P, De Koninck J: Imagery rehearsal therapy for frequent nightmares in children. Behav Sleep Med 7(2):81–98, 2009 19330581

Talbot LS, Maguen S, Metzler TJ, et al: Cognitive behavioral therapy for insomnia in posttraumatic stress disorder: a randomized controlled trial. Sleep 37(2):327–341, 2014 24497661

Tamanna S, Parker JD, Lyons J, et al: The effect of continuous positive air pressure (CPAP) on nightmares in patients with posttraumatic stress disorder (PTSD) and obstructive sleep apnea (OSA). J Clin Sleep Med 10(6):631–636, 2014 24932142

Yesavage JA, Kinoshita LM, Kimball T, et al: Sleep-disordered breathing in Vietnam veterans with posttraumatic stress disorder. Am J Geriatr Psychiatry 20(3):199–204, 2012 20808112

Zayfert C, DeViva JC: Residual insomnia following cognitive behavioral therapy for PTSD. J Trauma Stress 17(1):69–73, 2004 15027796

18

Self-Injurious Behaviors and Suicidality

Shayne N. Ragbeer, Ph.D.
Moira Kessler, M.D.

CHILDREN WITH CHRONIC histories of trauma and disruptions in significant attachment relationships often miss out on developmentally normative opportunities to learn adaptive self-soothing mechanisms. Moreover, trauma overwhelms the body's stress response system, making it more difficult to cope with daily stressors. Youth affected by trauma may in turn develop ineffective or even potentially harmful methods to regulate anxiety, distress, guilt, and shame; to communicate their emotional pain and seek assistance from others; or to feel "something" amid experiences of emotional numbness or "emptiness." This may involve inflicting physical pain on themselves or pervasive wishes to escape life's stressors entirely. Given this link, it is critical to include self-injury and suicidality in a broader discussion of assessing and treating children and adolescents exposed to trauma.

In this chapter, we review recent data regarding prevalence and risk factors of suicidality and self-injurious behavior (SIB) in young children and adolescents, including risk due to childhood traumatic experiences. We discuss developmental approaches to assessment and treatment of suicidality and self-injury and provide an overview of current empirical support for evidence-based psychotherapy models. We address potential challenges that may arise in treating children and adolescents with SIB and suicidal behavior, particularly in those affected by trauma. We offer two case examples highlighting developmental considerations and potential challenges. Finally, we discuss broader implications and future directions.

Prevalence Rates of Suicide and Nonsuicidal Self-Injury

In the United States, suicide is the second leading cause of death among adolescents (ages 15–24) and young adults (ages 25–34) and the third leading cause of death among 10- to 14-year-olds (Kann et al. 2016). In a nationally representative sample of U.S. high-school students, more than 17% endorsed seriously contemplating suicide, and more than 8% reported that they had attempted suicide at least once within the past year (Kann et al. 2016). Regarding SIB (see Table 18–1 for key terms and definitions), prevalence rates are more difficult to establish because of varying criteria for this behavior. Nonsuicidal self-injury (NSSI) refers to deliberate self-harm that inflicts pain or injury to the body without intent to die. Among adolescents, self-injurious behavior has also been observed among young children, including those with significant trauma histories. Younger children may present more commonly with biting, scratching with fingernails, hitting themselves, and banging their head.

Risk Factors for Suicide and NSSI

The Centers for Disease Control and Prevention outline several risk factors for suicide in the United States, including gender; age; race; history of suicide attempts; history of NSSI; and presence of a psychiatric disorder, including posttraumatic stress disorder (PTSD; Kann et al. 2016). (See Table 18–2 for a list of risk and protective factors.) On the basis of CDC reports (Kann et al. 2016), boys are more likely to complete suicide, whereas girls are more likely to attempt suicide. The most common method among 15- to 19-year-old males is firearms, whereas girls ages 10–19 and younger males are more likely to use hanging or suffocation. Young adults and older teens are more likely to complete suicide, whereas younger teens are more likely to attempt suicide.

TABLE 18–1. Definitions of key terms

Term	Definition	Examples
Self-injurious behavior (SIB)	Deliberate harm or injury or behavior with potential for injury afflicted on oneself	Cutting (e.g., on arms or inner thighs with razor, scissors, or box cutter; burning skin; scratching); does not include risk-taking behavior (e.g., substance use, speeding)
Nonsuicidal self-injury (NSSI)	SIB that is conducted without suicidal intent	Cutting behaviors where the goal is to reduce intense emotion and there is no intent to die
Passive suicidal ideation (passive SI)	Thoughts conveying a wish to be dead	"Everything would be better if I were dead"; "I wish I could go to sleep and not wake up"
Active suicidal ideation (active SI)	Thoughts about killing oneself, which may or may not include strong desires to die; thoughts about specific methods; thinking about plans or preparatory acts; or intent to actually act on thoughts	Fantasies of shooting self in the head or of jumping off a bridge or building: "I want to just kill myself"; "Maybe I'll get a gun"; "I could do it over the holidays when everyone is away"; "Everything will be better once I end all of this"
Other suicidal behavior	Carrying out plans or preparation	Buying gun, giving away possessions, preparing documents, writing suicide note

TABLE 18–1. Definitions of key terms *(continued)*

Term	Definition	Examples
Suicide attempt	Any behavior that either harms or has risk of harming oneself that is carried out with the intention to die as a result; it may or may not result in actual physical injury but does not result in death. A suicide attempt may be interrupted if someone is on the verge of carrying it out and is intercepted by himself or herself, another person, or another event.	Deliberately overdosing on prescribed or recreational drugs with intent to die; attempting to suffocate oneself
Suicide	Death by self-injury or behavior that was intended to be fatal	Act such as shooting oneself in the head, suffocation, intentional overdose, hanging, or jumping off tall structure that results in death

In terms of culture and ethnicity, indigenous groups identifying as American Indian or Alaska Native are currently at highest risk for both attempted and completed suicide, with a suicide rate that is approximately three to four times greater among 15- to 24-year-olds compared with other ethnic groups in the same age range. Individuals identifying as white or Hispanic have higher rates of suicide than those identifying as African American; however, individuals identifying as African American have higher rates of attempts than white individuals.

Maltreatment history confers high risk for suicidality and suicide attempts across diverse samples of adolescents (for a review, see Miller et al. 2013). Various forms of maltreatment, including childhood sexual abuse, physical abuse, emotional abuse, and neglect, are independently associated with suicidal ideation (SI) and suicide attempts and have an additive effect. Research suggests that emotional abuse (Miller et al. 2013), sexual abuse (Miller et al. 2013; Serafini et al. 2015), and exposure to a greater number of adverse events confer greater risk (for a review, see Serafini et al. 2015).

TABLE 18–2. Risk and protective factors for suicidality

Category	Factors not specific to age	Age-specific factors	
		Children (ages 5–9)	Adolescents
Gender	Boys more likely to complete suicide; girls more likely to attempt suicide	Boys more likely to complete suicide: 85% male vs. 15% female	Boys more likely to complete suicide: 70% male vs. 30% female (ages 12–14)
Age			Young adults and older teens more likely to complete suicide; younger teens more likely to attempt suicide
Culture/ethnicity	American Indian and Alaska Natives at highest risk; Hispanic population has higher rates of suicide than non-Hispanic black population; black population has higher rates of attempts than non-Hispanic white population	Black children complete suicide at a rate of 36.8%	Black adolescents complete suicide at a rate of 11.6%
Psychiatric disorders	Active psychiatric disorders such as PTSD, depressive disorders, anxiety disorders, ADHD, disruptive behavior disorders, bipolar disorder, eating disorders, schizophrenia, alcohol and substance use, personality traits (formerly Cluster B or Cluster C)	ADHD (60%) most significant mental health predictor vs. depression (33.3%)	Depression (almost 66%) most significant mental health predictor vs. ADHD (29%) for ages 12–14

TABLE 18–2. Risk and protective factors for suicidality *(continued)*

Category	Factors not specific to age	Age-specific factors	
		Children (ages 5–9)	Adolescents
Social stressors	Childhood trauma, sexual abuse (increased further if by family member), greater number of adverse events in childhood, being LGBTQ, bullying, parental psychopathology, recent discharge from a psychiatric hospitalization, relationship breakup or conflicts, disciplinary actions, recent suicide by peer or in the media, family stressors	Other, nonromantic relationships (e.g., peer relationships)	Stressors related to romantic relationships (ages 12–14)
Prior behaviors	Aggressive or violent behaviors, suicide attempts (increases with number of attempts), NSSI, impulsive behaviors		
Current symptoms	Hopelessness, sleep disturbance, suicidal ideation		
Protective factors	Family adaptability and cohesion, good problem solving		

Note. ADHD=attention-deficit/hyperactivity disorder; LGBTQ=lesbian, gay, bisexual, transgender, and queer/questioning; NSSI=nonsuicidal self-injury; PTSD=posttraumatic stress disorder.

The relationship between childhood sexual abuse and suicidality appears to be stronger when the abuser is a family member. This is also associated with more severe suicidal behavior, such as actual attempts (Serafini et al. 2015). Often, risk is elevated in association with high levels of worthlessness and hopelessness, as well as impulsivity, all of which are common among young children affected by trauma.

Psychiatric disorders associated with trauma, such as PTSD, depressive disorder, anxiety disorders, and alcohol or drug use disorder, are risk factors for suicidality and self-injury. Other disorders, including bipolar disorder, disruptive behavior disorders, eating disorders, and schizophrenia, are also associated with higher risk. Although depression is strongly associated with higher rates of suicidality across several periods of the lifespan, it is a less significant predictor among younger children. Indeed, in children ages 5–11, attention-deficit/hyperactivity disorder is the most common mental health correlate of suicide (Sheftall et al. 2016). Younger children may often lack the necessary executive functioning abilities to actually plan and carry out a lethal suicide attempt, and there are a lower prevalence of psychopathology and lower suicidal intent in this developmental period. However, younger children may also have less developed problem-solving skills and higher impulsivity, which could increase risk for harming themselves in the face of a stressor.

Precipitants of acute suicidal thoughts also tend to differ across developmental periods. For instance, clinicians may consider factors such as parental psychopathology as a more significant risk factor for young children and bullying as more significant for school-age children and events such as breakups or relationship conflicts as precipitants among adolescents.

The majority of adolescents and young adults who die by suicide have no documented history of prior suicidal behavior; however, SI, prior attempts, and engagement in NSSI are significant predictors of suicide attempts (Castellví et al. 2017). Additionally, impulsivity, sleep disturbance, a history of learning difficulties, a history of aggressive or violent behavior, and recent discharge from a psychiatric hospitalization may be important indicators of risk in clinical samples.

Prevention of Suicide and NSSI

There are various ways to approach suicide prevention in children and adolescents; we focus on prevention within a clinical setting. Advising families to restrict lethal means within the home is a critical aspect of prevention (Zalsman et al. 2016). Means may include guns, medications, sharp objects, and household chemicals. Research also supports the use of psychiatric medication in suicide prevention (Zalsman et al. 2016). There is evidence for the use of lithium for mood disorders, clozapine for psychotic disorders, and antidepressants for depression. Although there is a black box warning for increased suicidality when antidepressants are started with adolescents, evidence suggests that cautious treatment with antidepressants for depression is still warranted. Given the evidence to support various psychotherapies, which are discussed in the next section, another critical prevention strategy involves making sure children and adolescents at risk are identified, are connected to treatment, and are adherent.

Developmental Approaches
Preschool and School-Age Children
Assessment

Regardless of risk or intent, verbalization of SI by a young child is a clear indication of emotional distress. Although there is a need for more literature outlining evidence-based guidelines for assessing suicidality in preschool or school-age children, there are general principles that may guide a clinician in the assessment and management of such symptoms and behaviors. For instance, it is important to understand the meaning of the SI or statements to the child, as well as his or her understanding of death and dying. Until about ages 6–8 years, children often do not begin to comprehend the permanence of death or that a person who has died is no longer able to think, feel, or engage in the world. Full understanding of the finality of death, and their own vulnerability to it, often does not develop until adolescence. However, exposure to the death of a close loved one during childhood may accelerate this development, and there is variability due to other factors such as individual differences in cognitive development. Additionally, it is important to ask clarifying questions in multiple ways to ensure that children comprehend questions and concepts and that the clinician fully understands the meaning of the child's statements. Taking breaks during an assessment may be helpful. It is also important to interview children alone, where they may feel freer to respond openly than they would in the presence of their caregivers.

Exploring caregivers' experiences in relation to death may also be important in understanding the context of the child's statements. Moreover, assessing caregivers' reactions to these statements may help to elucidate the function of the child's statements and may clarify which behaviors of the caregivers may reinforce repeated statements. In turn, caregivers may have difficulty tolerating such verbalizations from their children, and their responses may serve to inhibit a child's expression.

Suicide assessment of young children may include the use of an existing structured interview tool such as the Child Suicide Risk Assessment (Larzelere et al. 2004). Assessment measures should supplement data obtained from directly observing and interviewing the child; interviewing the child's caregivers; and obtaining additional collateral information from teachers, guidance counselors, and other adults who interact with the child on a regular basis. Collateral information may also include school report cards, the child's medical chart, and records from child protective services or other involved systems that can provide information on the child's functioning over time. Multiple forms of information help to provide a comprehensive history in order to more accurately identify risk factors and evidence of prior suicidal or self-injurious thoughts or behavior.

Evidence-Based Interventions

Initial investigations into the feasibility of adapting interventions for preadolescents have not determined specific efficacy in reducing suicidality or self-harm in this developmental period. The Collaborative Assessment and Management of Suicidality (CAMS) treatment approach has been examined through case studies of younger children (Ridge Anderson et al. 2016). Briefly, CAMS is a clinical intervention developed by David Jobes that involves a therapeutic framework in which the patient and clinician use significant collaboration in order to perform assessment and to develop the treatment plan (Jobes 2012). The intervention uses the treatment alliance to increase motivation in the patient and also uses a suicide status form as a multipurpose tool. However, these findings are preliminary, and follow-up efficacy and effectiveness studies are needed to determine the generalizability of these interventions. Identifying other early indicators of adolescent suicidality and SIB could also help with creating earlier prevention and intervention programs targeting such behavior in childhood.

Clinical Vignette 1

Jude is a 6-year-old African American boy who lives with his foster mother. He attends first grade and has an Individualized Education Program (IEP) for a previously diagnosed mixed receptive-expressive language disorder. He was referred for treatment of disruptive and oppositional behavior at school. Jude entered foster care as a toddler after his biological mother's parental rights were terminated because of significant physical neglect and lack of supervision in the context of chronic substance use. A year after he entered the foster care system, his maternal grandparents initiated court proceedings seeking visitation rights, which were soon granted. During visits, Jude was allegedly exposed to excessive punishment by both grandparents on several occasions. For instance, his grandfather reportedly punched and slapped him with a belt buckle to the point of leaving marks and bruises, and his grandmother locked him in dark closets for long periods of time, subjecting him to both physical and emotional maltreatment, respectively. When Jude disclosed these incidents to his foster parent, she reported this information to the court, and visits were terminated while the grandparents underwent investigation.

Subsequently, Jude's biological father was granted visits with him. One day at school, Jude and his class were learning about natural disasters and ways to remain safe during them. Jude said, "I wish the hurricane could just come get me." The teacher reported this to Jude's foster mother and therapist. When the therapist asked Jude what he meant, he explained that he felt as if "everyone is always telling me what to do. I don't want to listen anymore." Further exploration revealed that during visits with his biological father, Jude would at times go to his maternal grandparents' house. Jude disclosed that the grandparents no longer physically hurt him, and they were helping his father to pay some bills in exchange for bringing him to see them. Jude reported they had all told him he could not share this secret, and although he did not like the situation, he felt he had to protect his family from getting in trouble. He verbalized that keeping the secret had become "too hard" for him. Appropriate officials were notified, and visits were paused while the matter was examined. Therapy continued to focus on developing Jude's ability to identify and express his feelings so he could more effectively communicate when he was overwhelmed. Significant psychoeducation and cognitive restructuring around his sense of "responsibility" to protect his biological family were also focal components of therapy. Jude also identified various "safe" adults with whom he could be honest and could disclose difficult situations impacting him.

In this case, Jude's passive suicidal statement was a means of expressing his wish to escape from an overwhelming situation and a way to share his feelings while maintaining the secrecy he felt obligated to keep. Although he did not specifically express a wish to be dead or intent to kill himself, Jude had multiple risk factors, including his history of physical and emotional maltreatment. Additionally, his expressive and receptive language difficulties may have complicated his ability to convey the meaning of his statements. By paying attention to Jude's meaning, his therapist was able to clarify the situation and improve his treatment, and Jude was removed from an inappropriate environment.

Adolescents

Assessment

Assessing and treating adolescents at risk for suicide involves an awareness of acute and chronic risk factors and careful assessment of these factors in the individual. A careful mental status examination should include the presence, frequency, and severity of a patient's SI because greater severity and frequency of SI are associated with increased suicidal risk. The clinician should note the thought process and content of the patient's SI, assessing whether the thought process is future oriented and goal directed. It is imperative in clinical practice that the individual's unique history and mental status be considered when conducting assessments of an adolescent's imminent or more chronic risk of suicide. When assessing and monitoring suicide risk, it is essential for clinicians to consider other contextual and interpersonal factors in addition to being aware of general risk and protective factors. As with treatment of children, working collaboratively with the adolescent, caregivers, and other active members of their systems can be pivotal in developing comprehensive safety plans and methods of assessing ongoing risk.

It is critical to ask questions directly even in the face of a clinician's fears or discomfort. Importantly, there is no evidence in the literature to suggest that asking directly about suicide will trigger suicidal thoughts, behavior, or NSSI that was not already present. In practice, using such tools as the Linehan Risk Assessment and Management Protocol (LRAMP; Linehan et al. 2012) and the Columbia Suicide Severity Rating Scale (CSSRS; Posner et al. 2011) is important in helping clinicians more easily identify relevant risk factors and in aiding clinicians in assessing a patient's level of risk. Of note, these tools do not replace a comprehensive interview, during which careful attention is paid to recent events that may precipitate more acute risk. However, after conducting a comprehensive interview, a clinician may use these measures as checklists to determine the number of risk factors an adolescent has and may use these data in determining level of risk.

The CSSRS has strong convergent and divergent validity, shows good sensitivity and specificity, includes sensitivity to change over time, and has good internal consistency. The CSSRS provides a tool to identify risk and protective factors, taken from medical records or interviews with the individual and his or her family, and helps to determine level of risk for suicide on the basis of the integrated data. The LRAMP is a semistructured checklist that also lists indicators of imminent suicide risk, which allows a clinician to tally a patient's risk factors, and provides guidance in conducting and documenting a comprehensive assessment of acute or imminent risk. The LRAMP is typically conducted at the beginning of treatment and can be used in an ongoing manner if there are subsequent incidents of self-harm, suicide attempt, or suicide threats or an increase in SI. The protocol serves as the clinician's aid in determining a treatment plan, such as whether or not hospitalization is justified, and provides important guidance for safety planning.

Evidence-Based Interventions

There is a growing body of evidence-based treatments (EBTs) that show efficacy in treating suicidality and NSSI among adolescents in outpatient settings. There is no current evidence to suggest that hospitalization or residential care is superior to outpatient treatment of suicidality, and, in fact, several theoretical models recommend maintaining outpatient-based care to the extent that is possible. We focus on EBTs that can be used on an outpatient basis. Pilot and preliminary randomized controlled trials (RCTs) among youth reviewed by Glenn et al. (2015) showed initial evidence that treatments such as integrated cognitive-behavioral therapy (I-CBT) by Esposito-Smythers and colleagues, attachment-based family therapy (ABFT) by Diamond and colleagues, interpersonal psychotherapy for adolescents (IPT-A) by Mufson and colleagues, and mentalization-based treatment for adolescents (MBT-A) by Rossouw and Fonagy may be efficacious in targeting suicidality and self-harm. However, at the time of the review, the efficacy of these treatments in reducing suicidality and/or self-harm had been examined only in a single RCT. More robust data from at least two independently conducted RCTs with an active comparison group are required to determine that these are well-established treatments for suicidality and self-harm (Glenn et al. 2015).

I-CBT adds parent training to traditional individual CBT strategies (e.g., addressing cognitive distortions, problem-solving) and family CBT strategies (e.g., behavioral contracting) and is conducted over a 12-month period. The first 6 months involve weekly sessions, the next 3 months move to biweekly sessions, and the final 3 months are a "maintenance" period of monthly sessions. I-CBT has been associated with reductions in suicide attempts compared with treatment as usual (TAU; Esposito-Smythers et al. 2011). These reductions in suicide attempts are possibly associated with the addition of the parent training component and with reductions in substance use, but this needs to be replicated in studies in which adolescents in TAU are receiving equivalent doses (see Esposito-Smythers et al. 2011).

Family-based therapies (FBTs) target family functioning as a mechanism of reducing self-injurious thoughts and behaviors and use traditional family therapy techniques, including building effective communication skills and problem solving. ABFT specifically employs more emotion-focused, process-oriented strategies in addition to CBT techniques to enhance relationship functioning among family members. ABFT has shown significant reductions in SI compared with a TAU protocol with referrals and monitoring. The Resourceful Adolescent Parent Program, another FBT that used parent training only, included a four-session psychoeducational program to reduce adolescent suicide risk through more effective parenting strategies and by decreasing family conflict. This program led to significant reductions in adolescent self-injury overall, including both suicidal behavior and NSSI, and the effects were mediated fully by improvements in family functioning (Diamond et al. 2002). However, it is unclear whether ABFT is effective in treating suicidal behavior and if FBT parent training is efficacious in treating SI, suicidal behavior, and nonsuicidal behavior independently.

IPT-A focuses on the reciprocal influences of depressive symptoms and interpersonal functioning on each other and targets the adolescent's interpersonal communication and problem-solving skills as a vehicle for reducing depressive symptoms. It typically consists of 12 weekly individual sessions, with adjunctive parenting work as needed. There is support for IPT-A being significantly associated with greater reductions in SI compared with TAU in an intensive delivery (2 weekly sessions for 6 weeks in school) among adolescents with depression (Tang et al. 2009). More RCTs are required to provide additional support for this link, as well as to help determine whether IPT-A is associated with reductions in suicidal behavior in addition to suicidal thoughts.

Mentalization-based treatment for adolescents (MBT-A) is a year-long manualized intervention that includes weekly individual and monthly family therapy sessions. MBT-A conceptualizes self-injurious behavior as a response to stress in the context of poor mentalization skills (i.e., the ability to understand the link between one's own and others' behaviors and feelings and cognitions). The model therefore aims to build mentalization skills and self-control in order to reduce self-injury. Adolescents receiving MBT-A have shown significantly greater reductions in deliberate self-harm posttreatment compared with those receiving TAU, and effects were mediated through increased mentalization skills and lower attachment avoidance (Rossouw and Fonagy 2012). Like the other interventions, there were several limitations, and additional RCTs with more diverse samples are required to further support the efficacy of this intervention.

Dialectical behavior therapy for adolescents (DBT-A), developed by Miller and colleagues (see Chapter 12, "Eye Movement Desensitization and Reprocessing and Dialectical Behavior Therapy"), includes the components of standard DBT for adults plus various adaptations that involve caregivers, including a multifamily skills group as well as a skills module called "Walking the Middle Path" that is focused on addressing difficulties within adolescent-family relationships. Evidence from predominantly female outpatient and clinical samples suggests that DBT-A is associated with significant reductions in SI, suicidal behavior, NSSI, and thoughts of NSSI, but either the majority of these studies were conducted without control groups or similar reductions were shown in TAU groups (for a review, see Glenn et al. 2015). Mehlum and colleagues (2016) conducted a randomized trial comparing DBT-A with enhanced usual care and examined 1-year follow-up data. At the end of the 19-week trial, DBT-A was superior to the control group in terms of reducing SI and self-harm. At 1-year follow-up, DBT-A maintained lower levels of self-harm, but there were no longer differences between the two groups with regard to SI because of improvements in the enhanced usual care group. This suggests that DBT-A may have an advantage in maintaining long-term reductions in self-harm and leads to quicker reductions in SI. Furthermore, a more recent independent trial has also shown efficacy for DBT-A in reducing suicide attempts and self-harm in a primarily female, high-risk sample of adolescents (McCauley et al. 2018). Although these data were not available at the time of the review by Glenn and colleagues (2015), current evidence (McCauley et al. 2018; Mehlum et al. 2016) supports DBT-A as an efficacious and established empirically supported treatment for suicidality and self-harm in youth. Further investigation is important to demonstrate robust effects and generalizability across diverse samples in clinical practice.

Many of these interventions target problem-solving skills and relationship effectiveness, thus addressing and building up abilities in areas identified as protective factors. Additionally, these interventions have been adapted to be developmentally informed, drawing on the importance of the family system's involvement in symptom reduction and quality of life improvement. However, many of these interventions remain understudied and require greater replication in larger-scale RCTs with diverse populations to better establish their efficacy and effectiveness in reducing suicidality and SIB in adolescents.

Clinical Vignette 2

Manuela is a 16-year-old lesbian Latina in the tenth grade, living with her mother and her mother's partner. At initial evaluation, Manuela's mother, Ms. R, reported she had noticed several cuts on Manuela's left forearm. Manuela explained that she had been cutting herself with a razor and disclosed that this behavior had begun in middle school when an older male cousin sexually assaulted her for the first time. For the next several years, Manuela had frequent contact with her cousin, and the abuse continued.

The cousin's family moved to another state when Manuela entered high school, at which time contact was naturally discontinued. Since then, Manuela reported she had continued to cut herself at times to "make myself feel better" and that she had recently been cutting more frequently after hearing about the sexual assault of a peer.

When Ms. R learned of the abuse and cutting behaviors, she notified the school guidance counselor, who helped notify child protective services, connected the family to legal services, and referred Manuela for therapy. Manuela met criteria for PTSD and had subthreshold symptoms of depression. Although Manuela denied any suicidal intent, she endorsed passive SI, sometimes wishing she could "just disappear forever." Manuela stated she would never do something lethal because she "would be too afraid" and denied ever making a plan. Given the chronic nature of her SI and recent acute exacerbation of her NSSI, Manuela was referred to a comprehensive outpatient DBT-A program. Although she continued to experience intermittent passive SI, it became much less frequent and much milder in intensity, and she stopped cutting herself for several months.

Manuela's emotion regulation skills improved and safety concerns diminished, but she continued to experience symptoms of PTSD such as anhedonia, restricted range of affect, and nightmares about her sexual abuse. When Manuela and her mother were approaching 6 months in the DBT-A program, Manuela and her team decided to shift to trauma-focused treatment. A week later, the individual therapist received a phone call from Manuela's school. Two students found Manuela standing on the railing of a 10-floor fire escape looking down. She had been crying and told the other students she wanted to jump. Manuela was taken to the hospital and was kept for observation in the psychiatric emergency room for 48 hours. At discharge, Manuela denied suicidal intent, agreed to stay safe, and collaborated on an updated safety plan.

When Manuela returned to therapy, the clinician used behavior analysis to help identify factors contributing to the recent escalation of suicidal behavior. Manuela reported that her primary emotion had been fear: "I thought I was ready for trauma treatment, but I just am not ready to go there." Manuela had thought that if she were in the hospital or having repeated safety concerns, she would not have to begin trauma treatment. Her ability to identify, validate, and tolerate her fear was pivotal in influencing her choices over the next few weeks. She was aware of her wish to avoid trauma treatment, but she was also aware that avoiding it would heighten her anxiety and would keep her feeling afraid. Manuela decided that she did not actually want to die and in fact wanted to live a happier life and that addressing her PTSD would be the most effective way to achieve this goal.

Manuela then maintained a month with no acts of self-harm or severe SI. She transitioned into trauma-focused therapeutic work. Although exposure and creating narratives around her trauma was terrifying to her, Manuela realized that addressing the trauma would help her "feel better" in the way that accepting and tolerating her emotions had helped her in DBT. Nine months later, Manuela endorsed mildly depressed mood, had improving grades, and was developing friendships and a romantic interest at school. She did not resume cutting, and her passive SI was infrequent and transient.

Manuela presented with several risk factors for attempting suicide, such as chronic NSSI; history of repeated sexual abuse by a family member; and such demographic characteristics as her age and her identification as lesbian, Latina, and female. In terms of protective factors, her mother was supportive and committed to treatment, and the family member who had abused her was no longer present, thus lowering her risk of revictimization. In addition, her cognitive functioning allowed her to participate in problem solving and to retain acquisition of new skills. Nonetheless, Manuela's case provides a picture of how a clinician may address an adolescent with a trauma history presenting with NSSI and suicidal behavior, understand risk factors, and formulate a treatment plan that is effectively tailored to keep adolescents safe while meeting their emotional needs.

Overcoming Potential Challenges

When assessing and treating NSSI and SI, managing safety and risk are both critical and challenging given that current predictors of risk are not robust. Moreover, although NSSI does not have suicidal intent, it remains a significant safety risk, especially in the context of substance use, and may unintentionally lead to more severe, permanent, and even lethal consequences.

When addressing these behaviors in youth exposed to trauma, a clinician must balance the need to maintain safety prior to addressing trauma with the need to address the underlying persistent symptoms of untreated posttraumatic stress reactions. Although it is important that youth are stable enough and developing adequate coping skills to be able to successfully engage in trauma work, it is also important not to reinforce the avoidance of trauma, which in turn maintains anxiety, or to inadvertently reinforce the suicidal thoughts, suicidal behavior, or NSSI. It is important to be mindful that the clinician and the patient may have varying, and seemingly conflicting, treatment goals. Whereas the clinician's primary priority is to maintain safety, the patient's goal may be to reduce pain at any cost. As such, there is a fine balance between prioritizing safety while supporting a patient's autonomous goals and maintaining rapport. EBTs such as DBT-A have considered the need to address such issues and aim to balance validation with necessary change. Further investigation into treatment of youth with trauma is needed, as well as youth exposed to trauma in diverse underrepresented groups, who may be at even greater risk for suicidality and SIB.

It is important that clinicians of all levels of experience in working with suicidality and self-injury be mindful of anxiety and/or increased stress that may be experienced when working with high-risk youth and managing risk on a constant basis. It is critical to ensure that a clinician's own reactions do not interfere with conducting comprehensive assessments or making appropriate decisions to focus on trauma with an adolescent who has chronic risk. Seeking consultation and supervision from colleagues and mentors and ensuring a therapist feels supported and is attending to personal self-care are important aspects of ensuring that a patient receives optimal care.

Sociocultural and Policy Implications

In addition to ensuring that mental health providers thoroughly assess and treat NSSI and suicidal behavior, it is important that caregivers, schools, the broader health care network, and other systems are informed about risk factors and signs of self-harm or suicide in youth. With significant media attention to suicide, which is often misinformed, mental health professionals may need to adopt a role of advocacy and dissemination of education to broader systems. Because portrayals of mental health care may be inaccurate, practitioners may need to provide psychoeducation that guides adolescents toward appropriate help. Connectedness to parents may be a protective factor, so educating parents about risk factors, warning signs, and how to talk to children about suicide is an important area for prevention.

The dissemination of prevention efforts specifically targeted to diverse groups at increased risk is particularly critical. It is imperative that more specific factors often not captured by broad, overinclusive demographic categories be examined. For instance, general categories used to identify ethnic differences may not capture important specificity related to country or region of origin, religion, multicultural identity, race, acculturation, and/or immigration experiences. Additionally, further investigation is necessary to inform considerations for youth of all genders and gender identities, including youth identifying as transgender, gender nonconforming, and gender nonbinary. Overall, it is critical to expand empirical evidence to include diverse and intersectional identities across neurodevelopment, intellectual and physical ability, culture, gender identity, and sexual orientation, among myriad other considerations. Moreover, addressing disparities in access to mental health care by augmenting the ability of professionals in primary care and school settings to identify and address the needs of youth at risk for suicide is an important direction for the future (see Asarnow and Miranda 2014).

Conclusion

Clinical practice with children and adolescents engaging in NSSI or suicidal behavior is challenging and poses additional considerations for work with youth exposed to trauma. Although researchers have investigated predictors of suicide and there are evidence-based treatments associated with the reduction of NSSI, SI, and suicide attempts, considerable work must be done to augment our predictive abilities and interventions. There is a paucity of research examining SI in preschool and school-age children. We recommend further research into earlier indicators of preadolescent and adolescent suicide risk and development of preventative interventions that target reducing risk at younger ages. Moreover, we should continue examining unique predictors affecting at-risk and often underrepresented groups to ensure that interventions are tailored to their individual needs.

Researchers and clinicians in mental health are well positioned to help disseminate policies that address the needs of youth at risk for NSSI and suicide and that promote the use of a trauma-informed lens within schools, primary care settings, and policy. Advocacy, public education, and evidence-based assessment and treatment are all important areas on which we should continue to focus.

KEY CONCEPTS

- A history of trauma is associated with an increased risk of nonsuicidal self-injury (NSSI) and suicide risk in children and adolescents, with sexual abuse and exposure to a greater number of adverse events being associated with highest risk.

- In assessing risk in children and adolescents engaging in NSSI or expressing suicidal ideation, it is important for the clinician to clarify the patient's understanding of death and his or her meaning in the statements. Additionally, clinicians should work to understand their personal reactions and the reactions of caregivers in response to suicidal risk.
- In assessing risk in children and adolescents engaging in NSSI or expressing suicidal ideation, clinicians should consider both acute risk factors and long-term risk factors in an effort to minimize risk of acting on these thoughts or continuing to act on these behaviors.
- There are limited data and a need for further research into evidence-based treatments to target NSSI and suicidal ideation in youth, especially in children.
- For adolescents, there is emerging promising evidence for using such treatments as attachment-based family therapy, mentalization-based treatment for adolescents, interpersonal psychotherapy for adolescents, and integrated cognitive-behavioral therapy to target symptoms, including NSSI and suicidal ideation. Dialectical behavior therapy is the first established treatment for suicidality and self-injurious behavior among adolescents. More research is needed and continues to be done.

Discussion Questions

1. What are the key components that should be considered when assessing a child or an adolescent with a trauma history for suicidal risk?

2. What are ways to balance the need to minimize safety risk and the need to minimize avoidance of addressing trauma in children and adolescents?

3. How should evidence-based treatments vary between children and adolescents to improve efficacy?

4. What is the role of mental health providers and researchers in disseminating accurate information about suicide risk and informing public prevention policies?

5. What are ways that you can improve your personal practice to be more sensitive and attuned to patients with a trauma history?

CHAPTER

19

Substance Use

Michael D. De Bellis, M.D., M.P.H.
Kate B. Nooner, Ph.D.

Definitions of Substance Use Disorders

Traumatic stress in childhood, particularly chronic interpersonal stress such as child maltreatment or witnessing family or community violence, greatly increases the risk for late childhood–, adolescent,- and young adult–onset substance use disorder (SUD; De Bellis 2001a; Kilpatrick et al. 2000). Having posttraumatic stress disorder (PTSD) in youth secondary to these types of interpersonal traumatic stressors also greatly increases the risk for adolescent-onset SUD (Kilpatrick et al. 2000). Child- and adolescent-onset SUD is defined as alcohol, marijuana, nicotine, or other substance use disorders. According to the *Diagnostic and Statistical Manual of Mental Disorders*, 5th Edition (DSM-5; American Psychiatric Association 2013), an SUD is diagnosed when one suffers from at least two of the following symptoms: 1) using a substance in larger amounts and over a longer period than intended; 2) a persistent desire or unsuccessful efforts to control one's substance use; 3) spending a great deal of time engaged in efforts to obtain the substance, use the substance, or recover from its effects; 4) craving for the substance; 5) recurrent use resulting in

389

et al. 2016). The ventral medial prefrontal cortex is a complex brain structure with many functions, including emotion regulation, decision making, assignment of value to context, danger prediction, fear learning, fear generalization, and the mediation of extinction learning and retention.

These stress-sensitive brain regions (amygdala, hippocampus, anterior cingulate cortex, and ventral medial prefrontal cortex) are integral for processing traumatic events in humans and animals because of their richness in glucocorticoid receptors and the tightly regulated connections between these cortical and limbic regions. Glucocorticoid receptors are essential for gene transcription. One of their roles in the brain is to bind to the major stress hormone cortisol, which is made in the adrenal cortex and is vital for stress regulation, body and brain development, metabolism, and immune response. When glucocorticoid receptors bind with cortisol, this has an impact on gene transcription, which has been found to be related to alterations in the aforementioned stress-sensitive brain structures following trauma (De Bellis and Zisk 2014). Trauma and stress contribute to increases in cortisol levels that can influence gene expression, which in turn can influence the way the brain responds to substances.

These neurobiological mechanisms can increase the risk of SUD and are an area of active research. The orbital frontal cortex in particular becomes dysregulated in youth with PTSD and youth and adults with SUD. This highlights the neurobiological underpinnings that are common to PTSD and SUD (Figure 19–1) (for a review, see De Bellis et al. 2013).

Self-Medication Mechanisms for Substance Use Disorder in Youth With PTSD Symptoms

PTSD is considered to be a disorder of recovery in which the prefrontal cortex is not able to dampen amygdala arousal in the face of traumatic reminders; PTSD symptoms can occur expectedly and precisely or unexpectedly and imprecisely. The traumatic reminder can be an external or internal conditioned stimulus that activates unwanted and distressing recurrent and intrusive memories of the traumatic experience(s) (e.g., the unconditioned stimulus). Accordingly, this activation causes PTSD symptoms (e.g., the unconditioned response). Youth may or may not be consciously aware of the association that triggers the PTSD symptom and may use substances in a range of unhealthy ways to try to curtail PTSD symptoms.

For example, a youth who experiences domestic violence may feel disproportionately angry and aggressive when he hears loud voices. He may then impulsively self-medicate with drugs that temporarily dampen the biological stress systems, such as alcohol, marijuana, or benzodiazepines

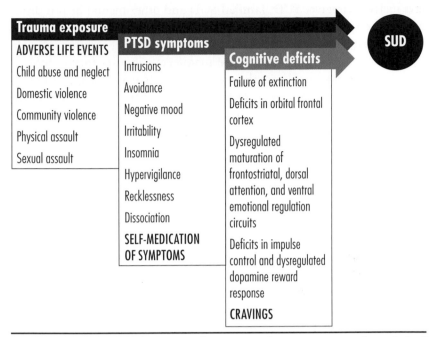

FIGURE 19–1. **Developmental traumatology conceptual model of trauma, posttraumatic stress disorder, and substance use disorder**

(e.g., alprazolam). Another youth may develop maladaptive use of alcohol or marijuana as a way to try to decrease insomnia-related PTSD symptoms. A youth whose major traumatic stress symptoms involve emotional numbing or anhedonia may consume stimulants, such as methylphenidate, cocaine, or hallucinogens, to relieve her sense of "nonbeing." Thus, youth with trauma history and PTSD symptoms are likely using substances to self-medicate their PTSD symptoms (De Bellis et al. 2013).

A youth may develop problematic substance use because he or she uses these substances to decrease unwanted PTSD symptoms; however, using substances in this manner may interfere with healthy functioning and will ultimately lead to an SUD. Trauma-focused cognitive-behavioral therapy is an evidence-based treatment for youth with PTSD that can assist youth in becoming more aware of PTSD-SUD associations so they can learn control in order to cope with PTSD and SUD symptoms without engaging in substance use or other harmful behaviors (Cohen et al. 2004).

Genetic and Learning Factors

There are other factors, particularly those related to genetics and family systems, that contribute to SUD in youth with trauma histories. These factors include caregiver SUD, familial SUD and other mental health disorders, poverty, and dysfunctional family dynamics (De Bellis 2001a, 2001b). They involve both genetics and learning (e.g., alcohol and substance use as coping skills) and are major contributors to youth SUD. These factors may complicate the successful treatment of youth with trauma history and SUD and need to be addressed in treatment. Research is under way to examine whether these factors are independent, additive, or amplifying and to determine how youth can become resilient to SUD despite extreme childhood stressors.

Clinical Presentations

Patients with SUD who have experienced trauma can present to clinicians in two ways: with PTSD symptoms or with a primary SUD. A patient who presents with SUD needs to be assessed for trauma history because trauma history will influence the course of treatment. This topic was comprehensively reviewed in *Substance Abuse Treatment for Persons With Child Abuse and Neglect Issues* (available for free at www.ncbi.nlm.nih.gov/books/NBK64901). This guideline is part of the Treatment Improvement Protocol (TIP) Series, which consists of evidence-based best practice guidelines for the treatment of substance abuse, provided as a service of the Substance Abuse and Mental Health Services Administration's (SAMHSA) Center for Substance Abuse Treatment. The guideline offers practical techniques on methods to assess trauma and deal with trauma issues in adult survivors of childhood trauma (Resource and Consensus Panel 2000), and much of this information is also important for clinicians who treat adolescents. Detailed discussion of assessment and treatment of individuals who present with SUD is beyond the scope of this chapter; we recommend that clinicians and researchers who treat youth in this area review the TIP guidelines and related materials. In this chapter, we focus on individuals who present with PTSD symptoms and need evaluation or treatment for SUD.

Preschool and School-Age Children

All youth should be assessed in a developmentally appropriate manner for alcohol and substance use, including in very young children if clinically indicated. Although it is unusual for preschool and school-age children to consume alcohol or drugs, the clinician can use developmentally tailored clinical tools to ask a young child about his or her knowledge of these issues, such as showing clinically appropriate photographs of beer bottles, wine glasses, cigarettes, or joints and asking the child if he or she has seen and/or can name the item. If the child can name the item, then the clinician can ask if the child ever saw an adult use these items or if the child ever drank or put these objects in his or her mouth. If the child responds in the affirmative to these questions, the clinician should follow up appropriately according to the clinical guidelines of the setting that the child is in and in full accordance with mandatory child abuse reporting laws for the region.

Follow-up for these questions should also involve the caregiver and could include a home visit or child protective services depending on the clinician's professional judgment. For example, a child may be brought to the emergency department because of alcohol or drug poisoning. This typically occurs because of a caregiver's failure to supervise (e.g., caregivers are intoxicated and leave alcoholic beverages in reach of a hungry child), and this warrants a child protective services report. It is important to remember that clinicians are mandated reporters. If a clinician thinks that a caregiver may have problematic substance use or a child may have inappropriate exposure to substances, the clinician is required to report; the role of investigation falls to the department of social services and law enforcement.

School-Age Children and Adolescents

Youth should be assessed for alcohol and substance use as part of the standard mental health assessment by simply asking them how many times they have used alcohol, cigarettes, marijuana, or other drugs to get high. This can be done in the form of a semistructured interview, such as those mentioned in Chapter 3, "Assessment of Individuals," or according to the guidelines of the clinical setting in which the child or adolescent is being evaluated. In substance use assessments with adolescents, clinicians are generally bound by the confidentiality guidelines of eminent danger, which means that an adolescent's report of substance use can remain confidential from caregivers as long as it is not eminently dangerous. Clinicians should be clear with adolescents and caregivers at the outset so that confidentiality and its limits are known before any clinical evaluation. In addition, clinicians should look to the laws of their specific region to know the exact rules and ages for confidentiality, eminent danger, and reporting with minors. Youth are usually more honest with these questions if the clinician can explain to them and their caregiver before the assessment what will remain confidential and under what conditions the clinician has the obligation to breach their privacy. Interviews or other clinical assessments should specifically ask about over-the-counter drugs, drugs the parents may have in the home, and substances used or obtained by friends.

Older grade-school children who have histories of trauma and neglect often are seen for a variety of SUDs, including alcohol, marijuana, tobacco, cocaine (crack), and opioid dependence. In the primary author's experience, maltreated youth have been introduced to substances by receiving them from older youth, adolescents, or young adults as "payment" for being forced to "run drugs" in their neighborhood. These youth usually have extensive histories of school absenteeism and other internalizing and externalizing behavior problems. On the basis of the primary author's experience, another concern when youth in this age group have an SUD is sexual abuse. Perpetrators of sexual abuse may give substances to seduce, sedate, or otherwise influence their victims to cooperate with inappropriate sexual behaviors. As stated, these cases warrant child protective services involvement, a team approach, and intensive treatment for trauma and SUD. Older youth and adolescents with trauma histories may begin to use substances to self-medicate PTSD symptoms.

If a youth answers yes to any substance use questions asked during assessment, appropriate follow-up should include questions related to amount of, duration of, setting for, and reasons for use and willingness to have a urine toxicology screen. It is useful to ask these questions using a structured, evidence-based format so that the clinician is thorough and consistent in evaluation. Some examples of instruments that are not costly to use are the substance use disorder section of the Kiddie Schedule for Affective Disorders and Schizophrenia—Present and Lifetime Version (K-SADS-PL) for DSM-5 (Kaufman et al. 2016) and the substance use assessment battery of the PhenX Toolkit's Substance Abuse and Addiction Collections (available at www.phenxtoolkit.org/index.php?pageLink=about).

Some important questions that can be asked when a youth gives a positive response are "How often are you using the substance?" "How much of the substance are you using?" "Are you using alone? Or with friends?" "Why do you use?" "What does the substance do for you? How does it make you feel?" Another good screening question a clinician can ask a youth is "If we did a urine toxicology screen today, what drugs would show up positive?" However, all clinicians should consider seeking guidance from their treatment setting (e.g., checking their clinic's operating procedures and/or holding a case conference so all relevant treatment providers can have input and make recommendations) before conducting a detailed clinical evaluation or treatment pertaining to PTSD and SUD. These cases are complex and may activate PTSD symptoms and increases in SUD self-medication behaviors; for these reasons, treatment usually requires a team approach and case management.

As part of this clinical evaluation, it is important to ascertain the patient's safety. Is the substance being used in dangerous situations? Is substance dependence present? It is also important to address suicidal ideation because substances may have been used in an overdose attempt. For outpatients, clinical consultation with a supervisor may be needed if the clinician feels that either talking to the youth's caregiver or hospitalization is indicated.

It is important to handle the assessment in a nonjudgmental way and to conduct the interview showing concern for the youth's physical and mental health. When having to discuss substance use with a caregiver who may be unaware of the situation, it is important to have an understanding of how the caregiver will respond to the child's behaviors. In the first author's experience, when the youth and clinician talk to the parent together, give psychoeducation about substance use, and come up with a safety and treatment plan at the time of this discussion, the parents are usually upset but grateful for the information and assistance. When it comes to highly sensitive issues such as PTSD and SUD, if the clinician works with parents and youth in this manner, youth are usually relieved to find that their parent is more concerned about their health and well-being than angry with them.

It should be noted that the information presented here represents a general overview and should not be taken as direct clinical recommendations for working with youth with PTSD and/or SUD. Clinicians should use the information here in collaboration with evidence-based practice, appropriate supervision, regional and national laws, and the guidelines and regulations at their specific treatment setting.

Adolescents and Transitional-Age Youth

SUD is three times more common in adolescents and young adults with trauma history than in those without trauma histories (Kilpatrick et al. 2000). Additionally, substance use starts younger in youth with trauma histories than in youth without such histories. In the first author's clinical experience, maltreated youth can present with SUD as young as 9 years. Therefore, it is important to ask about tobacco, alcohol, marijuana, and other drug use in elementary-age youth with trauma histories.

and adolescents. Clinicians who specialize in trauma-focused therapies can follow evidence-based guidelines, which can include adding developmentally appropriate coping skills that prevent SUD in their practice, thus leading to primary SUD prevention in youth.

Clinicians should always evaluate for alcohol and substance use and SUD before starting treatment because these issues will further complicate treatment and may lead to treatment dropout. Failure to routinely screen for alcohol and substance use and SUD can therefore limit evidence-based treatment planning. In this chapter, we described several well-established measures for assessing alcohol and substance use and SUD in children, adolescents, and young adults. Appropriate assessment of alcohol and substance use and SUD will lead not only to more informed and comprehensive differential diagnosis, including dual diagnosis, but also to the opportunity to provide appropriate evidence-based treatments or referrals for intervention for youth with trauma histories.

Evidence-based assessment, as a standard practice within mental health settings, can also help to destigmatize the experience of substance use and trauma. Clinicians can provide psychoeducation by explaining that self-medication with substances for trauma symptoms occurs in all segments of the population. Normalization of SUD symptoms associated with trauma and PTSD symptoms can help the patient and family understand that the child's responses are understandable in response to complex trauma; it can also help deflect anger or disappointment a caregiver may be experiencing while fostering a collaborative treatment approach. It is strongly recommended that the clinician provide hope by explaining empirically supported treatments that are available to address complex PTSD with SUD. The National Child Traumatic Stress Center maintains a detailed listing of empirically supported treatments and promising practices to address trauma and SUD in children and adolescents (National Child Traumatic Stress Network 2008).

KEY CONCEPTS

- Substance use disorders (SUDs) are more common and can be more treatment resistant in adolescents and adults who have experienced childhood trauma or maltreatment, particularly if they also have posttraumatic stress disorder (PTSD).

- Substance use assessment for children, adolescents, and adults with trauma histories should be part of a comprehensive mental health evaluation.

- PTSD symptoms in children and adolescents that are left untreated can contribute to later SUDs.
- Evidence-based treatment for youth with PTSD, SUDs, and dual diagnosis are critical for preventing long-term sequelae and intergenerational transmission of trauma.

Discussion Questions

1. In what ways is substance use different in youth with trauma histories than youth without trauma histories?

2. What are the most effective and efficient means to assess youth substance use in clinical practice?

3. What are the most effective and efficient means to treat youth substance use?

4. What barriers exist to assessing youth substance use and trauma histories?

Suggested Websites for Additional Information

American Academy of Child and Adolescent Psychiatry: www.aacap.org
National Child Traumatic Stress Network: www.nctsn.org
Seeking Safety: www.seekingsafety.org
Substance Abuse and Mental Health Services Administration: www.samhsa.gov

References

American Psychiatric Association: Diagnostic and Statistical Manual of Mental Disorders, 5th Edition. Arlington, VA, American Psychiatric Association, 2013

Brown SA, Brumback T, Tomlinson K, et al: The National Consortium on Alcohol and NeuroDevelopment in Adolescence (NCANDA): a multisite study of adolescent development and substance use. J Stud Alcohol Drugs 76(6):895–908, 2015 26562597

Bukstein OG, Bernet W, Arnold V, et al; Work Group on Quality Issues: Practice parameter for the assessment and treatment of children and adolescents with substance use disorders. J Am Acad Child Adolesc Psychiatry 44(6):609–621, 2005 15908844

20

Full Spectrum of Care

Laura D. Heintz, Psy.D.

TRAUMA IS NOT a new concept. Trauma is part of the human condition; most people will experience a sudden loss or tragic event of some sort in their lives that triggers a survival response. That response is natural, yet, depending on the severity, duration, and symptoms of the response, the individual may require professional support to move through the aftereffects. However, until recently, trauma treatment seemed applicable to only a small portion of the population. Posttrauma responses were first recognized as posttraumatic stress disorder (PTSD) in survivors of war or catastrophic events. Not all symptomatology rises to the level of PTSD, but changes in behavior and other symptoms after a traumatic event or enduring chronic stress and chaos can be seen in individuals, groups, and communities.

It is now understood that trauma-informed care is necessary in the treatment of mental health challenges in children and adults. Trauma-informed care must begin with safety (Substance Abuse and Mental Health Services Administration 2014). Children and youth who remain in an unsafe or unpredictable environment and live in fear for their physical or emotional safety will not be able to change the coping behaviors or begin to heal until they feel a sense of safety. Depending on the youth's behaviors, devel-

the interventions. The family is at the center of the development of the treatment goals and is absolutely necessary for treatment plans to be successfully implemented and completed.

Understanding the therapeutic service relationship goes hand in hand with the understanding of services. Trust and engagement will likely not be present when services begin but must be developed over time. Collaboration and partnership in the treatment process allow for sustained progress and engagement throughout treatment. Child and family teaming is an example of a structure that supports family-centered practice and helps build trust and facilitates engagement in treatment. Extensive training should be provided to the designated facilitator, who is responsible for facilitating collaboration between the child welfare worker, behavioral health practitioners, families, natural supports, and the youth to plan, coordinate, and monitor the mental health treatment plan. In child and family team meetings, the facilitator of the meeting engages the youth and family in the process of envisioning where they desire to be at the end of service and defining their goals. These meetings include critical members of the treatment team, including the youth and primary caregivers, therapist, social worker, probation officer, and/or other identified key natural support people such as a teacher. The whole team regularly meets to determine goals, review progress toward goals, define skill-building focus areas, identify key intervention strategies, and assign responsibility. The team evaluates progress together, holds one another accountable, and celebrates successes. This process in itself reduces isolation, builds trust, improves communication, and helps develop problem-solving skills. Everyone on the team is obligated to honor the family-centered principles and holds one another accountable to those principles (Figure 20–1).

In order to identify natural supports for the youth, which is especially important for foster youth and for transitional-age youth, clinicians have used family connection maps in practice (Figure 20–2). The maps are completed in child and family team meetings and are color coded to identify heart connections, mentors and teachers, spiritual leaders, and those who understand the family culture. These connection maps are a form of genogram and focus on biological relatives and nonrelated people to whom the youth considers himself or herself to be connected. A person identified on the map can serve in one or multiple roles.

Developmental Factors

The response to trauma will vary for every person depending on the severity or duration of the trauma in conjunction with the youth's age and the cop-

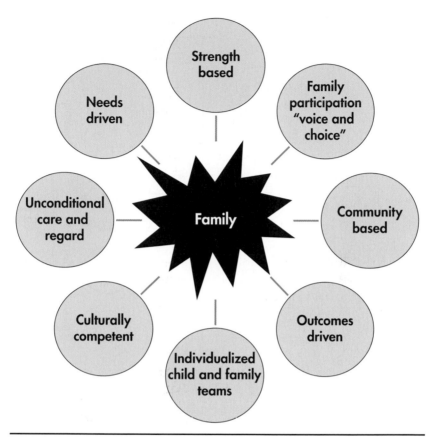

FIGURE 20–1.   Family-centered principles diagram.

Source.   Stanford Youth Solutions. Used with permission.

ing skills of the primary caregiver. Thus, individualized treatment approaches are needed. Trauma-informed care is intended to promote healing by addressing the fundamental needs of the individual, as well as identifying his or her strengths and natural support system. Trauma-informed care does not necessarily reference specific trauma treatments; instead it is an approach that can be provided in multiple settings along the full spectrum of care. In addition, there is a commitment to identify and address the trauma as early as possible. Treatment is focused on understanding the connection between the presenting symptoms and behaviors and the youth's past trauma history. At every level of treatment, first and foremost, there must be a commitment to do no harm. This commitment is more difficult than one may think. As the trauma symptoms and behaviors increase in severity, frequency, or duration and manifest in harmful

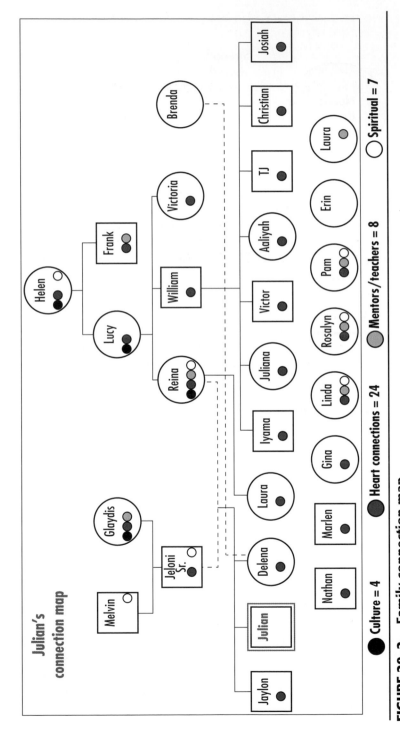

FIGURE 20–2.   Family connection map.

Source. Stanford Youth Solutions. Used with permission.

behaviors, often the treatment plan includes safety interventions that may cause additional trauma (Frueh 2005).

Developmental Approaches

The treatment of severe and chronic trauma needs to be flexible. Trauma treatment for youth must be tailored to the youth's age and developmental level: for young children, treatment relies primarily on nonverbal approaches, and for older youth, treatment consists of a combination of verbal and nonverbal interventions. Specialized techniques include several different activities including, but not limited to, play, art, music, dance, storytelling, narrative, and role-playing. Trauma-specific therapy can be provided in the home, school, clinical office, community (place of worship or neighborhood center), or a group home or residential treatment setting. Therapeutic services must take into account the unique culture and preferences of the youth and his or her family. Whatever a person's age, treatment is not one size fits all. Clinicians must take into account the needs of the whole person—including the individual's developmental stage and cognitive abilities, trauma symptoms, and familial and social support system—throughout the full spectrum of care (Figure 20–3).

Parenting Support Through Early Home Visiting

Ideally, the earlier a parent or caregiver is provided support, the more likely he or she will be to provide a safe, nurturing environment conducive to the child's healthy development. Home visiting is a prevention strategy used to support pregnant moms and new parents to promote infant and child health; foster educational development and school readiness; and help prevent early trauma, especially child abuse and neglect. High-quality home visiting programs offer vital support to parents as they deal with the challenges of raising young children (David and Olds 2002). Participation in these programs is typically voluntary. Home visitors may be trained nurses, social workers, child development specialists, or parent partners, depending on the model. Their visits focus on linking pregnant women with prenatal care and community resources, promoting strong parent-child attachment, and supporting parents' role as their child's first and most important teacher.

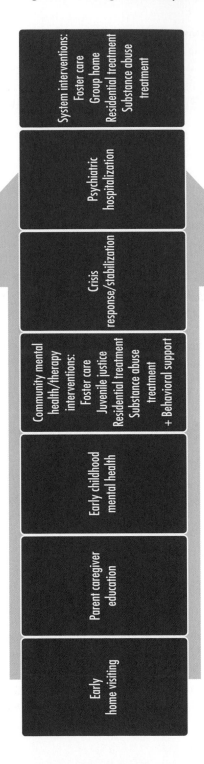

FIGURE 20–3.   Spectrum of care diagram.

Parent Education

Parenting education programs provide a structured curriculum that focuses on enhancing parenting practices and behaviors, such as developing and practicing positive discipline techniques, learning age-appropriate child development skills and milestones, promoting play and positive interactions between parents and children, and skill building to better access community services and supports. There are several evidence-based parent education programs that focus on varying youth developmental stages from early childhood to transitional-age youth (Gateway 2013). Both individual and group learning opportunities are available. Many of the programs provide structured group sessions and applied in-home assignments to increase parents' skill, knowledge, and confidence.

Early Childhood Mental Health

Early childhood mental health reflects both the social-emotional capacities and the primary relationships in children from birth through age 5 years. Because young children's social experiences and opportunities to explore the world depend on their caregivers, the child's relationships are central to infant and early childhood mental health. Early childhood mental health consultation programs are gaining popularity as an effective way of supporting professional consultants and caregivers to foster healthy early childhood development (Brennan 2008). An array of childhood mental health services are offered for at-risk young children (ages 0–5 years) and their families in center-based child care programs, family child care homes, and homeless shelters. Services are provided by various community-based mental health agencies. Core services may include the following: child assessment via observation, case and program consultation, direct therapeutic services to youth and their families with a focus on attachment and safety, therapeutic play groups, early referrals for specialized services, and parent education with support groups.

Community Mental Health

Community mental health is a decentralized service delivery of mental health support. Community-based care is designed to supplement and decrease the need for more costly inpatient mental health care delivered in hospitals or congregate care settings. Community mental health care is intended to be more accessible and responsive to local needs because it is based in a variety of community settings rather than aggregating and isolating patients and patient care in central hospitals. Therapeutic services include evidence-based therapy for the youth, for both the youth and his or her family, or in a group setting. Services are provided in a clinic, in school, or within the family home. More intensive therapeutic services, consisting of more frequent and longer sessions, can be provided if the youth displays more intense symptoms and behavior is impaired. Paired with therapy, a skill-building specialist may provide rehabilitation services to improve the youth's day-to-day functioning. Family partners and youth advocates can provide additional peer-to-peer support to meet the needs of the entire family system by ensuring access to community resources and advocacy. Support groups for both youth and caregivers are sometimes provided in addition to the therapy.

Behavioral Services

Behavioral services are considered an adjunct mental health service because these services do not address the underlying trauma. The specific purpose of this intervention is to target a behavior that jeopardizes the current stability of the placement of the youth in school, a group home, a foster home, or the family home. The service includes the provision of a behavioral analyst and is expected to be short term, 3–4 months. The behavioral analyst completes a functional behavioral assessment that is intended to identify the triggers of problematic behaviors and the environmental reinforcements for the youth. The behavioral analyst then develops a behavior intervention plan with the youth and caregiver based on the findings of the assessment. The analyst supports the caregiver or adult and the youth in the implementation of the plan. Often, this may require daily observation for hours at a time to collect data for the assessment and intensive coaching of youth and caregiver throughout the day during implementation. The analyst's presence is reduced until it is completely terminated as the problematic behavior is reduced and replaced with a more acceptable behavior.

Interventions Within the Spectrum of Care

Child Protective Services

Safety is of utmost importance when providing mental health services. Child protective services may need to intervene because of continued neglect, violence, or other safety issues that are persisting within the youth's living environment. The removal of a youth from his or her family and home is in itself a traumatic event. In addition, separating siblings or placing a youth in a shelter, group home, or stranger foster home is also traumatic. Placements with kin or extended family members can mitigate some trauma (Doyle 2007). Only very recently has it been recognized that foster youth should be provided professional support for the trauma of removal and disruption. In California, state Assembly Bill (AB) 403, known as Continuum Care Reform, provides the statutory and policy framework to ensure that services and supports provided to foster youth are tailored toward the ultimate goal of stable, permanent family. Services must include trauma-informed mental health services, as determined by a comprehensive needs assessment.

Juvenile Justice

Trauma is pervasive in the life of youth in the juvenile justice system. Studies from a number of psychological journals report that between 75% and 93% of youth who enter the juvenile justice system annually are estimated to have experienced some degree of traumatic victimization (Justice Policy Institute 2010). Not only do many of these youth have extensive trauma histories, but the nature of the system makes them vulnerable for continued traumatic experiences. Often, youth who commit crimes and enter the juvenile justice center have trauma histories that are overlooked. Youth in correctional facilities face significant challenges related to their incarceration and justice involvement, including separation from their families, communities, school, and other positive social networks. There is risk of retraumatization by staff and other youth in these correctional facilities.

Substance Abuse Treatment

The relationship between trauma and substance abuse is complex and requires a multifaceted treatment approach.

> Many factors influence whether an adolescent tries drugs, including the availability of drugs within the neighborhood, community, and school.... The family environment is also important: Violence, physical or emotional abuse, mental illness, or drug use in the household increases the likelihood an adolescent will use drugs. (National Institute on Drug Abuse 2014, p. 3)

Through brain science, it is known that the teenage years are a vulnerable time for developing lifelong challenges with substance use. Although some areas of the brain have already developed, the higher-level functions of the brain are still developing (Figure 20–4). The parts of the brain that process feelings of reward and pain—crucial drivers of drug use—are the first to mature during childhood (National Institute on Drug Abuse 2014). However, the prefrontal cortex, which controls higher-level cognitive functioning, and its connections to other brain regions continue to develop into a person's mid-20s. The prefrontal cortex is responsible for assessing situations, making sound decisions, and controlling our emotions and impulses.

When substance use disorders occur in adolescence, they can interfere with normal brain maturation. These potentially lifelong consequences make addressing adolescent drug use an urgent matter. Engaging youth in substance abuse treatment is only part of a recovery process. The mental health needs of the youth must be addressed as well as the family and social system dynamics. Often, substance abuse treatment is paired with individual, group, or family therapy in the context of the community or in a congregate care setting, such as a group home or residential treatment program.

Foster Care, Treatment Foster Care, and Residential Care

Standard foster care is used when the priority is removal of the youth from an unsafe environment. The intervention is considered to be necessary to allow for the child's healthy development. Treatment foster care, which is also referred to as therapeutic foster care, is specialized foster care oriented toward trauma treatment. In treatment foster care, foster parents are provided with specialized training to care for a wide variety of youth, usually those with significant emotional, behavioral, or social issues and/or medical needs. Specialized foster parents typically receive additional supports, such as a behavioral specialist, that help to address behaviors that jeopardize the safety or healthy development of the youth. Treatment foster care is designed to provide safe and nurturing care to youth in a more structured home environment than typical foster care, and it can be a cost-effective alternative to residential treatment.

Residential treatment is typically used when the youth's behaviors and trauma symptoms are too difficult to handle in a family home. Often, foster youth with significant safety behaviors are placed in residential treatment. Youth who are not foster youth may also be placed in residential

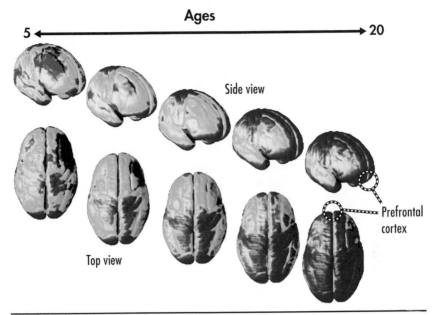

Ages

5 ← → 20

Side view

Top view

Prefrontal cortex

FIGURE 20–4. **Images of brain development in healthy children and teens (ages 5–20 years).**

Mature brain regions at each developmental stage are indicated from lightest to darkest shading to demonstrate the brain's progressive development. The prefrontal cortex, which governs judgment and self-control, is the last part of the brain to mature.

Source. Reprinted from Gogtay N, Giedd JN, Lusk L, et al: "Dynamic mapping of human cortical development during childhood through early adulthood." *Proceedings of the National Academy of Sciences of the United States of America* 101(21):8174–8179, 2004. Copyright (2004) National Academy of Sciences, U.S.A. Used with permission.

treatment. Residential treatment is focused on maintaining safety while also providing therapeutic support. It is considered an intervention for stabilization, with the intent of returning the youth to a family living environment once treatment is complete.

There is a distinction between residential treatment and group home care. Unfortunately, group homes have been used historically to house foster youth or probation youth with trauma histories. Group homes do not necessarily have a mental health treatment modality, which can lead to youth growing up in a group home without addressing their trauma history or mental health needs. Through the passage of Continuum of Care Reform, group homes in California will be phased out, and short-term residential treatment will be used to stabilize youth, with a goal of transitioning youth back into family homes.

Crisis Stabilization

Mobile mental health crisis response teams are composed of mental health professionals and practitioners who are trained to intervene in a mental health crisis. These professionals can meet a youth at home, at school, or wherever a crisis occurs. The teams meet face to face with the youth in crisis to assess and de-escalate the situation. Additional services may include placement in a crisis stabilization unit, rapid access to psychiatrists, health care navigators, and referrals to community mental health providers. Teams can also contact emergency law enforcement services when necessary. Mobile response teams are being used in some communities but are not present in every community.

Crisis residential treatment is a temporary alternative for youth experiencing an acute psychiatric episode or intense emotional distress who might otherwise face voluntary or involuntary hospitalization. It is a residentially based alternative to psychiatric hospital care that provides crisis stabilization, medication monitoring, and evaluation to determine the need for the type and intensity of additional services within a framework of peer support and trauma-informed approaches to recovery planning. Crisis residential treatment often includes treatment for co-occurring disorders based on either a harm-reduction or an abstinence-based approach to wellness and recovery. The goal of the program is to rapidly assess a youth's symptoms and situation while quickly initiating interventions to enable the youth to return home safely. There are very few crisis residential services for youth in the state of California.

Crisis residential treatment is also referred to as hospital diversion. Hospital diversion is helpful when a youth is experiencing acute stress due to emotional, behavioral, social, and/or family problems. Youth participate in an intensive, targeted assessment so that service providers can understand their immediate needs. As additional information is uncovered, it is incorporated into the overall evaluation and treatment stabilization plan.

Hospitalization

Inpatient hospitalization is a frontline treatment intervention for depressed youth despite the lack of evidence supporting this approach and growing evidence of negative effects. In fact, hospitalization is a traumatic experience. Community mental health providers consider hospitalization a failure in the treatment plan. Safety plans developed through the child and family team process are used with the intent of maintaining safety while the youth remains in the community. These safety plans are proactively developed with the family and include strength-based ways to respond to a crisis or potential crisis that are focused on maintaining the safety of the youth, family, and the community. Because of confidentiality laws, it is extremely challenging to coordinate after care while a youth is in the hospital.

Developmental Implications

Because childhood is marked with rapid developmental changes that are foundational to the full growth of the individual, it is a time of great opportunity and vulnerability. During this time, youth are especially vulnerable to the impact of trauma. The individual impact of trauma is influenced by multiple factors, including but not limited to the unique personality and coping skills of the youth; the level of support from caregivers; the frequency, duration, and type of trauma; and the developmental age of the youth.

The age of the youth when the trauma occurs is an important factor because trauma has a physical impact on the brain. An individual's brain has a neurophysiological and neuroendocrine response to perceived threats. Early trauma has the greatest potential impact because of the fact that it can actually affect the growth and functioning of the brain (Perry 2000). Trauma that occurs during the time of preverbal development requires innovative treatment approaches because standard treatment requiring verbal processing does not address those deep trauma wounds.

Ages 0–5 Years

Early childhood trauma generally refers to the traumatic experiences that occur when children are 0–5 years old. Because the reactions of infants and young children may be different from those of older youth and they may not be able to verbalize their reactions to threatening or dangerous events, many people assume that young age protects children from the impact of traumatic experiences. This is a false assumption. Early trauma can have a long-lasting impact on the child's mental health. Young children who experience trauma are at particular risk because their rapidly developing brains are very vulnerable. Early childhood trauma has been associated with reduced size of the cerebral cortex. This area is responsible for many complex functions, including memory, attention, perceptual awareness, thinking, language, and consciousness (Perry 2000).

The treatment of mental health disorders in the first years of life has focused primarily on enhancing the quality of the emotional relationship between the young child and the caregivers. The focus is on the caregiver-child relationship and the caregiver responses to the child's behaviors. The transactional nature of the caregiver-child relationship contributes to the child's ability to respond to stressors and learn emotional regulation. The caregivers' strengths are used as the foundation for building new parental competencies to meet the needs of the young child.

It is important to understand that both caregiver-child attachment and trauma exposure must be considered in the assessment and treatment of infants and toddlers with mental health and relationship problems. The quality of attachment is an important factor in children's capacity to process and resolve traumatic experiences. At the same time, traumatic events often have a damaging effect on the quality of existing attachments. Consistent with trauma treatment throughout the developmental stages, environmental safety must be ensured first.

Ages 6–11 Years

When addressing youth trauma, it is critical that the youth is residing in a safe, consistent, loving environment. Not only will the youth need mental health therapeutic support, but the primary caregiver will also need support and education. Like younger children, youth who range in age from 6 to 11 years also require treatment that involves the primary caregiver because both the young person and his or her caregiver must learn new skills in the areas of coping, communication, and emotional regulation techniques.

If behaviors escalate and there is danger to self or others, then crisis stabilization or even psychiatric hospitalization may be necessary. On discharge back to the home and community, there must then be a safety plan in place that both the youth and the caregiver have played a critical role in developing. If the youth cannot successfully maintain safety in the family home, then a residential treatment placement may be necessary. Unfortunately, when a youth is removed from his or her home and community and is placed in a congregate care setting, he or she experiences additional trauma from both the separation and the new living environment. The focus must be on continuing to strengthen the family and the youth's skills in the areas of emotional regulation techniques, communication, and coping.

Ages 12–17 Years

Youth who range from ages 12 to 17 years may exhibit varying responses that require flexibility in treatment such as individual therapy and substance abuse counseling, peer group therapy, or family therapy in the home or clinic. If behavior persists or increases, a higher level of care may be necessary, such as crisis stabilization or psychiatric hospitalization for self-harm or aggressive behaviors or a residential care setting for self-harm, extreme aggression, or antisocial behaviors. Engagement of the adolescent is still dependent on caregiver engagement. Ideally, engagement of the primary caregiver or parent is desired; however, if the primary caregiver is unable to provide the support, an additional support person can be used. This support person should be identified through consultation with the adolescent and primary caregiver. Through the therapeutic process, the caregiver or other identified support will have an opportunity for psychoeducation, skill building, and support from the professionals.

Ages 16–24 Years

When individuals enter adulthood (ages 16–24 years, referred to as transitional-age youth), there is a need for services that focus on navigating the adult world. These individuals want to be as autonomous as possible, but healing from trauma requires the support of others. Although youth voice and family voice should be at the center of treatment throughout the developmental phases, it is absolutely critical for the youth's voice to be the driver of services in the transition age range. These youth not only give their own treatment consent; they also need to be encouraged to advocate for what they need in order to develop living skills. The team process continues to be a valuable tool in the engagement, planning, and implementation of treatment, and outcomes will be determined by the youth and the support system that he or she has built.

Importance of Screening

No matter when the youth enters the system of care, it is critical that at least a brief screening for trauma is completed, such as the Life Events Checklist for DSM-5 or PTSD Checklist—Civilian Version (Weathers et al. 2013). Until recently, this was an uncommon practice. For organizations that are trauma informed, thorough trauma screenings such as the UCLA Child/Adolescent PTSD Reaction Index for DSM-5 (Pynoos and

Steinberg 2013) or the Traumatic Events Screening Instrument (Ribbe 1996) are standard practice and are completed on intake.

When a youth has externalizing behavior, that behavior, rather than the underlying trauma, may become the focus of treatment. If only the behavior is addressed, treatment is incomplete. Many youth diagnosed with a substance abuse issue have significant trauma histories that go untreated. Misdiagnosis often occurs without proper trauma screenings, which could lead to inappropriate or contraindicated interventions. For example, a child with significant trauma history may be diagnosed with attention-deficit/hyperactivity disorder (ADHD) and prescribed a medication for the ADHD. However, ADHD medication is contraindicated for hyperactive symptoms caused by trauma.

In addition to trauma history screening, it is critical to determine if the youth is still in a dangerous environment. It is impossible to truly address what are considered dysfunctional behaviors if they are still necessary for a youth's current perceived or actual survival. Caregivers should be included in the assessment process in order to get a complete view of the youth's current situation. It is important to note that the screening and assessment process can be destabilizing because emotions such as fear, guilt, shame, and/or anger can arise. The clinician must provide support, practice emotional regulation techniques with the youth, and follow up with the family to ensure the stabilization of the youth.

Environment

When treating a youth with past trauma, it is necessary that the youth is currently in a safe, supportive environment. Involving the entire household in treatment and ensuring ongoing safety in the environment is as critical as addressing the past trauma. Continued reality may reinforce past trauma responses. Additional stressors such as poverty, unstable housing, and too much responsibility or chaos in the home can continue to impact the youth. Although removal from an unsafe environment is traumatizing in itself, it may be necessary in order for treatment to begin. For example, a young person with a past history of violence may still live in an area where gangs are prevalent, or domestic violence may be ongoing. Dangers are present in the home and in the neighborhood, and addressing these dangers should be the first priority when working with the youth.

When trauma is ongoing or at high risk of reoccurrence, the therapist should engage multisystem interventions. Wraparound support consists of intensive community-based mental health services that support the stabilization of the whole family system. For example, the child and family team may identify that the caregiver needs substance abuse treatment and supports the family in securing treatment. A youth who is experiencing gang violence or bullying while traveling to and from school may need a ride to school. In this case, the wraparound child and family team may approve repair of the family car so that a caregiver can provide safe transportation for the youth. When wraparound support is necessary, it is critical that the basic safety issues are addressed immediately. The safety plan is critical for each and every youth and family served. In addition, the philosophy of wraparound support is that the process is family centered. Every aspect of the process involves the youth and family. Wraparound services are often used after transitioning a youth from residential treatment or a group home back into a family home in the community.

Strengths-Based Practice

Effective trauma-informed care and family-centered practice are founded on the premise that the strengths of youth and their caregivers can and should be leveraged. Through the assessment process, the clinician starts with an understanding that the youth is managing as well as he or she can and that there are areas where the clinician can enhance support, improve stability, and help increase knowledge and develop skills that leverage the youth's existing strengths and facilitate healing and recovery. Strengths-based practice involves building on the strengths of the youth, his or her family, and the community. Treatment is approached in a collaborative way with a focus on partnership.

When assessing the youth, the clinician must also understand the strengths of the family. It is important to identify the caregivers, others living in the home, and significant people in the community who are connected to the family, including, but not limited to, kin. The fundamental premise is that the family cares for the youth and wants the youth to be successful. Clearly identifying what successful treatment goals will look like during the assessment and treatment planning (i.e., the child and family team meeting) will engage the family in the treatment and recovery process. Engaging the caregivers in the therapeutic process, including strengthening communication skills and providing safe, nurturing structure in the living environment are essential aspects of the therapeutic interventions.

Overcoming Potential Challenges

The effects of trauma seem to be cumulative, meaning that additional trauma impacts the effects of a past trauma. If a youth has been exposed to trauma over time, additional trauma exposure will exacerbate the trauma symptoms. In addition, even though safety must be given the highest priority, interventions themselves may compound trauma. Chronic trauma impacts normative development. If a youth must make adaptations to his or her neurobiological system—a chronic state of fight-or-flight responses—there will be more challenges in overcoming the trauma symptoms. The fight-or-flight state may become the norm. Youth exposed to chronic trauma may display overreactivity, aggression, inability to relax, difficulty concentrating, and relationship dysfunction (Perry and Pollard 1995).

If a youth was struggling with preexisting mental health vulnerabilities prior to the trauma exposure, trauma symptoms can be more severe. It is important to address the mental health challenges in order to strengthen the youth's ability to cope. If the mental health challenges are unrecognized, treatment will likely be less effective. Therefore, a thorough, comprehensive assessment is necessary to identify underlying mental health issues.

Important Factors in Recovery Prognosis

Social Support

Youth who have a strong support system, including supportive, caring family and friends, are likely to be more resilient when dealing with a trauma exposure. On the other hand, if a youth lives in a dangerous, unpredictable, stressful environment without nurturance and support, the youth's recovery and development will be negatively impacted. Families are the most important support system for all youth facing trauma-related symptoms. Supporting the family in developing additional skills and providing psychoeducation regarding the impact of trauma and the need for safety in the therapeutic process is critical. Engaging the community in enhancing safety and providing mentorship to youth are also important.

Psychotropic Medication

The use of psychotropic medication for youth is controversial. Medication should not be the first treatment intervention if at all possible, especially for young children. However, when trauma symptoms are severe and debilitating and/or when there are comorbid mental health challenges that can be treated with medication, then there may be a need for medication. Psychiatrists may prescribe medication to address specific target symptoms that affect self-regulation and daily functioning and monitor these symptoms over time. However, medication alone is not adequate treatment to address the trauma and the corresponding trauma symptoms.

Sociocultural and Policy Implications

The Adverse Childhood Experiences study highlights the fact that childhood trauma is associated with medical and physical health consequences (Felitti et al. 1998). Youth who enter the child protective system by definition have suffered trauma. Neglect (physical, emotional, medical, and/or educational) is the most common form of maltreatment. Physical and emotional neglect are most damaging when they occur over time in the early life of youth. Infants who do not receive emotional and physical stimulation, such as being held and spoken to, may fail to thrive, which means that they do not develop and grow, or they may even die. Children younger than 3 years who are subjected to sustained neglect are at high risk of developing challenges with attachment and self-regulation. These children may demonstrate hyperactivity or aggression and may have other behavioral challenges. It is critical that identification be done as early as possible with a thorough assessment and that comprehensive interventions are in place. A history of trauma is also presvalent among youth in the juvenile justice system (Ford et al. 2007). Many of these youth do not receive necessary trauma-informed mental health treatment. There is beginning to be recognition of the need to treat the trauma in order to reduce the risk of recidivism.

Conclusion

Along the spectrum of mental health care for youth, there are complex factors to consider when determining the level of care and any additional interventions. Acknowledgment that the clinician must assess for historical and current trauma should be kept at the forefront of care. The guiding principles of trauma-informed practice (Substance Abuse and Mental Health Services Administration 2014) and family-centered practice (VanDenBerg 2007) are important within the context of the full spectrum of care. Individualized care and flexibility in the type of care are necessary to ensure that needs are met and the strengths of the youth and their support system are maximized.

KEY CONCEPTS

- Trauma has significant effects on child and adolescent brain and development.

- Effective whole-family engagement and support can play an important role in treating childhood trauma.

- Empowerment of youth in the treatment planning process is important in supporting recovery.

- Clinicians should identify strategies for delivering treatment and services that are strengths based, youth and family centered, individualized, collaborative, culturally reflective, trauma informed, and outcome focused.

- The individual impact of trauma is influenced by multiple factors, including, but not limited to, the unique personality and coping skills of the youth; the level of support of caregivers; the frequency, duration, and type of trauma; and the developmental age of the youth.

Discussion Questions

1. When a youth has externalizing harmful behavior, what should a practitioner do to determine treatment?

2. How can providers incorporate trauma awareness, knowledge, and skills into all of an organization's culture, practices, and policies?

3. How can providers and county partners within the systems of care be more effective at implementing trauma-informed practices across sectors?

4. What possible strategies could you identify to ensure safety of a youth through treatment other than removal from his or her family?

5. What are some strategies providers can use in providing support to the *whole family* impacted by trauma rather than providing services only to the youth identified as needing treatment?

Suggested Readings

D'Andrea W, Ford J, Stolbach B, et al: Understanding interpersonal trauma in children: why we need a developmentally appropriate trauma diagnosis. Am J Orthopsychiatry 82(2):187–200, 2012 22506521

Felitti VJ, Anda RF, Nordenberg D, et al: Relationship of childhood abuse and household dysfunction to many of the leading causes of death in adults: the Adverse Childhood Experiences (ACE) Study. Am J Prev Med 14(4):245–258, 1998

van Der Kolk B: The Body Keeps the Score: Brain, Mind, and Body in the Healing of Trauma. New York, Viking Penguin, 2014

References

Brennan EM: The evidence-base for mental health consultation in early childhood settings: research synthesis addressing staff and program outcomes. Early Educ Dev 19(6):982–1022, 2008

David L, Olds JR: Home visiting by paraprofessionals and by nurses: a randomized controlled trial. Pediatrics 110(3):486–496, 2002 12205249

Doyle JJ: Child Protection and child outcomes: measuring the effects of foster care. Am Econ Rev 97(5):1583–1610, 2007 29135212

Felitti VJ, Anda RF, Nordenberg D, et al: Relationship of childhood abuse and household dysfunction to many of the leading causes of death in adults: the Adverse Childhood Experiences (ACE) Study. Am J Prev Med 14(4):245–258, 1998 9635069

Ford JD, Chapman JF, Hawke J, et al: Trauma among youth in the juvenile justice system: critical issues and new directions. Delmar, NY, National Center for Mental Health and Juvenile Justice, June 2007. Available at: www.ncmhjj.com/wp-content/uploads/2013/10/2007_Trauma-Among-Youth-in-the-Juvenile-Justice-System.pdf. Accessed March 23, 2018.

Frueh KC: Special section on seclusion and retraint: patients' reports of traumatic or harmful experiences within the Psychiatric Setting. Psychiatr Serv 56(9):1123–1133, 2005 16148328

Gateway CW: Parent Education to Strengthen Families and Reduce the Risk of Maltreatment. Washington, DC, Child Welfare Information Gateway, 2013. Available at: www.childwelfare.gov/pubs/issue-briefs/parented. Accessed March 23, 2018.

Justice Policy Institute: Healing Invisible Wounds: Why Investing in Trauma-Informed Care for Children Makes Sense. Washington, DC, Justice Policy Institute, 2010

National Institute on Drug Abuse: Principles of Adolescent Substance Use Disorder Treatment: A Research-Based Guide. Bethesda, MD, National Institute on Drug Abuse, January 14, 2014. Available at: www.drugabuse.gov/publications/principles-adolescent-substance-use-disorder-treatment-research-based-guide. Accessed March 23, 2018.

Perry B: Traumatized children: how childhood trauma influences brain development. Journal of the California Alliance for the Mentally Ill 11(1):48–51, 2000

Perry B, Pollard RA: Childhood trauma, the neurobiology of adaptation, and "use-dependent" development of the brain: how "states" become "traits." Infant Mental Health 16(4):271–291, 1995

Pynoos RS, Steinberg AM: The UCLA PTSD Reaction Index for DSM-5. Los Angeles, CA, Behavioral Health Innovations, 2013

Ribbe D: Psychometric review of Traumatic Event Screening Instrument for Children (TESI-C), in Measurement of Stress, Trauma, and Adaptation. Edited by Stamm BH. Lutherville, MD, Sidran Press, 1996, pp 386–387

Substance Abuse and Mental Health Services Administration: Guiding Principles of Trauma-Informed Care. Rockville, MD, Substance Abuse and Mental Health Services Administration, 2014. Available at: www.samhsa.gov/samhsaNewsLetter/Volume_22_Number_2/trauma_tip/guiding_principles.html. Accessed March 23, 2018.

VanDenBerg J: High fidelity wraparound. Centennial, CO, Vroon VDB, 2007. Available at: www.yftipa.org/files/file/pa-counties/member-criteria/Appendix%20A%20HFW%20overview.pdf. Accessed March 23, 2018.

Weathers FW, Blake DD, Schnurr PP, et al: The Life Events Checklist for DSM-5 (LEC-5)—Standard, 2013. Washington, DC, National Center for PTSD. Available at: www.ptsd.va.gov/professional/assessment/te-measures/life_events_checklist.asp. Accessed March 23, 2018.

21

Integrated Models

David S. Grunwald, M.D., M.S.
Steven Sust, M.D.

THERE IS A SUBSTANTIAL unmet need for mental health care of children and adolescents in the United States. According to the American Academy of Child and Adolescent Psychiatry, nearly one out of every five children in the United States suffers from a mental illness, and only 20% of these children receive treatment. Half of all lifetime mental illnesses emerge by age 14, and three-quarters begin by age 24. Furthermore, the average delay between onset of symptoms and the initiation of treatment for children has been shown to be between 8 and 10 years (Martini et al. 2012).

Adding to this problem of access to care, there are well-documented shortages of child and adolescent psychiatrists (CAPs) in the United States. Most states are experiencing severe shortages, with between 1 and 17 psychiatrists per 100,000 children. A 2016 report from the U.S. Department of Health and Human Services (Health Resources and Services Administration 2016) projects significant shortages of other behavioral health practitioners as well. These shortages tend to be particularly acute in rural and low-income areas (Tyler et al. 2017). In addition to shortages and unequal regional distribution of CAPs, several other factors contribute to the underutilization of mental health services by parents and children, including stigma, cost, and cultural barriers (Gabel 2010).

Primary care providers (PCPs) play an important role in the care of children with emotional, behavioral, and developmental disorders. Approximately 75% of children and adolescents with psychiatric disorders are seen in the pediatrician's office, and about half of all pediatric office visits involve behavioral, emotional, developmental, psychosocial, and/or educational concerns. Given their position on the front line, it is not surprising that pediatricians and family medicine practitioners are frequently charged with the role of identifying, diagnosing, and treating psychiatric disorders in children and adolescents. However, the treatment of mental health issues, including trauma, is challenging and time consuming, and PCPs may find the work to be burdensome without sufficient support, training, knowledge of local resources, and access to specialists. These mounting challenges are helping to drive innovation in the delivery of mental health care, such as various models of integrating primary care and psychiatric care. Given the widespread prevalence of trauma and its ramifications, the development of trauma-informed integrated care models, in particular, will be necessary to ensure that such integrated systems will be effective.

Integrated Care Overview

The American Academy of Pediatrics and the American Academy of Child and Adolescent Psychiatry both have advocated for the integration of elements of mental health care into the primary care setting. There are different models and names for this type of collaboration, including integrated care, collaborative care, and the pediatric medical health home. Although there are some differences between these approaches to integrating care, common themes among these models include striving to provide care that is accessible, continuous, comprehensive, family centered, coordinated, compassionate, and culturally informed. Other less comprehensive models seek to bridge the gap in assisting PCPs to get their patients access to mental health care. All of these models of care are discussed in more detail in the next section of this chapter. Whatever model a clinic, hospital, or health system chooses to implement, there is now a substantial body of evidence that individuals with mental health needs, including those affected by trauma, benefit significantly when primary care practices reflect these characteristics (Martini et al. 2012).

More than 80 randomized controlled trials show integrated care to be more effective than usual care for adults. These findings are further substantiated by several meta-analyses. Integrated care has been shown to be effective for many different psychiatric disorders, including anxiety, depression, and posttraumatic stress disorder (PTSD), and also has been shown to be more cost-effective compared with nonintegrated care. Work from Osofsky et al. (2017), who studied 340 patients over 16 months in rural Louisiana primary care clinics with integrated behavioral health, found 1) significant improvement in PTSD symptoms, 2) four tracks of symptom severity courses (stable low, steep decline, stable high, and increasing symptoms), and 3) a significant effect of previously experienced adverse experiences on the track of symptom severity (Osofsky et al. 2017). Integrated and collaborative care has been studied more extensively within the adult population, but there is a growing body of literature supporting this type of care within the pediatric setting. A recent meta-analysis of randomized controlled trials comparing integrated care programs with usual pediatric primary care found that treatment interventions targeting mental health problems and using collaborative models improved outcomes when compared with usual care, including statistically significant improvements in outcomes of patients with depression, anxiety, and behavioral disorders but not substance use disorders (Asarnow et al. 2015).

The general principles of integrated care apply to both the pediatric and adult populations. However, delivery of integrated care within the pediatric setting differs from integrated care with adults in several ways. In pediatric integrated care, there is an increased sensitivity to how children are developing, both mentally and emotionally. Families play a crucial role in pediatric settings, and treatment emphasizes coping and adjustment techniques in addition to standard care. There is more need for the ongoing evaluation for intellectual disability and developmental delays when working with younger populations (www.nimh.nih.gov/health/statistics/autism-spectrum-disorder-asd.shtml). Another crucial element of integrated care that differs within the pediatric population is the need for consideration of child development. Approaches to care and interventions need to be tailored appropriately along the developmental continuum for children, adolescents, and their families, including careful attention to such factors as attachment, emotional regulation, identity, and cognition (Saxe et al. 2006).

Given the aforementioned shortage of CAPs, regional consultation models have been developed in a number of areas that make it easier for pediatricians to consult with their child psychiatry colleagues in a timely fashion. One of the best established models of consultation is the Massachusetts Child Psychiatry Access Project (MCPAP). The MCPAP model uses regional teams, each of which consists of child psychiatrists, licensed therapists, care coordinators, and administrative support. Pediatricians who use the program can access prompt assistance for any patient with a mental health concern via phone consultation with a CAP. Depending on the clinical indication, MCPAP is then able to provide in-person clinical assessment, short-term therapy, or a facilitated connection to a community resource (Straus and Sarvet 2014).

Colocation generally refers to a model in which both mental health specialists and primary care providers are able to practice at the same physical site. Colocation can improve access, decrease barriers to care coordination, and help streamline billing.

Collaborative Care, developed at the University of Washington's Advancing Integrated Mental Health Solutions (AIMS) Center (https://aims.uw.edu), is one of the most rigorously studied and well-vetted models of integrated care. The principles of Collaborative Care are helpful in illustrating components that are often shared by other integrated care modalities. The five principles of collaborative care are patient-centered team care, population-based care, measurement-based treatment to target, evidence-based care, and accountable care.

Patient-centered team care requires the collaboration of primary care and behavioral health providers via the use of shared care plans that incorporate patient goals. Providing both physical and mental health care at a familiar location makes patients feel more comfortable and reduces duplicate assessments. Population-based care involves sharing a defined group of patients tracked in a registry to help follow patient outcomes in an organized fashion. Measurement-based treatment to target includes designing a unique treatment plan for each patient, which helps to articulate personal goals and clinical outcomes that are routinely measured by evidence-based tools such as the Patient Health Questionnaire (PHQ-9) depression scale. The broader use of evidence-based care is an additional principle of Collaborative Care that helps guide clinicians to choose treatments that are proven to work in primary care settings, such as cognitive-behavioral therapy, parent management training, and medications. Finally, adhering to the principle of accountable care helps ensure that providers are reimbursed for quality of care and clinical outcomes, not just the volume of care provided (http://aims.uw.edu/collaborative-care/financing-strategies-collaborative-care).

Heath et al. (2013, p. 5) built on previous literature to devise an integration framework "designed to help organizations implementing integration to evaluate their degree of integration across several levels and to determine what next steps they may want to take to enhance their integration initiatives." The framework contains six levels of collaboration and integration (Figure 21–1).

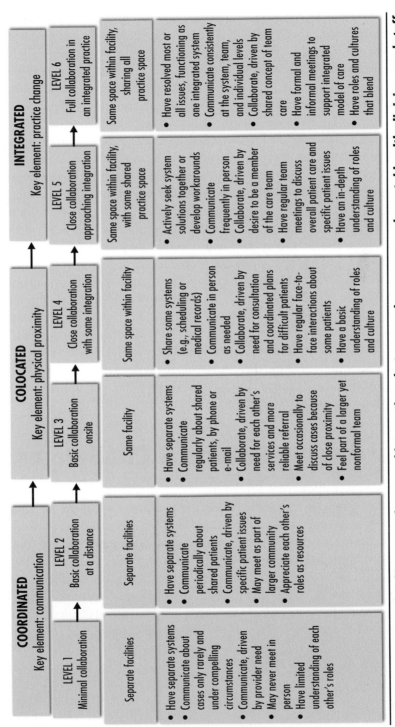

FIGURE 21–1.   Levels of integrated care and interactions between primary care and mental health clinicians and staff.

Source.   Adapted from Heath B, Wise Romero P, Reynolds K: A Review and Proposed Standard Framework for Levels of Integrated Healthcare. Washington, DC, SAMHSA-HRSA Center for Integrated Health Solutions, 2013.

The first two levels of integrated care involve minimal collaboration and collaboration at a distance, respectively. At these levels, communication between mental health providers and PCPs is rare and generally is done only for especially challenging cases. The key distinctions between level 1 and level 2 are frequency and type of communication. Level 3 consists of basic collaboration on site. At this level, the proximity of providers from different specialties allows for greater ease of collaboration. However, there are still significant barriers to care integration. For example, clinicians may be using different record systems, and there may be no dedicated time for intradepartmental collaboration. At level 4, there is more sharing of the same systems, and interactions between specialties are more frequent. However, each provider can still practice independently without communicating with others. Thus, colocation reduces time spent traveling from one clinician to another but does not guarantee integration of care. Levels 5 and 6 involve the greatest amount of practice change, which results in a blending or blurring of cultures in which no one discipline predominates. Level 5 entails close collaboration that approaches an integrated practice, in which a unified team seeks system solutions to reduce barriers to care integration for a broader range of patients. Finally, level 6 involves the greatest amount of practice change, in which providers and patients view the operation as a single health system treating the whole person. At this level, the principle of treating the whole person is applied to all patients, not just targeted groups (Heath et al. 2013).

Overcoming Potential Challenges

Making the transition from a more traditional model of care to a fully integrated care practice can be a challenging endeavor. It requires substantial planning, resources, workforce development, and plenty of patience. The process often demands significant changes in the culture of the practice environment, which can be stressful on employees and those in leadership positions as they adapt from the prior model of care delivery to the new model being implemented. The AIMS Center website (https://aims.uw.edu) offers anticipatory guidance about common challenges that are encountered in this process, as well as strategies to ease the transition (Table 21–1).

Overall, the primary literature is limited with regard to specific studies of integrated care programs directed at childhood trauma. Specific recommendations about developing trauma-informed systems of care in the pediatric setting come from a policy briefing by Lang et al. (2015). The

TABLE 21–1. Challenges in moving from a traditional model of care to fully integrated care

Challenge	Response
Limited appreciation of core principles of collaborative care	Educate employees and leadership about Collaborative Care and how it may differ from care as usual. Address the common misconception that Collaborative Care is the same as colocated care. Provide orientation to all team members. Promote clear vision of goals for program.

Vision not aligned with resources	Encourage leadership buy-in.
	Collaborative Care may require additional staff.
	Ensure adequate staffing based on expected patient caseload.
	Consider practical needs such as patient registry, private space to see patients, computers, and a telephone.
	Limit screening to behavioral health issues the organization has resources to address.
	Address funding concerns:
	  Anticipate costs for both short-term start-up and long-term sustainability.
	  Consider creative partnerships.
	  Assess billing practices.
	  Identify referral resources and partners (e.g., for social needs).

Limited time and resources to build a team	Identify facilitator or champion to lead this process. Leadership should advocate for time to complete assessment and participate in facilitated team building. Schedule adequate time for team building and give the work group a clear timeline. Consider using a facilitated process (such as the AIMS team building tool) to build the team and develop workflow.

TABLE 21–1.   Challenges in moving from a traditional model of care to fully integrated care *(continued)*

Challenge	Response
Inadequate skills in effective teamwork	Plan training and practice specific collaborative care skills (e.g., integrated care planning).
	Train together:
	Ideally, all team members participate in training as group.
	Each member should understand the model of the program and individual roles and responsibilities.
	Consider online programs for training.
	Review program effectiveness in regularly scheduled QI meetings after program launch and identify needs for additional training and resources.
Individual concerns about scope of practice	Seek to understand concerns of providers.
	Acknowledge strengths of team members and apply those skills to new roles.
	Clearly define roles through team building within scope of practice for each provider.
	Provide training to support team in performing in new roles.
	Focus on patient outcomes and collaborative care tasks to reach those outcomes.
Team burnout	Focus on good team communication.
	Publicly share success stories.
	Regularly review workflow and revise as needed.
	Consider team reflection to address inevitable challenges.

Note.   AIMS=Advancing Integrated Mental Health Solutions; QI=quality improvement.
Source.   Adapted from Advancing Integrated Mental Health Solutions Center at University of Washington: Implementation Guide Step 4: Launch Your Care: Address Unanticipated Challenges, created by the University of Washington AIMS Center, 2018. Available at:https://aims.uw.edu/collaborative-care/implementation-guide/launch-your-care/address-unanticipated-challenges.

authors made a broad range of suggestions, including the engagement of leadership at the state level to support trauma-informed systems for children and families. The development of a statewide plan could help to ensure that trauma-informed care programs are coordinated with current system integration efforts. The authors also recommended attempting to identify opportunities for blended funding across child-serving systems for trauma-focused prevention and early intervention services. An example of this could be using the same source to fund trauma screening completed by both pediatric and behavioral health providers. At the individual program level, Lang and colleagues emphasized the risks of secondary trauma in care providers who work with young people affected by trauma. Given the unique occupational hazards of this work, the authors recommended the development of a plan to promote wellness and address secondary traumatic stress for all staff who interact with children exposed to trauma (Lang et al. 2015).

Sociocultural and Policy Implications

Unmet Child Mental Health Needs and Effects on Other Systems

Prevention and early intervention were found to be efficacious in many serious mental illnesses such as PTSD, and more recent research has also found efficacy for schizophrenia and bipolar disorder. The classic 1999 Centers for Disease Control and Prevention Adverse Childhood Experiences (ACE) study investigated the effects of childhood toxic stress and trauma on general health (Felitti et al. 1998). The results showed a positive correlation between childhood adversity and longitudinal medical comorbidities and even early death. Furthermore, the ACE Study suggested that early toxic stress and trauma lead to correspondingly earlier involvement with other systems such as juvenile justice and child welfare, which then leads to further distancing from the educational system and thus to high school dropout. In considering the subsequent socioeconomic costs of untreated stress and trauma, the ACE Study stimulated research into the justice and education system.

More recently, the juvenile justice system has focused on the rehabilitation of juvenile offenders given the astronomic costs of adult incarceration in the United States. Recent work investigating mental illness in the juvenile justice system estimated that 40%–80% of those youth met criteria for a diagnosable mental disorder, and an additional 10% met criteria for a substance use disorder (Underwood and Washington 2016). Various evidence-based treatment models have been used with the individual and/or family, such as cognitive-behavioral therapy, integrated co-occurring treatment, and functional family therapy, but the time-intensive multisystemic therapy (MST) had particularly good evidence supporting its efficacy in reducing juvenile justice recidivism. A 2004 meta-analysis noted that MST was highly efficacious in treating juvenile offenders' antisocial behaviors and preventing rearrests but noted that there were significant differences in effect size between MST practitioners (i.e., graduate students versus community therapists), which highlighted the difficulty of implementing MST in a community (i.e., nonacademic) setting (Curtis et al. 2004).

Schools also increasingly recognized the significant role of toxic stress and anxiety in educational outcomes. A 2011 retrospective study of factors associated with school dropout noted that childhood trauma, mental illness with externalizing behavior, and substance abuse were significantly associated with school dropout. Not surprisingly, dropping out of school was also found to be associated with incarceration (Porche et al. 2011). Moreover, effects of childhood adversity on income have been shown to decrease average income at age 50 years by 28% (Goodman et al. 2011).

Clinical Vignette

Mateo, a 6-year-old (primarily Spanish speaking) Latino, was referred by a clinic pediatrician to Integrated Behavioral Health Services (IBHS) for worsening school avoidance. Mateo's mother, Elena, reported that she and her son were undocumented immigrants and that they had left El Salvador 1 year ago after she had been a victim of intimate partner violence from Mateo's father. Elena reported that the border crossing with others was distressing for them both, and after reaching the United States, she sought out support from family members already residing in the San Francisco Bay Area, where they helped her apply for asylum. Elena reported that the transition into living in the Bay Area was challenging. She and Mateo did not speak English. She had to wear a Department of Homeland Security ankle bracelet and was required to follow up weekly with an immigration case worker. However, she also reported feeling grateful to be together with family.

During this time, Elena noted that Mateo had difficulty sleeping at night alone and had frequent nightmares; new-onset separation anxiety from his mother; irritability; low frustration tolerance; and social isolation, with worsening anxiety around strangers. Elena hoped that these problems would decrease with time, but she noted that Mateo was struggling with transitioning into his kindergarten class because of his profound separation anxiety, such that she had to spend the whole day with Mateo at school. After 2 weeks, school staff advised Elena to follow up with her son's pediatrician, who referred him for an evaluation by the IBHS therapist and child psychiatrist.

A detailed trauma history was explored in the initial IBHS evaluation. In addition to the challenges that Elena and Mateo faced as immigrants,

Elena recalled an incident about 1 year ago in which Mateo described what appeared to be a sexual assault by an older cousin. Mateo started in weekly therapy, which included an evidence-based modality to address childhood PTSD. The child psychiatrist started guanfacine 0.5 mg every night to target hyperarousal and insomnia, with good effect. The prescribing of this medication was eventually handed over to the pediatrician, with ongoing consultation as needed by the child psychiatrist. Over the next few months, Mateo's anxiety symptoms improved such that he was able to participate and learn in class without his mother being present, and Elena was able to get a job cleaning homes during the day.

Sustainability

With the growing evidence supporting integrated behavioral health care over the past 10 years, the U.S. Centers for Medicare and Medicaid Services (CMS) enacted initial funding for integrated behavioral health. In January 2018, CMS released a fact sheet expounding on the University of Washington Improving Mood—Promoting Access to Collaborative Treatment (IMPACT) model plus newly approved Current Procedural Terminology (CPT) billing codes to support that model of care (U.S. Centers for Medicare and Medicaid Services 2018). However, the IMPACT integrated care model was studied primarily in adults. Thus, broad-based longitudinal support for integrated behavioral health in pediatric populations was limited despite the growing recognition of value in addressing child mental health problems. Two notable exceptions are the MCPAP and Seattle Children's Hospital Partnership Access Line, which both provide telephone child psychiatry consultation to state primary care providers for children with regard to behavioral health questions (Straus and Sarvet 2014).

Conclusion

The major psychiatric disorders have an onset prior to adulthood. Given the increasing awareness of child and adolescent mental health needs, coupled with a limited supply of child psychiatrists, primary care providers are now in a transitional role around management of their patients' mental health treatment. Moreover, a comprehensive review of research on behavioral health models in pediatrics found statistically significant chances of clinical improvement when targeting depression, anxiety, and behavioral disorders (Asarnow et al. 2015). Although specific studies of integrated care programs directed at childhood trauma are currently limited, multiple converging lines of scientific evidence, public health data, and socioeconomic reports, when taken together, support the role of integrated care systems in mitigating the consequences of untreated toxic stress and trauma. Although initial reports with regard to the use of integrated care in the treatment of childhood trauma are promising, more research and advocacy are necessary in order to continue to advance this field and improve outcomes for children in this country and globally.

KEY CONCEPTS

- Integrated care is a practical and cost-effective way to deliver mental health care within primary care settings and has a substantial and growing evidence base.

- The unmediated effects of trauma and toxic stress, which begin to accrue in childhood and adolescence, are increasingly being identified as contributors to lifelong physical and mental health sequelae. Trauma-focused integrated care is an emerging paradigm that shows promise in delivering more effective care to children and teenagers with a history of trauma.

- Implementation of integrated care within a traditional primary care setting requires a significant amount of practice change. There is a continuum that typical clinics may travel along as they transition from nonintegrated care, to colocated care, and finally to fully integrated care.

- In addition to affecting personal wellness, untreated toxic stress can also lead to maladaptive coping strategies that interfere with school engagement and to diversion into an increasingly costly justice system. Thus, integrated behavioral health presents an opportunity for meaningful policy making and secondary prevention.

Discussion Questions

1. Describe key differences between various models and levels of integrated care.

2. How might the needs of children and families affected by trauma differ from those of adults, and how might this alter the design of an integrated care program for children and adolescents?

References

Advancing Integrated Mental Health Solutions Center at University of Washington: Address unanticipated challenges, in Implementation Guide Step 4: Launch Your Care. Seattle, WA, AIMS Center, 2018. Available at: https://aims.uw.edu/collaborative-care/implementation-guide/launch-your-care/address-unanticipated-challenges. Accessed March 24, 2018.

Asarnow JR, Rozenman M, Wiblin J, et al: Integrated medical-behavioral care compared with usual primary care for child and adolescent behavioral health: a meta-analysis. JAMA Pediatr 169(10):929–937, 2015 26259143

Curtis NM, Ronan KR, Borduin CM: Multisystemic treatment: a meta-analysis of outcome studies. J Fam Psychol 18(3):411–419, 2004 15382965

Felitti VJ, Anda RF, Nordenberg D, et al: Relationship of childhood abuse and household dysfunction to many of the leading causes of death in adults: the Adverse Childhood Experiences (ACE) study. Am J Prev Med 14(4):245–258, 1998 9635069

Gabel S: The integration of mental health into pediatric practice: pediatricians and child and adolescent psychiatrists working together in new models of care. J Pediatr 157(5):848–851, 2010 20633899

Goodman A, Joyce R, Smith JP: The long shadow cast by childhood physical and mental problems on adult life. Proc Natl Acad Sci USA 108(15):6032–6037, 2011 21444801

Health Resources and Services Administration/National Center for Health Workforce Analysis; Substance Abuse and Mental Health Services Administration/Office of Policy, Planning, and Innovation. National Projections of Supply and Demand for Selected Behavioral Health Practitioners: 2013–2025. Rockville, MD, Health Resources and Services Administration, November 2016. Available at: https://bhw.hrsa.gov/sites/default/files/bhw/health-workforce-analysis/research/projections/behavioral-health2013-2025.pdf. Accessed March 24, 2018.

Heath B, Wise Romero P, Reynolds K: A Review and Proposed Standard Framework for Levels of Integrated Healthcare. Washington, DC, SAMHSA-HRSA Center for Integrated Health Solutions, 2013

Lang JM, Campbell K, Vanderploeg JJ: Advancing Trauma-Informed Systems for Children. Farmington, CT, Child Health and Development Institute of Connecticut, 2015

Martini R, Hilt R, Marx L, et al: Best Principles for Integration of Child Psychiatry Into the Pediatric Health Home. Washington, DC, American Academy of Child and Adolescent Psychiatry, June 2012. Available at: www.aacap.org/App_Themes/AACAP/docs/clinical_practice_center/systems_of_care/best_principles_for_integration_of_child_psychiatry_into_the_pediatric_health_home_2012.pdf. Accessed March 24, 2018.

Osofsky HJ, Weems CF, Hansel TC, et al: Identifying trajectories of change to improve understanding of integrated health care outcomes on PTSD symptoms post disaster. Fam Syst Health 35(2):155–166, 2017 28617017

Porche MV, Fortuna LR, Lin J, et al: Childhood trauma and psychiatric disorders as correlates of school dropout in a national sample of young adults. Child Dev 82(3):982–998, 2011 21410919

Saxe GN, Ellis BH, Kaplow JB: Collaborative Treatment of Traumatized Children and Teens. New York, Guilford, 2006

Straus JH, Sarvet B: Behavioral health care for children: the Massachusetts Child Psychiatry Access Project. Health Aff (Millwood) 33(12):2153–2161, 2014 25489033

Tyler ET, Hulkower RL, Kaminski JW: Behavioral Health Integration in Pediatric Primary Care: Considerations and Opportunities for Policymakers, Planners, and Providers. New York, Milbank Memorial Fund, March 2017. Available at: www.milbank.org/publications/behavioral-health-integration-in-pediatric-primary-care-considerations-and-opportunities-for-policymakers-planners-and-providers. Accessed March 24, 2018.

Underwood LA, Washington A: Mental illness and juvenile offenders. Int J Environ Res Public Health 13(2):228, 2016 26901213

U.S. Centers for Medicare and Medicaid Services: Medicare Learning Network Fact Sheet on Behavioral Health Integration Services. January 2018. Available at: www.cms.gov/Outreach-and-Education/Medicare-Learning-Network-MLN/MLNProducts/Downloads/BehavioralHealthIntegration.pdf. Accessed June 29, 2018.

22

Global Mental Health and Trauma

Christina Tara Khan, M.D., Ph.D.

What Is Global Mental Health?

The term *global mental health* was first used in the literature by Surgeon General Dr. David Satcher (2001) to describe a field within public health (Cohen et al. 2014). Since then, there has been increased recognition of the contribution of mental illness to the global burden of disease, with mental and nervous disorders among the leading causes of disability around the world (GBD 2015 Disease and Injury Incidence and Prevalence Collaborators 2016; World Health Organization 2008). There has been a surge of interest in this emerging field in the past decade, with special topic issues and reports published by journals and professional organizations and priority funding from governments, academic institutions, nongovernmental organizations, and foundations. Global mental health aims to improve identification and treatment of mental health problems, decrease stigma, increase access to services, and reduce human rights abuses of people experiencing neuropsychiatric conditions around the world.

Trauma has been an important focus of global mental health work around the world. From war and conflict to poverty and gender-based violence, widespread trauma of various forms has impacted the mental health and well-being of individuals around the world (Table 22–1). Hu-

TABLE 22–1. Types of trauma encountered in global mental health work

Type of trauma	Examples
Interpersonal trauma	Loss of a parent, domestic violence, physical assault or abuse, human trafficking, genital mutilation, sexual assault or rape, psychological abuse and intimidation
War or conflict	War, postconflict devastation, displacement
Accidents and injuries	Road traffic accidents, workplace injuries
Natural environmental disasters	Hurricanes, tsunamis, earthquakes, floods, extreme weather conditions due to climate change
Unnatural environmental disasters	Nuclear warfare, oil spills
Secondary trauma	Vicarious victimization of aid workers and medical and social services personnel

man security threats and limited enforcement of human rights have further contributed to the psychological sequelae of trauma in all age populations. Although a variety of approaches have been employed to address the mental health of vulnerable pediatric populations affected by traumatic events, to date, the evidence base for interventions in pediatric global mental health is quite limited. In this chapter, I provide a brief overview of fundamental concepts pertinent to work in global mental health, review broad types of trauma experienced by children and youth globally, and review the current evidence base on interventions for children and adolescents impacted by global trauma.

Human Rights Framework: Key Considerations

Work in global health requires recognition of health as a human right. A human rights framework means respect, freedom, and dignity for all people. Protection of international human rights formally came about with the founding of the United Nations, although movements around the world had embraced the basic principles of a human rights approach (Table 22–2) long before formal recognition in the Universal Declaration of

TABLE 22–2.   Basic principles of human rights

Principle	Definition
Universality	Every person, by virtue of being human, is entitled to the protection of human rights, without exception.
Nondiscrimination	Human rights must be guaranteed without discrimination of any kind. This includes both purposeful discrimination and implicit or institutional bias.
Transparency	Governments must be open about information related to decision making regarding resources, including how public institutions that protect human rights, such as schools and hospitals, are organized and run.
Indivisibility	Human rights are indivisible and interdependent. If a government violates protection of one human right, this affects the ability of the affected individuals to exercise other rights.
Participation	People have the right to participate in how decisions are made about their rights. This includes the civil right to participate in the election of public officials and to provide input on lawmakers' decisions about human rights.
Accountability	Governments must be held accountable for the enforcement of human rights. This includes not only making laws and policies about rights but also putting in place appropriate mechanisms to ensure those standards are met.

Source.   Adapted from National Economic and Social Rights Initiative 2018.

Human Rights (United Nations 1952). The basic principles of human rights are interdependent and rely on government policy and protection to guarantee dignity and freedom for all people. In practice, the right to mental health has not been protected in many countries, despite the World Health Organization's slogan "No health without mental health." Barriers have included lack of policies and laws, low priority within national health policy, limited resources, training and workforce deficits, and stigma and discrimination.

Human Security

Human security broadly refers to any threat to human dignity and livelihood. More narrowly, it is often focused on violent threats to individuals and communities associated with war, genocide, and the displacement of populations. Human security threats can have widespread deleterious effects on mental health and well-being and affect millions of children around the world.

War and Conflict

War and related disasters have existed since the beginning of humankind. There is evidence of increasing numbers of children and youth exposed to war and violent conflicts, with nearly 250 million youth globally, or approximately 1 in 10 individuals younger than age 18, living in countries or regions impacted by war or conflict (United Nations Children's Fund 2016). The impact of war on psychological well-being is broad and includes emotional, behavioral, and mental health effects. Children exposed to war and violent conflict are at increased risk for posttraumatic stress disorder (PTSD), anxiety, depression, and behavioral problems, among other health effects. Some outcomes are immediate and short term, whereas others may result in long-term or even lifelong illnesses. Many children recover from trauma in the short or intermediate term with no overt impact on their emotional and behavioral well-being. A portion of these children will exhibit a delayed PTSD response, with emerging mood, anxiety, sleep, or concentration difficulties appearing later in adolescence or adulthood. The impact of risk and protective factors varies depending on the traumatic exposure and characteristics of each individual's psychosocial environment.

Postconflict Regions

Many nations are now postconflict and are experiencing the aftereffects of violence. These effects include both mental and physical health problems, which are often intricately linked. Poverty and malnutrition are often a major problem in postconflict settings and can be associated with the development or progression of emotional, behavioral, and mental health conditions. The United Nations and other humanitarian organizations are routinely involved in peace-building efforts to try to support coordinated recovery from conflict and prevent relapse into renewed war.

Mental health concerns are now being recognized as an important development issue in conflict-affected regions. Traditionally, attention to mental health in postconflict reconstruction and reconciliation efforts was limited to short-term interventions in the immediate aftermath of disaster (e.g., critical incident debriefing). Research has demonstrated, however, that these short-term efforts may be harmful (Rose et al. 2003), and there is increasing recognition that the psychological impact of trauma can be and often is long lasting. For example, studies with child survivors of the Nazi Holocaust and the Cambodian Pol Pot genocide showed that individuals may experience symptoms of PTSD as many as 40–50 years after the traumatic experience (Port et al. 2001; Sack et al. 1999). As such, in recent years there has been increasing attention to mental health and well-being in the aftermath of trauma for communities affected by conflict and war.

Gender-Based Violence and Interpersonal Trauma

Gender-based violence has been used as a tool of war and systematic oppression. This type of violence does not obey the protective effects of education, wealth, and other indicators of economic development; all over the world women and children are victimized in crimes perpetrated because of gender. In a multicountry study by the World Health Organization (García-Moreno et al. 2005), prevalence estimates of intimate partner physical and sexual violence in mainly low-income countries ranged from 15% to 71%. Up to 40% of women reported sexual violence as their first sexual encounter, often as a minor. In high-income countries, estimated prevalence of sexual violence is 23.2% (World Health Organization Media Centre 2016). Silence commonly follows sexual victimization (Priebe and Svedin 2008), with risk for internalization of shame (Feiring et al. 2002) and increased risk of revictimization (Walker et al. 2017). The mental health consequences of interpersonal violence are broad and include low self-esteem, depression, suicide, substance abuse, revictimization and retaliatory violence, and, commonly, PTSD.

In addition to the psychological consequences, violence has the capacity to affect an individual's overall health and susceptibility to illness and disease. Adults with a history of childhood trauma are more likely to suffer from a variety of physical health problems (Felitti et al. 1998). Violence has been associated with more somatic complaints, more frequent visits to health facilities, chronic pain syndromes, and more distress when seeking care (Khan et al. 2014). Exposure to multiple adverse childhood experiences is a significant risk factor for diverse health conditions, including metabolic and cardiovascular diseases, cancer, substance abuse, and mental illness (Hughes et al. 2017).

Human Trafficking

Human trafficking is estimated to be the second-largest criminal industry worldwide, second only to illicit drug dealing. It is estimated that 21 million men, women, and children around the world are victims of human trafficking (United Nations Office on Drugs and Crime 2012). In the United States, as many as 17,500 individuals are trafficked into the country each year, and an estimated 100,000 children with U.S. citizenship are victims of trafficking, with an additional 200,000 considered at risk. Victims are trafficked by force, fraud, or coercion, and the majority of victims are women and girls. Environments affected by war, postconflict aftermath, or military presence facilitate the sex trafficking of the most vulnerable amid violent conflict, including women and girls, the poor, the elderly, and people with mental illness. Serious psychological harm may result from childhood sexual exploitation, including the onset of depression, PTSD, and attachment and personality disorders. Although there are very few systematic data on the mental health outcomes of human trafficking, one clinical study compared children who were sexually abused with children who were victims of commercial sexual exploitation and found that youth exploited for commercial sex reported higher rates of PTSD symptoms, conduct symptoms, sexualized behaviors, and substance abuse (Cole et al. 2016).

Accidents and Injuries

Road traffic accidents and injuries are the leading cause of death among people ages 15–29 years. Around the world, about 1.25 million people die each year from road traffic crashes, and the majority (90%) of these are in low- and middle-income countries (World Health Organization 2017). In addition to the loss of life, traffic accidents cause considerable economic loss to individuals, families, and nations, with significant disability and lost productivity for those who are injured and for family members who take off time to care for the injured. Risk factors for accidents are many and include substance abuse and distracted driving as well as the nonuse of motorcycle helmets, seat belts, and child restraints.

Environmental and Natural Disasters

Natural disasters have a significant impact on health and well-being. In recent years, hurricanes, tsunamis, earthquakes, and other extreme weather events have affected the lives of millions of people around the world, leading to substantial loss of life and morbidity among those who survive. Individuals and families living in poverty and the mentally ill are especially vulnerable to the economic and social devastation that can result from natural disasters. The public health impact of disasters such as the Indian Ocean tsunami of 2004, Hurricane Katrina in 2005, and the Haiti earthquake of 2010 has highlighted the importance of attention to mental health in the wake of catastrophic events. Poorly coordinated services may result in limited effectiveness of available aid and may even increase risk of harm to individuals and communities impacted by the traumatic event (Davis et al. 2006). Looting, squatting, and crime commonly increase in response to resource limitations following disaster, with the potential for the most vulnerable members of society, including children and those living with mental illness, to be targeted through assault, intimidation, and rape.

Secondary Trauma and Vicarious Traumatization

Secondary trauma refers to negative psychological symptoms related to repeated or extreme exposure to aversive details of traumatic events through occupational exposure. Any human services professional who attends to the adversity or trauma experienced by others is at risk for secondary trauma. Police officers, humanitarian aid workers, nurses, and physicians are a few examples of professionals who may experience secondary trauma as a result of their daily activities. In particular, work with vulnerable populations and children in conflict settings holds a high propensity for vicarious traumatization; the shattering of beliefs about justice and human rights can lead to anger, confusion, and even a posttraumatic-like syndrome, similar to the process experienced in primary trauma (Newell and MacNeil 2010). Secondary trauma and vicarious traumatization may manifest first with low-level symptoms of professional burnout and may progress to more severe and longer-lasting symptoms with associated impairment. In settings characterized by chronic conflict and devastation, it is important to monitor professionals for secondary trauma symptoms and implement a rotation of duties or intermittent work schedule that protects aid workers from excessive exposures. Aid organizations are beginning to recognize the importance of interventions to address secondary traumatic stress in refugee and conflict settings (Chatzea et al. 2017).

Sociocultural and Policy Implications

Given the breadth of traumas described in the previous section and their impact on overall health, one might expect a far-reaching response from governmental and humanitarian agencies, including financial and logistical support for addressing pediatric global mental health. However, there is a surprising lack of information and resources dedicated to addressing the psychological consequences of childhood trauma. Most governments globally have limited budgets for mental health (<2% of the national health budget in the majority of low- and middle-income countries), and the resources that do exist rarely support community mental health. Strategies for improving attention to pediatric global mental health despite this resource constraint include direct care or trauma-informed interventions financed by nongovernmental organizations; implementation research to determine the effectiveness of interventions; mental health care integration into existing systems of care and augmentation of resources for mental health through task sharing or shifting; mental health policy development; and improving mental health financing and partnerships (Khan et al. 2016).

Clinical Vignette

Resources for community mental health in Guatemala are scarce. As in many low- and middle-income countries, the national health budget devoted to mental health is less than 2%, and the majority of these funds (~94%) go to a single psychiatric hospital in the capital, Guatemala City, where extensive human rights abuses have been documented. The majority of trained mental health personnel reside and work in the capital, leaving only a handful serving the more than 13 million who reside outside the Guatemala City metropolitan area. In 2017, there were six attending psychiatrists working outside Guatemala City, and none of them had child and adolescent training (personal communication, Dr. Lourdes Trigueros, Pan American Health Organization/World Health Organization, and Dr. Mayra Becker, Guatemalan Ministry of Health, July 2017). Attention to pediatric mental health is severely limited, with usually only the most severe problems coming to the attention of primary care professionals or traditional healers.

Populations in the west central highlands of Guatemala have experienced widespread trauma and human security threats, from poverty and malnutrition to genocide of the Maya populations during the 36-year-long civil war, to multiple recent natural disasters and gang-related violence. For many years, there was limited to no mental health infrastructure in this region, with only one public sector psychiatrist working part time in Sololá province and no regular psychologists or trained therapists. In 2013, ALAS Pro Salud Mental (www.alasprosaludmental.org/home) was founded in this region with the mission to provide education, outreach, and access to mental health care for those who could not otherwise afford it. Resources and services include community sensitization to mental health through school and community workshops, a regular Maya language radio program, and annual educational and advocacy events; training of nonspecialist health workers to participate in mental health care delivery (Rissman et al. 2016); consultation clinics in primary care centers throughout the state; and partnerships with universities to help build resources for mental health research and care (Khan et al. 2016). Today, approximately 300 of the estimated 725 persons living with moderate to severe mental illness in the state of Sololá are receiving care through ALAS (B.R. Sampathi, J.R. Paiz, G. Bontemps, et al.: "Addressing mental health inequities in rural Guatemala through a collaborative community-based intervention," submitted to *International Journal for Equity in Health*, 2018). Nevertheless, there is no trained child and adolescent provider in the state, and the mental health needs of children remain severely underserved.

Evidence-Based Interventions

Interventions for trauma in children exposed to war and disaster include a variety of therapeutic modalities such as cognitive-behavioral therapy, exposure therapy, narrative therapy, psychodynamic psychotherapy, eye movement desensitization and reprocessing, supportive psychotherapy, debriefing, and family therapy. Although many of these interventions have been implemented in diverse settings around the world, there is yet very limited research evidence for their effectiveness in international settings. A Cochrane systematic review of 51 randomized controlled trials from around the globe (Gillies et al. 2016) examined the evidence for interventions focused on the prevention of PTSD. The review found that the likelihood of being diagnosed with PTSD was significantly reduced for children receiving a psychological therapy compared with control subjects for up to 1 month following treatment, but this effect was not significant in the medium (1–12 months) or long (>12 months) term. There was also moderate evidence that cognitive-behavioral therapy might be more effective than other psychological therapies in reducing symptoms of PTSD in youth exposed to trauma for up to 1 month following the start of treatment. Nevertheless, the confidence in these findings was limited by the low quality of the included studies and the heterogeneity between studies. Indeed, the number of studies relative to existing programs and interventions is remarkably low, in no small part due to limited research infrastructure in disaster, postconflict, and other low-resource settings. There is a strong need for further empirical inquiry into interventions for global childhood trauma to improve understanding and evidence for how best to approach these problems.

Conclusion

Global mental health is a diverse field with an overarching aim to improve the mental health of populations around the world. Traumatic events play a substantial role in the mental health conditions experienced by children and youth globally, and a human rights approach is essential for engaging in this work. Historically, there have been many challenges in addressing the psychological consequences of trauma, with limited resources and limited research on existing programs. With increasing recognition of the importance of mental health to overall health, there is an opportunity to implement creative strategies to build mental health infrastructure in low-resource settings. Utilization of existing systems of care through behavioral health integration is an important step in building capacity to improve pediatric global mental health.

KEY CONCEPTS

- Trauma is a large contributor to the global burden of disease and must be taken into account when considering the health and well-being of populations.

- A human rights framework is essential in order to address the potential impact of stigma and discrimination when working in global mental health.

- Human security concerns are a major contributor to traumatic events and have serious psychological consequences for both affected individuals and the practitioners caring for them.

- There is a limited evidence base on interventions for pediatric global trauma.

- Mental health integration into existing systems of care can help build capacity for mental health care in regions where there is no existing mental health infrastructure.

Discussion Questions (See Case Vignette)

1. Given the history of the region, what are some of the mental health problems we might expect to see in children and adolescents in this part of Guatemala?

2. What are some potential resources for building capacity for child and adolescent mental health care?

3. How might ALAS Pro Salud Mental increase its reach beyond the state of Sololá?

Suggested Readings

Gillies D, Maiocchi L, Bhandari AP, et al: Psychological therapies for children and adolescents exposed to trauma. Cochrane Database Syst Rev 10:CD012371, 2016 27726123

Patel V, Minas H, Cohen A, et al: Global Mental Health: Principles and Practice. New York, Oxford University Press, 2014

References

Chatzea V-E, Sifaki-Pistolla D, Vlachaki S-A, et al: PTSD, burnout and well-being among rescue workers: seeking to understand the impact of the European refugee crisis on rescuers. Psychiatry Res 262:446–451, 2017 28923435

Cohen A, Patel V, Minas H: A brief history of global mental health, in Global Mental Health: Principles and Practice. Edited by Patel V, Minas H, Cohen A, et al. New York, Oxford University Press, 2014, pp 3–26

Cole J, Sprang G, Lee R, Cohen J: The trauma of commercial sexual exploitation of youth: a comparison of CSE victims to sexual abuse victims in a clinical sample. J Interpers Violence 31(1):122–146, 2016 25381275

Davis T, Rogers H, Shays C; Select Bipartisan Committee to Investigate the Preparation for and Response to Hurricane Katrina: A Failure of Initiative: Final Report of the Select Bipartisan Committee to Investigate the Preparation for and Response to Hurricane Katrina. 109th U.S. Congress 2nd Session. Washington, DC, U.S. Government Printing Office, 2006. Available at: http://govinfo.library.unt.edu/a257.g.akamaitech.net/7/257/2422/15feb20061230/www.gpoaccess.gov/katrinareport/mainreport.pdf. Accessed July 20, 2018.

23

Technology-Facilitated Interventions

Pamela J. Shime, J.D., M.A.

BY THE SUMMER OF 2017, 71% of young people ages 15–24 years worldwide were online (United Nations Children's Fund 2017). As 2017 drew to a close, more than 5 billion people around the globe—66% of the world's population—were using a mobile device (Sivakumaran and Iacopino 2018). In the United States, at least 98% of 18- to 24-year-olds own smartphones (Nielsen 2016). The number of their peers from developing countries who are in the same situation is increasing exponentially (Poushter et al. 2018). As a new digital generation begins to populate the health care workforce and patient base, the accelerated integration of technology into mental health is inevitable.

Technology has the potential to not only scale but also revolutionize or, in tech parlance, *disrupt*, how we deliver, consume, and research mental health care and pediatric traumatic stress assessment and treatment. The new paradigm that emerges will fundamentally alter how children with traumatic stress and their families access and experience mental health services. Mobile sensors, virtual reality, artificial intelligence, and robots, among other innovations, will by their very nature transform established approaches to pediatric traumatic stress clinical care and research.

In this chapter, I canvass the striking opportunities and challenges at the intersection of technology and traumatic stress clinical care. I explore the technologies that are transforming assessment and treatment of traumatic stress and identify next-stage technologies that show promise for this population and the practitioners who serve them. I close with recommendations for our profession in an era of groundbreaking change, so that we may harness digital mental health's overwhelming promise and skirt its notable pitfalls.

Developmental Approaches

It is too early in the development of technology-facilitated assessment and treatment of pediatric traumatic stress to be able to discuss available technology for different developmental stages from infancy to early adulthood. There is not yet a sufficient number of technology-provided services for each developmental group. This presents the field with an important opportunity.

We are at an early enough stage that, as these technologies are being designed, we may still integrate a developmental approach. Such an approach would centrally incorporate the ways in which technology interacts with young brains at each developmental stage. This will be especially important for young people living with traumatic stress, who may already have had their healthy development at least partially derailed as a result of trauma's impact on brain architecture and function.

There are clear ethical challenges with respect to testing the impact of technology on developing brains. As researchers design studies of technological interventions for young people living with traumatic stress, we will need to develop guidelines that inform study protocols and ensure ethical approaches to investigating the developmental effects of technology-facilitated assessment and treatment.

Children today are growing up on "screens." They are the most technology-literate age group, and this will remain the case over time. Each new generation grows up on and with technology that is new to their parents, for whom it is never as familiar. Therefore, clinicians and researchers in the area of pediatric traumatic stress need to involve youth when designing interventions.

Technology Meets Trauma: Opportunities and Challenges

Why Technology?
Ten Technology Transformations

Young people living with traumatic stress, their families, and their clinicians stand to make significant gains as technology meets trauma. Technology will allow clinicians to aspire to achieve, in unprecedented ways, their patients' "physical, mental and social well-being," the World Health Organization's definition of health (World Health Organization 1948).

In 2015, Thomas Insel, then director of the National Institute of Mental Health (NIMH), wrote,

> The biomarkers for depression and psychosis and post-traumatic stress disorder are likely to be objective measures of cognition and behavior, which can be collected by smartphones. Some of our most effective interventions are psychosocial treatments that can be delivered or extended by smartphones and tablets. Most important, the sensors and the interventions can be integrated into a closed loop so that care is continuous and iterative. Increasing symptoms, suicidal impulses, and paranoid thoughts lead immediately to an intervention. (Insel 2015)

In an elegant articulation of the ways in which technology will transform pediatric traumatic stress assessment and treatment, Insel (2015) described what he saw as a necessary shift in mental health care "from episodic to continuous, reactive to proactive, and physician-centered to patient-centered."

Space and time in mental health practice have long been significantly constrained in the larger scope of patients' and therapists' lives—on average, one "therapy hour" a week in the same room. The challenges inherent in patient self-report based on memory are mitigated somewhat in pediatric practice when parents and guardians are surveyed, but the flaws inherent in self-report from memory often extend to their responses as well.

Technology breaks this mold. No longer are clinicians, young people, and families reliant on self-report once a week in a therapy room. Assessment and treatment now operate across time and space, accessed without interruption via computers, tablets, mobile devices, wearables, and emerging technologies, including Alexa and Google Home, voice-activated "home assistants." Continuous monitoring and assessment of the biological and other markers of traumatic stress, such as increased heart rate on encountering a trigger, reduced social media engagement, or unusually rapid keystrokes on texts and posts, enrich what clinicians know about their patients and when they receive that information.

Technology further allows for much more of a dynamic interplay between assessment and treatment of pediatric traumatic stress. A continuum of care can now mean not only ongoing assessment but also immediate delivery of an evidence-based intervention that is responsive to up-to-date tracking data and analysis. Interventions include connecting young people living with traumatic stress with avatar therapists, peers, or actual therapists via chat, videoconference, or phone conversation, either regularly or when continuous assessment data indicate that urgent care is required. The ability to identify and quickly intervene at crisis points will be life saving for young people living with traumatic stress, whose suicide rates are disproportionately high.

Our field faces a number of challenges that technology is especially equipped to meet. There is an urgent workforce challenge—by numbers alone, we have the capacity to reach only a minority of those who require assessment and treatment. In the United States, 43 states have a severe shortage of child psychiatrists, and none of the other states has a supply proportional to the current challenges of child and adolescent mental health. Further, there are insufficient data on how many of the existing mental health providers provide interventions that are evidence based, that is, having demonstrated efficacy in replicated, rigorous research studies. In addition, the stigma attached to mental health; the limited resources of affected families; and generational, social, and cultural biases against seeking care for mental health issues dramatically limit the reach of critically necessary clinical care for young people living with traumatic stress and other mental health challenges.

With technology, we can reach young people where they live—on their devices—with much reduced (if any) stigma and provide them with evidence-based interventions and increased equity of access. Integration of technology into pediatric trauma assessment and treatment will help clinical practitioners, patients, and families realize new and increased levels of each of 10 tech transformations in pediatric trauma and mental health care.

Ten Tech Transformations
1. *Equity of access* to clinical care through expanded reach, meeting young people where they live—on their devices
2. *Efficacy of clinical care* via scaling of evidence-based assessments and treatments and user-centered digital mental health for generations raised in the new millennium
3. *Data-driven clinical care* as a result of the extraordinary unprecedented capacity of technology-facilitated mental health tools to collect, analyze, and model extensive data points over time
4. *Precision mental health care*, comprising prescription of digital and other interventions (e.g., playing a therapeutic digital game three times per week for 3 months) on the basis of much-improved knowledge regarding individual biomarkers that correlate with responsiveness to particular treatments
5. *Complementary physical and mental health care* that mirrors the lived experience of the mind-body connection, as opposed to the silos within and between mental and physical health care
6. *Seamless continuum of care*, from prevention to monitoring to identification of and immediate responsiveness to a need for urgent care
7. *Continuity of care* 24 hours a day, 7 days a week
8. *Patient-centered assessment and treatment* flowing from the iterative user-centered design process employed in the technology sector
9. *Patient engagement* through mental health games and continuous access to "quantified self" monitoring and tracking data and responsive interventions (i.e., the ongoing collection, reporting, and analytics of personal physiological, behavioral, and other data through the use of technology, including fitness and/or sleep trackers, health apps, exercise logs, mood charts, and productivity journals) (Wolf 2009)
10. Evidence-based interventions that integrate the *social and emotional dimensions* of mental health care, at least in part through social media platforms

Why Not? Ten Digital Dangers

Artificial intelligence is the development of "intelligent" machines, which are able to mimic human intelligence, as demonstrated through a capacity for decision making, facial and voice recognition, and world-class chess play, among other abilities. It is one of the most highly anticipated technological developments of our time.

During fall 2016 and winter 2017, the technology sector's heavyweights joined forces with the American Civil Liberties Union to establish the Partnership on Artificial Intelligence to Benefit People and Society. Amazon, Apple, Facebook, Google, Microsoft, and IBM, along with artificial intelligence (AI) organizations, formed the partnership in order to anticipate and prevent, as much as possible, the risks inherent in the development of AI. Their concerns include safety, transparency, fairness, and the impact of AI on individuals and society. The emergence of the partnership was a groundbreaking, high-powered nod to the significant ethical concerns that accompany the rapid development of new technologies, with which it is impossible for industry guidelines, government regulations, and the law to keep pace.

These ethical concerns are amplified in the public sector and perhaps especially in health care, at the heart of which is the Hippocratic Oath. For vulnerable young people who are living with traumatic stress, ethical breaches could serve to retraumatize them and drastically set back treatment, recovery, and healthy development (Torous and Roberts 2017). Medical groups are collaborating to attempt to avoid these risks. The American Heart Association, the American Medical Association, DHX Labs (originally the Digital HealthX Group), and the Healthcare Information and Management Systems Society have formed Xcertia, a new nonprofit that is developing guidelines on the quality, safety, and effectiveness of mobile health apps. There is also now a Smartphone App Evaluation Task Force at the American Psychiatric Association that publicly reviews apps and wearable sensors to address similar concerns.

It is a challenge for clinicians and researchers to keep up with the rapid pace of technological change in a field in which training rarely includes knowledge or skills related to technology-facilitated interventions. The groups mentioned above are doing important work, but because of the constant infusion into the market of emerging technologies and mental health applications, even they risk stumbling.

There are two levels of ethical concerns for clinicians and researchers in pediatric mental health care, as well as health care in general. First, as with any untested assessment battery, treatment modality, or research methodology, new digital tools must be designed, developed, and disseminated according to ethical standards. Second, at another level, technology presents unprecedented ethical challenges for professionals in the field of pediatric traumatic stress and mental health care. These often unforeseeable ethical complications require new ways of thinking and practicing if we are to successfully anticipate and prevent breaches.

The integration of technology into traumatic stress clinical care poses challenges in addition to ethics. Researchers studying smartphone administration of basic psychiatric assessment scales found that this delivery mode may result in "significantly different scores" from those that result from in-person assessment with the same scales (Torous et al. 2015). These findings merit further investigation and explanation as we begin to rely more and more on technological delivery of formal assessments and continuous monitoring of patients. We are early in the study of this area and need to explore how and why smartphone assessments may produce different results from those conducted in person.

Below is a list of 10 digital dangers that have emerged for clinicians and researchers working with young people living with traumatic stress and other mental health conditions. It is likely that this taxonomy will change over time as technology continues to surprise us in both exciting and troubling ways.

Ten Digital Dangers
1. *The developing brain:* A primary question when working with children, adolescents, and young adults is whether the intervention has a detrimental impact on the developing brain. It is too early to know, for example, what effects extended immersion in virtual reality may have on the developing brain. The stakes are high, and much more research is necessary.
2. *Patient safety and security:* Current laws do not address the novel risks that accompany digital mental health, such as the safety of data from hacking and exposure.
3. *Patient privacy:* New laws and regulations are necessary for the unprecedented privacy issues that arise in the context of technology, including patients' control of their own data.

Ten Digital Dangers *(continued)*
4.   *Regulation:* There is currently little to no regulation of digital health tools. Regulation is necessary with respect to corporate interests in access to data, as well as funding and influence in research and development. It is still unclear whether cognitive-behavioral therapy provided through a mobile game should be subject to regulation. The U.S. Food and Drug Administration focuses on patient risk and diagnosis or treatment that should be delivered by an expert in person but instead is provided via technology. As technology evolves, however, so will the areas of risk and quality of care. A broader and deeper conversation is required here.
5.   *Standards of care:* There is an urgent need for standard-of-care protocols in the world of digital mental health care. This includes guidelines for supervision of technology-facilitated clinical care and oversight of direct-to-patient digital mental health care. In addition, many young people living with traumatic stress experience co-occurring conditions, such as anxiety or depression. The mental health needs related to these conditions will also need to be incorporated into digital interventions and standards of care in evidence-based ways.
6.   *Evidence basis:* There are two challenges here. The first is that we are very early in establishing an evidence basis for technological interventions in the face of mental health apps flooding the market. Second, there is an unbridgeable gap between the time required to conduct scientific and medical research and the speed with which technology becomes obsolete. The chasm between these two timelines will necessitate solutions that are scientific and also allow for development of technologies that are not obsolete on their release.
7.   *Ongoing equity challenges:* The digital divide—the gap between those who have access to devices and the Internet and those who do not—is an ongoing challenge for digital health. Bridging this gap requires culturally appropriate tools, technology that serves diverse disabled communities, and linguistically accessible interventions (for speakers of a range of languages, as well as patients who are functionally illiterate).

Ten Digital Dangers *(continued)*
8. *Reimbursement:* Insurance industry reimbursement models have not yet integrated the existence of mental health games, apps, or technologies. This is a significant access issue in the United States. If American insurance companies do not reimburse for prescribed technological mental health tools, there will be a structural disincentive for digital health tool developers, who operate primarily in the private sector. Companies will invest in development of products that generate revenue. This will mean that digital mental health tools that could be life changing for children living with traumatic stress may not be developed. These consequences will be felt both inside and outside the United States.
9. *Technology for older-generation devices:* The majority of people working in technology are in the private sector, and their training prepares them to design for, develop for, and disseminate to consumers who have the latest devices. Many young people, especially those in low-income communities around the world, use Android phones that are a few generations old. As a result, they are unable to access any applications designed exclusively for iPhones or iPads or applications designed for more recent Android devices. Developers need to be aware of these challenges or we will continue to fail to even approach equity of access to mental health care in the context of pediatric traumatic stress and beyond.
10. *The overpromise:* In the current climate of great technological promise, without regulation and accurate labeling and marketing, patient expectations could well exceed the power of digital interventions. The gap between those expectations and the capacity of technology will likely exist for some time and could result in troubling health consequences, especially for young people who have not developed the skills to make such assessments.

What's Out There? Eight Elements and Ten Tools

There is no stable of pediatric traumatic stress digital tools at this stage. The available tools include PTSD tools designed for adults (often veterans) or age-appropriate tools for young people that target traumatic stress and/or a range of mental health conditions that often co-occur with traumatic stress. There are 10 technological tools that may be deployed on their own or in combination for young people living with traumatic stress, their families, and their clinicians. Each of these tools will include one or more of the following elements, among others:

1. Surveys by voice, selecting an answer on a touch screen or with a mouse, or writing in answers
2. Interactive documentation by user of moods and psychological and other events through journaling or voice or video recording
3. Data collection, modeling, and analytics
4. Communication via online chat, video chat, or texting
5. Psychoeducation
6. Information and resources
7. Skill-building using games, videos, and exercises
8. Community-building, often using social media, for offline or online connection

Ten Tech Tools
1. *Websites*, such as Screening for Mental Health (SMH; https://mentalhealthscreening.org), were the first line of tech tools. SMH offers online screenings for a range of mental health issues, including PTSD, as well as education, assessment, and prevention programs in schools, workplaces, and other sites.
2. *Apps* are key tools in the context. One example is PTSD Coach (www.ptsd.va.gov/public/materials/apps/PTSDCoach.asp), designed, developed, and studied by the U.S. Department of Veterans Affairs for veterans with PTSD. The PTSD Coach app provides 1) psychoeducation about PTSD and its causes, symptoms, and management; 2) ongoing self-assessments; and 3) techniques for managing PTSD (Rodriguez-Paras et al. 2017). Digital health in particular is seeing more development of app suites that provide users with a range of app types that together provide holistic digital health care. Intellicare (https://intellicare.cbits.northwestern.edu), a suite of 13 mental health apps, is one example. These 13 apps provide social connection; management support for anxiety, sleep, exercise, and mood variation; activity encouragement and tracking; a negative thought challenger; and mindfulness training and support (Mohr et al. 2017). The apps are linked, and notifications are available app to app within the suite.
3. *Texting applications*, such as Crisis Text Line, provide anonymous 24-hour counseling. When a young person texts the number, an automated reply provides information and then queries, "What's on your mind?" Texts that indicate the person is in crisis receive immediate attention from a crisis counselor.

Ten Tech Tools *(continued)*

4. *Virtual worlds*, such as Second Life (https://secondlife.com), provide simulated environments in which young people living with traumatic stress can customize an avatar (electronic image) and engage in activities and social connection that may not be possible for them in the real world. In one study, researchers found that adults engaging in weight maintenance through Second Life had better results than those in an in-person weight maintenance group (Sullivan et al. 2013). Similarly, pediatric traumatic stress treatment in a virtual world could potentially yield better results than real world in-person treatment with all its attendant constraints.

5. *Games*, such as SPARX, a 3-D role-playing game based on cognitive-behavioral therapy, can be played in order to improve mental health. SPARX was the subject of a randomized controlled trial (Merry et al. 2012) and, as a result of the findings in that study, is now an evidence-based treatment for mild to moderate depression and anxiety in 12- to 25-year-olds. In the study by Merry et al. (2012), depressed young people who played SPARX were 170% more likely to overcome their depression than those in traditional therapy. SPARX, which stands for smart, positive, active, realistic X-factor thoughts, was developed by researchers and clinicians at the University of Auckland and is currently available only in New Zealand. It has the production value of a non–health care videogame and incorporates cultural references to the indigenous Maori population. Each SPARX player journeys through seven worlds on quests (approximately half an hour each), meeting other characters as a player-customized avatar. A guide explains the game initially and then, at the end, explicates how the player can use the skills learned in the game to overcome depression.

6. *Mixed reality*—augmented reality (AR) and/or virtual reality (VR)—is being studied in a number of areas relevant to pediatric traumatic stress. In AR, sensory information is overlaid onto the real-world environment. It is increasingly being accessed on mobile devices that project virtual images and/or text onto real environments (such as a projection of a calming image and mantra onto an anxiety-provoking environment for a young person living with traumatic stress). VR provides an immersive environment through use of both content and hardware (headsets and, recently, headset-free booths). VR exposure therapy (VRET) is used for people living with traumatic stress. VRET has been proven useful when employed predisaster in order to build resilience in children who live in disaster-prone areas (Botella et al. 2015).

Ten Tech Tools *(continued)*
7. *AI* can be used to help deliver treatment. Woebot, "an automated conversational agent (chatbot) who helps you monitor mood and learn about yourself" (https://woebot.io), is based on cognitive-behavioral therapy and delivered through Facebook Messenger. Woebot develops a personality; asks users daily how they are feeling and what's going on; provides support, psychoeducation, and helpful information; and, through AI, learns more about the user over time, applying that knowledge in order to personalize education, information, and support (Fitzpatrick et al. 2017).
8. *Avatars*, such as an artificially intelligent 3-D avatar on a television screen, can be used to administer assessment questionnaires. A recent study found that veterans with PTSD reported more symptoms to a virtual therapist than they did to a human therapist, perhaps because there is enhanced anonymity and less shame with an avatar (Lucas et al. 2017).
9. *Sensors* can be used to gauge (geo)location, sleep patterns, behaviors, movement, and biological markers, including physiological and neurological data such as heart rate and brain waves. They are often linked to tools that provide visualization, analysis, and information about the sensor-collected data. An example relevant for young people living with traumatic stress is Socialise (www.blackdoginstitute.org.au/research/key-research-areas/emental-health/socialise), developed and being studied by the Black Dog Institute in Australia, a leading mental health organization doing cutting-edge work in digital mental health. Socialise is an app that uses sensors to track social activity via smartphones. The app is a central component of a project with the goal of identifying young people with anxiety or depression, which co-occur with traumatic stress at a disproportionately high rate, and monitoring their symptoms during treatment.

Ten Tech Tools *(continued)*
10. *Platforms*, such as the Icahn School of Medicine's Rx Universe (http://apps.icahn.mssm.edu/rxuniverse), can efficiently deliver a range of information and services for providers and consumers of mental health care in the area of pediatric traumatic stress and beyond. Rx Universe is a delivery platform for mobile health technology that prescribes evidence-based digital health apps, often selected on the basis of specific patient data that correspond to the data of others who responded to that app. Rx Universe helps health care providers and consumers navigate the overwhelming world of digital health and the constant infusion of new apps into app stores. Through Rx Universe, the apps are prescribed directly and immediately to patient mobile devices. Rx Universe also incorporates patient education, surveys and monitoring, integrated wearables, telemedicine opportunities (video appointments with a mental health provider), appointment scheduling, patient social networks, and clinical trial recruitment.

What's Next? Five Emerging Innovations

AI is on the cusp of altering our experience of the world and digital mental health care. In addition to AI, there are five emerging technological innovations that will likely make important contributions to clinical care for pediatric traumatic stress. These tools will quickly render obsolete those that are currently operating at the cutting edge of technologies for mental health, presenting a new set of transformational opportunities in clinical care for pediatric trauma and, at the same time, posing a similarly unprecedented set of digital dangers.

Five Emerging Innovations
1. *Pervasive or ubiquitous computing:* This field envisions the integration of communication, task performance, AI, and other computing capacities into almost every element of our environment, including walls, lights, kitchen appliances, cars, sidewalks, robots, and even human bodies and skin (Tamburro 2016).

Five Emerging Innovations *(continued)*
2.   *Self-driving cars:* Car and technology companies have invested significantly in research on self-driving cars, which will be much more like a mobile living space than the transportation-focused vehicles with which we are familiar. Researchers are exploring the potential of the commute for stress management through immersion in virtual worlds, surrounding individuals in the car with relaxing images and sound or other evidence-based interventions. The spaces in the car could transform into spaces for clinical interventions, creative play, or work in addition to entertainment.
3.   *Wearable technology:* Under Armour has led the way in clothing and shoe technology, with sensors in shoes that provide real-time tracking along with a built-in memory; 3-D-printed shoe components; and sensors that measure breathing, heart rate, temperature, and speed while seamlessly attached to shirts. This technology has been used primarily for fitness purposes, but it has exciting potential for data collection and feedback in the context of clinical care for pediatric traumatic stress. Analytics regarding movement pace and measurements of breathing and heart rate could help identify significant changes related to rising stress in young people. The integration of this technology into clothing and shoes further reduces stigma and would provide invaluable data for mental health clinicians, consumers, and researchers.
4.   *Drones:* Drones could become companions for young people living with traumatic stress, helping to monitor challenges to safety and security while incorporating AI in order to develop a healthy relationship with a child who may not have experienced one in his or her family or community (Landay 2014). To date, drones have not been used this way.
5.   *Eye tracking:* Developments in eye tracking will allow us to assess how young people are responding to different elements of screens, images, text, and possibly the broader environment. This could be useful in identifying what triggers young people living with traumatic stress and when those triggers result in an especially strong reaction. Related innovations in gaze will mean that we are able to control devices, games, and components of the environment with our eyes. This has important implications for data collection, as well as treatment, including increasing a sense of mastery in children living with traumatic stress, an evidence-based intervention in the field.

Overcoming Challenges and Developing Patient-Centered Policies and Practices

Our approach as clinicians and community members to disruptive transformations in technology will determine whether those we serve receive the full benefit of digital mental health or whether, instead, young people who have already experienced trauma are unnecessarily exposed to new forms of risk and harm. It is still relatively early in this new field, but we are facing pressing standard-of-care, ethical, social, and policy challenges. To get out in front of both the potential and the challenges inherent in digital mental health care, clinicians and researchers in the field of pediatric trauma care must together create time and space at our institutions and among ourselves to reflect, anticipate benefits and risks, and develop systems and protocols to maximize the potential of new technologies and prevent or ameliorate the dangers.

The dizzying rate at which emerging technologies enter the market has further created an urgent need for new ways of collaborating across disciplines, including medicine, engineering, art, data science, design, policy, and law. To fully realize the power and potential of new technologies for children, adolescents, and families living with traumatic stress, patients, their families, and clinicians will also need to learn from each other. As we work together to stay ahead of the curve in this fast-paced area, there are 10 policy and practice priorities that need to be at the top of a patient-centered agenda.

Ten Policy and Practice Priorities

1. *Data:* One of the most important distinctions between in-person and technology-facilitated mental health care is the capacity of the latter to collect, analyze, and model data to increase our understanding of and ability to effectively treat mental health challenges such as pediatric traumatic stress. If we maximize the data potential in technology-facilitated pediatric traumatic stress clinical care, we will develop an unprecedented understanding of the mechanics of each patient's challenges and evidence-based interventions.

Ten Policy and Practice Priorities (continued)
2. *Developmental approach:* The interaction of technology with developing brains and bodies remains, for the most part, a mystery to us. If we require a developmental approach in our research, technology design and development, and teaching, we will elucidate the effects of different technologies on healthy development, as well as determine the most efficacious interventions for young people struggling with traumatic stress and their families.
3. *Sociocultural implications and equity of access:* Technology promises to help us achieve equity of access to evidence-based interventions for pediatric traumatic stress beyond anything we could have imagined before. However, we will need to attend to the digital divide between wealthy and low-income communities and developed and developing countries. There is also a risk that corporate interests will dominate technological innovation and the people we serve will become even more vulnerable. We will need to ensure further that the assessment and treatment we provide via technology is culturally appropriate and that diverse patients play a role in each design process.
4. *Ethical challenges:* Clinicians in the field of youth trauma are serving a particularly vulnerable population. It is essential that we ensure that we meet our ethical obligations in both our research and our clinical work.
5. *Standards of care:* Similarly, we must ensure that we establish high-quality standards of care in technology-facilitated pediatric traumatic stress clinical care. Apps will continue to flood the market, as will other technologies over time, and there will need to be guidelines and safeguards that protect patients from false advertising and the significant potential for harm in this area.
6. *Research studies:* Stakeholders in this area need to advocate for significant funding for technological research and clinical applications. In addition, traditional modes of research work on timelines that are incoherent in the face of the pace of technological change. This tension must be resolved by accommodating the pace of technological change without sacrificing essential components of the scientific process.

Ten Policy and Practice Priorities *(continued)*
7. *Safety, security, and privacy of patients and their data:* Technology-facilitated clinical care brings extraordinary benefits. However, if we cannot ensure the safety, security, and privacy of our patients and their data, we will fail to reap those benefits and instead will cause harm. Collaboration with experts in these areas in the world of technological innovation is necessary, and urgently so.
8. *Regulation and policy directions:* There is little sense of how, when, and why we need to regulate digital mental health care and technology-facilitated clinical care for children and adolescents living with traumatic stress. That work is necessary and cannot wait.
9. *Insurance industry:* Early collaboration with the insurance industry is essential if we are to develop clinical care for pediatric traumatic stress as an area of robust and fruitful innovation.
10. *Engagement of young people:* The more we involve young people as our advisors with respect to the direction of technological innovation in this field and the design and development of tools to help children and adolescents with traumatic stress, the more likely it will be that we will produce technologies that they will use and that will support their mental and emotional health.

Conclusion

The overwhelming promise and significant pitfalls that accompany technological innovation in digital mental health care constitute a call to action. This call to action requires us to urgently engage in and sustain collaborations and conversations that advance technological innovation in the field of pediatric traumatic stress. Those collaborations and conversations must be driven by and be true to the core value trifecta of scientific discovery, equity of access, and ethical policy and practice. If we achieve this, we will have the opportunity to achieve extraordinary breakthroughs for young people suffering from traumatic stress, their families, and the clinicians and researchers who serve them.

KEY CONCEPTS

- Technology will fundamentally transform clinical and research practice in mental health care in general and the assessment and treatment of pediatric traumatic stress in particular.

- The implications of this change in mental health care are centrally related to the ways in which technology provides patients and their families who are living with traumatic stress an unprecedented capacity to 1) attain equity of access and 2) collect and analyze new forms of data.

- The number of technological tools available to clinical practitioners is rapidly evolving. As such, there is an insufficient evidence base regarding the efficacy and dangers of these tools, in particular in the context of the developing brain.

- The pace of change in technology will mandate new forms of research that allow clinicians, researchers, and young people to harness new technologies with the potential to notably enhance assessment and treatment of pediatric traumatic stress.

- The overwhelming promise and significant pitfalls inherent in the integration of technology into pediatric trauma clinical and research practice constitute a call to action. This call to action requires us to develop new and unprecedented collaborations and strategies to ensure that we fulfill the promise and skirt the pitfalls.

Discussion Questions

1. What is the most significant challenge you face in your work with young people living with traumatic stress?

2. What technological tool mentioned in this chapter do you think could best help you overcome this challenge?

3. What is a risk that this tool could pose for you and/or your patients? What do you think would be the best approach for eliminating or mitigating the risk?

4. If you are unable to incorporate one of the technology-based mental health tools into your practice, why not? How could you make it possible to implement one of these tools?

5. How do you think your field or institution could contribute to maximizing the benefits of and minimizing the risks that accompany the integration of technology into clinical care for childhood traumatic stress? What is one step you can take in the next 48 hours to help advance that process?

Suggested Readings

Insel T: Look who is getting into mental health research. Bethesda, MD, National Institute of Mental Health, August 31, 2015. Available at: www.nimh.nih.gov/about/directors/thomas-insel/blog/2015/look-who-is-getting-into-mental-health-research.shtml. Accessed March 24, 2018.

Rodriguez-Paras C, Tippey K, Brown E, et al: Posttraumatic stress disorder and mobile health: app investigation and scoping literature review. JMIR Mhealth Uhealth 5(10):e156, 2017 29074470

Torous J, Roberts LW: The ethical use of mobile health technology in clinical psychiatry. J Nerv Ment Dis 205(1):4–8, 2017 28005647

References

Botella C, Serrano B, Baños RM, et al: Virtual reality exposure-based therapy for the treatment of post-traumatic stress disorder: a review of its efficacy, the adequacy of the treatment protocol, and its acceptability. Neuropsychiatr Dis Treat 11:2533–2545, 2015 26491332

Fitzpatrick KK, Darcy A, Vierhile M: Delivering cognitive behavior therapy to young adults with symptoms of depression and anxiety using a fully automated conversational agent (Woebot): a randomized controlled trial. JMIR Ment Health 4(2):e19, 2017 28588005

Insel T: Look who is getting into mental health research. Bethesda, MD, National Institute of Mental Health, August 31, 2015. Available at: www.nimh.nih.gov/about/directors/thomas-insel/blog/2015/look-who-is-getting-into-mental-health-research.shtml. Accessed July 9, 2018.

Landay J: Autonomous wandering interface (AWI)—concept video. YouTube, July 8, 2014. Available at: www.youtube.com/watch?v=cqU_hR2_ILU. Accessed March 24, 2018.

Lucas G, Rizzo A, Gratch J, et al: Reporting mental health symptoms: breaking down barriers to care with virtual human interviewers. Frontiers in Robotics and AI 4:51, 2017

Merry SN, Stasiak K, Shepherd M, et al: The effectiveness of SPARX, a computerised self help intervention for adolescents seeking help for depression: randomised controlled non-inferiority trial. BMJ 344:e2598, 2012 22517917

Mohr DC, Tomasino KN, Lattie EG, et al: IntelliCare: an eclectic, skills-based app suite for the treatment of depression and anxiety. J Med Internet Res 19(1):e10, 2017 28057609

Nielsen: Millennials are top smartphone users. Mobile Insights, November 2016. New York, Nielsen, 2016. Available at: www.nielsen.com/us/en/insights/news/2016/millennials-are-top-smartphone-users.html. Accessed July 9, 2018.

Poushter J, Bishop C, Chwe H: Social media use continues to rise in developing countries but plateaus across developed ones. Washington, DC, Pew Research Center, June 2018

Rodriguez-Paras C, Tippey K, Brown E, et al: Posttraumatic stress disorder and mobile health: app investigation and scoping literature review. JMIR Mhealth Uhealth 5(10):e156, 2017 29074470

Sivakumaran M, Iacopino P: The Mobile Economy 2018. London, GSMA Intelligence, 2018. Available at www.gsma.com/mobileeconomy/wp-content/uploads/2018/05/The-Mobile-Economy-2018.pdf. Accessed July 9, 2018.

Sullivan DK, Goetz JR, Gibson CA, et al: Improving weight maintenance using virtual reality (Second Life). J Nutr Educ Behav 45(3):264–268, 2013 23622351

Tamburro P: Corning's "A Day Made of Glass" finally became a reality. Los Angeles, CA, Mandatory Media, January 21, 2016. Available at: www.craveonline.ca/design/945283-cornings-day-made-glass-finally-became-reality. Accessed March 24, 2018.

Torous J, Roberts LW: The ethical use of mobile health technology in clinical psychiatry. J Nerv Ment Dis 205(1):4–8, 2017 28005647

Torous J, Staples P, Shanahan M, et al: Utilizing a personal smartphone custom app to assess the patient health questionnaire-9 (PHQ-9) depressive symptoms in patients with major depressive disorder. JMIR Ment Health 2(1):e8, 2015 26543914

United Nations Children's Fund: The State of the World's Children 2017: Children in a Digital World. New York, UNICEF, December 2017

Wolf G: Know thyself: tracking every facet of life, from sleep to mood to pain, 24/7/365. Wired, vol 365, June 22, 2009. Available at: www.wired.com/2009/06/lbnp-knowthyself. Accessed July 9, 2018.

World Health Organization: Preamble to the Constitution of the World Health Organization as adopted by the International Health Conference, New York, June 19–22, 1946; signed on July 22, 1946 by the representatives of 61 states (Official Records of the World Health Organization No 2, p 100) and entered into force on 7 April 1948

Index

Page numbers printed in **boldface** type refer to tables or figures.

477